Computational Methods for the Analysis of Genomic Data and Biological Processes

Computational Methods for the Analysis of Genomic Data and Biological Processes

Editors

Francisco A. Gómez Vela
Federico Divina
Miguel García-Torres

MDPI • Basel • Beijing • Wuhan • Barcelona • Belgrade • Manchester • Tokyo • Cluj • Tianjin

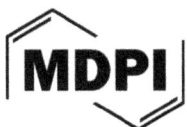

Editors
Francisco A. Gómez Vela
Universidad Pablo de Olavide
Spain

Federico Divina
Universidad Pablo de Olavide
Spain

Miguel García-Torres
Universidad Pablo de Olavide
Spain

Editorial Office
MDPI
St. Alban-Anlage 66
4052 Basel, Switzerland

This is a reprint of articles from the Special Issue published online in the open access journal *Genes* (ISSN 2073-4425) (available at: https://www.mdpi.com/journal/genes/special_issues/comput_genetics).

For citation purposes, cite each article independently as indicated on the article page online and as indicated below:

LastName, A.A.; LastName, B.B.; LastName, C.C. Article Title. *Journal Name* **Year**, *Volume Number*, Page Range.

ISBN 978-3-03943-771-9 (Hbk)
ISBN 978-3-03943-772-6 (PDF)

© 2020 by the authors. Articles in this book are Open Access and distributed under the Creative Commons Attribution (CC BY) license, which allows users to download, copy and build upon published articles, as long as the author and publisher are properly credited, which ensures maximum dissemination and a wider impact of our publications.

The book as a whole is distributed by MDPI under the terms and conditions of the Creative Commons license CC BY-NC-ND.

Contents

About the Editors vii

Francisco Gómez-Vela, Federico Divina and Miguel García-Torres
Computational Methods for the Analysis of Genomic Data and Biological Processes
Reprinted from: *Genes* **2020**, *11*, 1230, doi:10.3390/genes11101230 1

Celia Salazar, Osvaldo Yañez, Alvaro A. Elorza, Natalie Cortes, Olimpo García-Beltrán, William Tiznado and Lina María Ruiz
Biosystem Analysis of the Hypoxia Inducible Domain Family Member 2A: Implications in Cancer Biology
Reprinted from: *Genes* **2020**, *11*, 206, doi:10.3390/genes11020206 5

Omid Mahmoudi, Abdul Wahab and Kil To Chong
iMethyl-Deep: N6 Methyladenosine Identification of Yeast Genome with Automatic Feature Extraction Technique by Using Deep Learning Algorithm
Reprinted from: *Genes* **2020**, *11*, 529, doi:10.3390/genes11050529 25

Javed Zahoor and Kashif Zafar
Classification of Microarray Gene Expression Data Using an Infiltration Tactics Optimization (ITO) Algorithm
Reprinted from: *Genes* **2020**, *11*, 819, doi:10.3390/genes11070819 37

Mobeen Ur Rehman and Kil To Chong
DNA6mA-MINT: DNA-6mA Modification Identification Neural Tool
Reprinted from: *Genes* **2020**, *11*, 898, doi:10.3390/genes11080898 65

Xiangrui Zeng, Wei Zong, Chien-Wei Lin, Zhou Fang, Tianzhou Ma, David A. Lewis, John F. Enwright and George C. Tseng
Comparative Pathway Integrator: A Framework of Meta-Analytic Integration of Multiple Transcriptomic Studies for Consensual and Differential Pathway Analysis
Reprinted from: *Genes* **2020**, *11*, 696, doi:10.3390/genes11060696 77

Abdelaziz Ghanemi, Aicha Melouane, Mayumi Yoshioka and Jonny St-Amand
Exercise and High-Fat Diet in Obesity: Functional Genomics Perspectives of Two Energy Homeostasis Pillars
Reprinted from: *Genes* **2020**, *11*, 875, doi:10.3390/genes11080875 91

Thomas Vanhaeren, Federico Divina, Miguel García-Torres, Francisco Gómez-Vela, Wim Vanhoof, Pedro Manuel Martínez García
A Comparative Study of Supervised Machine Learning Algorithms for the Prediction of Long-Range Chromatin Interactions
Reprinted from: *Genes* **2020**, *11*, 985, doi:10.3390/genes11090985 107

Daria D. Novikova, Pavel A. Cherenkov, Yana G. Sizentsova and Victoria V. Mironova
metaRE R Package for Meta-Analysis of Transcriptome Data to Identify the *cis*-Regulatory Code behind the Transcriptional Reprogramming
Reprinted from: *Genes* **2020**, *11*, 634, doi:10.3390/genes11060634 125

Panagiotis C. Agioutantis, Heleni Loutrari and Fragiskos N. Kolisis
Computational Analysis of Transcriptomic and Proteomic Data for Deciphering Molecular Heterogeneity and Drug Responsiveness in Model Human Hepatocellular Carcinoma Cell Lines
Reprinted from: *Genes* **2020**, *11*, 623, doi:10.3390/genes11060623 139

Fernando Delgado Chaves, Francisco Gómez-Vela, Federico Divina, Miguel Garcia-Torres, Domingo Rodriguez-Baena and Pedro Manuel Martínez-García
Computational Analysis of the Global Effects of *Ly6E* in the Immune Response to Coronavirus Infection Using Gene Networks
Reprinted from: *Genes* **2020**, *11*, 831, doi:10.3390/genes11070831 161

Ruoyu Tian, Yidan Pan, Thomas H. A. Etheridge, Harshavardhan Deshmukh, Dalia Gulick, Greg Gibson, Gang Bao and Ciaran M Lee
Pitfalls in Single Clone CRISPR-Cas9 Mutagenesis to Fine-Map Regulatory Intervals
Reprinted from: *Genes* **2020**, *11*, 504, doi:10.3390/genes11050504 195

About the Editors

Francisco A. Gómez Vela received his Ph.D. in Computer Science from the Pablo de Olavide University of Seville, in addition to Computer Science Engineering from the University of Seville. His lines of research are focused on the treatment of information using intelligent techniques, applying machine learning and data mining techniques. He has focused mainly on the analysis of genetic and biomedical data in his research. His research is mainly based on the inference of biological models based on gene networks. In addition, he has recently focused on the research of new big data techniques for the exploitation of different types of data.

Federico Divina obtained his Ph.D. in Artificial Intelligence from the Vrije Universiteit of Amsterdam, and, after that, worked as a postdoc at the University of Tilburg, within the European project NEWTIES. In 2006, he moved to the Pablo de Olavide University. He has been working on knowledge extraction since his Ph.D. thesis at the Vrije Universiteit of Amsterdam. His main research interests focus on machine learning, and in particular on techniques based on soft computing, bioinformatics, and big data.

Miguel García-Torres is an Associate Professor at the Escuela Politécnica Superior of the Universidad Pablo de Olavide. He received his BS degree in physics and Ph.D. degree in computer science from the Universidad de La Laguna, Tenerife, Spain, in 2001 and 2007, respectively. After obtaining the doctorate he held a postdoc position in the Laboratory for Space Astrophysics and Theoretical Physics at the National Institute of Aerospace Technology (INTA). There, he joined the Gaia mission from the European Space Agency (ESA) and started to participate in the Gaia Data Processing and Analysis Consortium (DPAC) as a member of "Astrophysical Parameters", Coordination Unit (CU8). He has been involved in the "Object Clustering Analysis" (OCA) Development Unit since then. His research areas of interest include machine learning, metaheuristics, big data, time series forecasting, bioinformatics, and astrostatistics.

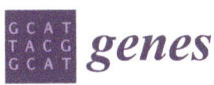

Editorial

Computational Methods for the Analysis of Genomic Data and Biological Processes

Francisco Gómez-Vela *, Federico Divina and Miguel García-Torres

Computer Science Division, Pablo de Olavide University, ES-41013 Seville, Spain; fdivina@upo.es (F.D.); mgarciat@upo.es (M.G.-T.)
* Correspondence: fgomez@upo.es

Received: 14 October 2020; Accepted: 14 October 2020; Published: 20 October 2020

Today, new technologies, such as microarrays or high-performance sequencing, are producing more and more genomic data. This fact has brought new opportunities and challenges in the fields of computational biology and bioinformatics, since this huge number of data need to be analysed in order to be exploited.

In this context, new computational methods and tools, such as machine learning approaches or gene expression analysis tools, could provide the solution to such issues.

The overall aim of this Special Issue is to compile the latest research and developments in the field of computational methods for the analysis of gene expression data and, in particular, with the modelling of biological processes.

Among all the submissions, eleven papers were accepted and published in this Special Issue. In this sense, machine learning-based approaches have received particular attention, such as the work presented by Vanhaeren et al. [1]. In this work, the authors used 1D sequencing signals to model cohesin-mediated chromatin interactions in two human cell lines and evaluate the prediction models obtained. To this end, they tested the performance of six popular machine learning algorithms: decision trees, random forests, gradient boosting, support vector machines, multi-layer perceptron and deep learning. The results obtained showed that gradient boost outperformed the other five methods, yielding accuracies of about 95%. Despite these results, the authors established that it was necessary to examine other cell lines and tissues to confirm the obtained observations.

In another article, Rehman and Chong [2] presented work where the authors propose a Convolution Neural Network (CNN) and Long Short-Term Memory (LSTM)-based tool named DNA6mA-MINT for DNA-6mA modification identification. The tool uses the CNN for feature extraction, while LSTM provides optimal interpretation for those features. The authors showed that the performance of their tool is superior to that achieved with existing state-of-the-art techniques on the "combined-species", *Mus musculus* genome, and rice genome datasets. Moreover, the authors carried out a performance analysis on 5- and 10-fold cross-validation in order to obtain a better comparative analysis. The tool is provided by a user-friendly web server, publicly available.

Another example of the use of CNN is the work by Mahmoudi et al. [3], where a new computational model for identifying N6-methyladenosine (m6A) post-transcriptional modification in RNAs is proposed. The technique, called iMethyl-deep, provides a novel computational method for identifying m6A *Saccharomyces cerevisiae* sites by using single-nucleotide resolution to convert RNA sequences into high-quality feature representations in the CNN. The model is able to extract the relevant features from the input samples. The results obtained show that iMethyl-deep outperforms state-of-the-art methods and achieves accuracies of 89.19% and 87.44% on the M6A2614 and M6A6540 benchmark datasets, respectively.

In the context of machine learning, Delgado-Chaves et al. [4] presented an analysis of the effects of the gene *Ly6E* in the immune response against the coronavirus responsible for murine hepatitis (MHV). With this aim, the work used different datasets from mice, with and without the ablation of the gene

Ly6E, to reconstruct computational gene co-expression networks, by using a machine learning-based algorithm called EnGNet. The authors carried out an integration of differential expression analyses and reconstructed network exploration, and significant differences in the immune response to the virus were observed in Ly6E compared to in wild-type animals. The obtained results show that Ly6E ablation in hematopoietic stem cells (HSCs) leads to a progressive impaired immune response in both the liver and spleen.

Zahoor and Zafar [5] propose a novel optimization algorithm inspired by the "infiltration tactics" of the war zone (ITO) for the task of classifying microarray datasets. The algorithm integrates parameter-free and parameter-based classifiers to provide a highly accurate and reliable binary classifier. The results are generated in two steps: (a) the Lightweight Infantry Group converges quickly to find non-local maxima and produces comparable results, and (b) the Follow-up Team (FT) applies advanced tuning to enhance the baseline performance. Each soldier is considered as a base model with its own independently chosen subset selection method (pre-processing, and validation methods and classifier). Therefore, successful soldiers are combined for optimal results. The performance of the algorithm was successfully tested using three mouse livers and a rat liver.

In this Special Issue, some tools are presented as well, such as in the work by Zeng et al. [6]. In this article, the authors present a new meta-analytic integration tool, called the Comparative Pathway Integrator (CPI), which is able to deal with multiples studies of different conditions. To do so, the tool uses an adaptive weighted Fisher's method to discover consensual and differential enrichment patterns, a tight clustering algorithm to reduce pathway redundancy, and a text-mining algorithm to assist the interpretation of the pathway clusters. The authors demonstrate its effectiveness by applying CPI to jointly analyse six psychiatric disorder transcriptomic studies. The results described show functions confirmed by previous biological studies as well as novel enrichment patterns. The tool is publicly available as a CPI R package.

Another interesting tool provided as an R package, named metaRE, was presented by Novikova et al. [7]. MetaRE is able to perform a systematic search for cis-regulatory elements enriched in the promoters of the genes significantly changed in their transcription in a reaction. metaRE extracts datasets of multiple expression profiles generated to test the response of the same organism and identifies simple and composite cis-regulatory elements that are systematically associated with the differential expression of genes. The authors tested metaRE's performance for the identification of low-temperature-responsive cis-regulatory code in *Arabidopsis thaliana* and *Danio rerio*. MetaRE was able to identify potential binding sites for known as well as unknown cold response regulators.

Computationally based analyses of biological processes are also included in this Special Issue. For example, the work by Agioutantis et al. [8] analysed 21 human hepatocellular carcinoma (HCC) cell lines (HCC lines) to explore intertumoral molecular diversity and pertinent drug sensitivity. This article proposes an integrative computational approach based on an exploratory and single-sample gene-set enrichment analysis of transcriptome and proteome data, and then a correlation analysis of drug-screening data. The presented results classified HCC lines into two groups. In particular, the lines were classified as poorly differentiated and well-differentiated, displaying lower/higher enrichment scores in a "Specifically Upregulated in Liver" gene set, respectively. It is worth mentioning that the analysis of correlation showed a differential effectiveness of specific drugs against poorly differentiated compared to well-differentiated HCC lines, which is possibly applicable in clinical research with patients with analogous features. As a result, this study may expand the knowledge of HCC lines and proposes a cost-effective computational approach to precision anti-HCC therapies.

The work by Tian et al. [9] addresses the effect that deleting single-nucleotide polymorphisms (SNPs) of genes affected by large-effect expression Quantitative Trait Loci (eQTL) may have on gene expression. To this end, CRISPR-Cas9 mutagenesis was used to delete SNPs, obtaining single-cell clones. The bottlenecks for the fine mapping of such SNPs were suggested to be the impossibility of targeting many SNPs and the clonal variability of single-cell clones, among others.

An analysis of the hypoxia inducible domain family member 2A (HIGD2A) was presented in Salazar et al. [10]. The protein HIG2A is produced by the HIGD2A gene, found in mitochondria and the nucleus, promoting cell survival in hypoxic conditions. The main objective of this study was to carry out a biosystem analysis of *HIGD2A* with the aim of discovering its implications in cancer biology. The authors used different public databases such Gene Expression Omnibus to evaluate some gene expression datasets. The results presented suggested that the gene's alterations are present in the different cancers studied.

Finally, Ghanemi et al. [11] presented a review about the therapeutic alternatives to exercise in obesity. The review focuses on a functional genomics perspective, in particular, finding potential therapeutic targets for obesity. The authors point out various approaches, identifying differential gene expression-based studies that aimed at finding genes that are differentially expressed under diverse conditions depending on physical activity and diet (mainly high-fat). The authors suggested that this area of functional genomics-related exploration will lead to novel mechanisms and also new applications and implications along with a new generation of treatments for obesity and the related metabolic disorders.

Funding: This research received no external funding.

Acknowledgments: We would like to thank all the authors and peer reviewers for their valuable contributions to this Special Issue. This issue would not be possible without their valuable and professional work. In addition, we would also like to take the opportunity to show our gratitude to the Genes editorial team for their work, due to which this Special Issue has been a success.

Conflicts of Interest: The authors declare no conflict of interest.

References

1. Vanhaeren, T.; Divina, F.; García-Torres, M.; Gómez-Vela, F.; Vanhoof, W.; Martínez-García, P.M. A comparative study of supervised machine learning algorithms for the prediction of long-range chromatin interactions. *Genes* **2020**, *11*, 985. [CrossRef] [PubMed]
2. Rehman, M.U.; Chong, K.T. DNA6mA-MINT: DNA-6mA modification identification neural tool. *Genes* **2020**, *11*, 898. [CrossRef] [PubMed]
3. Mahmoudi, O.; Wahab, A.; Chong, K.T. iMethyl-Deep: N6 methyladenosine identification of yeast genome with automatic feature extraction technique by using deep learning algorithm. *Genes* **2020**, *11*, 529. [CrossRef] [PubMed]
4. Delgado-Chaves, F.M.; Gómez-Vela, F.; Divina, F.; García-Torres, M.; Rodriguez-Baena, D.S. Computational analysis of the global effects of *Ly6E* in the immune response to coronavirus infection using gene networks. *Genes* **2020**, *11*, 831. [CrossRef] [PubMed]
5. Zahoor, J.; Zafar, K. Classification of microarray gene expression data using an infiltration tactics optimization (ITO) algorithm. *Genes* **2020**, *11*, 819. [CrossRef] [PubMed]
6. Zeng, X.; Zong, W.; Lin, C.W.; Fang, Z.; Ma, T.; Lewis, D.A.; Enwright, J.F.; Tseng, G.C. Comparative pathway integrator: A framework of meta-analytic integration of multiple transcriptomic studies for consensual and differential pathway analysis. *Genes* **2020**, *11*, 696. [CrossRef] [PubMed]
7. Novikova, D.D.; Cherenkov, P.A.; Sizentsova, Y.G.; Mironova, V.V. metaRE R package for meta-analysis of transcriptome data to identify the cis-regulatory code behind the transcriptional reprogramming. *Genes* **2020**, *11*, 634. [CrossRef] [PubMed]
8. Agioutantis, P.C.; Loutrari, H.; Kolisis, F.N. Computational analysis of transcriptomic and proteomic data for deciphering molecular heterogeneity and drug responsiveness in model human hepatocellular carcinoma cell lines. *Genes* **2020**, *11*, 623. [CrossRef] [PubMed]
9. Tian, R.; Pan, Y.; Etheridge, T.H.A.; Deshmukh, H.; Gulick, D.; Gibson, G.; Bao, G.; Lee, C.M. Pitfalls in single clone CRISPR-Cas9 mutagenesis to fine-map regulatory intervals. *Genes* **2020**, *11*, 504. [CrossRef] [PubMed]
10. Salazar, C.; Yañez, O.; Elorza, A.A.; Cortes, N.; García-Beltrán, O.; Tiznado, W.; Ruiz, L.M. Biosystem analysis of the hypoxia inducible domain family member 2A: Implications in cancer biology. *Genes* **2020**, *11*, 206. [CrossRef] [PubMed]

11. Ghanemi, A.; Melouane, A.; Yoshioka, M.; St-Amand, J. Exercise and high-fat diet in obesity: Functional genomics perspectives of two energy homeostasis pillars. *Genes* **2020**, *11*, 875. [CrossRef] [PubMed]

Publisher's Note: MDPI stays neutral with regard to jurisdictional claims in published maps and institutional affiliations.

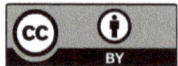

© 2020 by the authors. Licensee MDPI, Basel, Switzerland. This article is an open access article distributed under the terms and conditions of the Creative Commons Attribution (CC BY) license (http://creativecommons.org/licenses/by/4.0/).

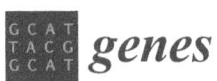

Article

Biosystem Analysis of the Hypoxia Inducible Domain Family Member 2A: Implications in Cancer Biology

Celia Salazar [1], Osvaldo Yañez [2], Alvaro A. Elorza [3,4], Natalie Cortes [5], Olimpo García-Beltrán [5], William Tiznado [2] and Lina María Ruiz [1,*]

[1] Instituto de Ciencias Biomédicas, Facultad Ciencias de la Salud, Universidad Autónoma de Chile, Santiago 8910060, Chile; celia.salazar@uautonoma.cl
[2] Computational and Theoretical Chemistry Group, Departamento de Ciencias Químicas, Facultad de Ciencias Exactas, Universidad Andres Bello, Santiago 8370251, Chile; osvyanezosses@gmail.com (O.Y.); wtiznado@unab.cl (W.T.)
[3] Institute of Biomedical Sciences, Faculty of Medicine and Faculty of Life Sciences, Universidad Andres Bello, Santiago 8370146, Chile; alvaro.elorza@unab.cl
[4] Millennium Institute on Immunology and Immunotherapy, Santiago 8331150, Chile
[5] Facultad de Ciencias Naturales y Matemáticas, Universidad de Ibagué, Carrera 22 calle 67, Ibagué 730002, Colombia; natalie.cortes@unibague.edu.co (N.C.); jose.garcia@unibague.edu.co (O.G.-B.)
* Correspondence: lina.ruiz@uautonoma.cl; Tel.: +56-2-2303-6662

Received: 8 January 2020; Accepted: 13 February 2020; Published: 18 February 2020

Abstract: The expression of *HIGD2A* is dependent on oxygen levels, glucose concentration, and cell cycle progression. This gene encodes for protein HIG2A, found in mitochondria and the nucleus, promoting cell survival in hypoxic conditions. The genomic location of *HIGD2A* is in chromosome 5q35.2, where several chromosomal abnormalities are related to numerous cancers. The analysis of high definition expression profiles of *HIGD2A* suggests a role for HIG2A in cancer biology. Accordingly, the research objective was to perform a molecular biosystem analysis of *HIGD2A* aiming to discover HIG2A implications in cancer biology. For this purpose, public databases such as SWISS-MODEL protein structure homology-modelling server, Catalogue of Somatic Mutations in Cancer (COSMIC), Gene Expression Omnibus (GEO), MethHC: a database of DNA methylation and gene expression in human cancer, and microRNA-target interactions database (miRTarBase) were accessed. We also evaluated, by using Real-Time Quantitative Reverse Transcription Polymerase Chain Reaction (qRT-PCR), the expression of *Higd2a* gene in healthy bone marrow-liver-spleen tissues of mice after quercetin (50 mg/kg) treatment. Thus, among the structural features of HIG2A protein that may participate in HIG2A translocation to the nucleus are an importin α-dependent nuclear localization signal (NLS), a motif of DNA binding residues and a probable SUMOylating residue. *HIGD2A* gene is not implicated in cancer via mutation. In addition, DNA methylation and mRNA expression of *HIGD2A* gene present significant alterations in several cancers; *HIGD2A* gene showed significant higher expression in Diffuse Large B-cell Lymphoma (DLBCL). Hypoxic tissues characterize the "bone marrow-liver-spleen" DLBCL type. The relative quantification, by using qRT-PCR, showed that *Higd2a* expression is higher in bone marrow than in the liver or spleen. In addition, it was observed that quercetin modulated the expression of *Higd2a* gene in mice. As an assembly factor of mitochondrial respirasomes, HIG2A might be unexpectedly involved in the change of cellular energetics happening in cancer. As a result, it is worth continuing to explore the role of *HIGD2A* in cancer biology.

Keywords: *HIGD2A*; cancer; DNA methylation; mRNA expression; miRNA; quercetin; hypoxia

1. Introduction

Mitochondria are crucial for virtually all aspects of malignant transformation and tumor progression, counting since the proliferation of transformed cells, the resistance of these cells to hostile environmental surroundings, the interaction of transformed cells with the tumor stroma, and their dissemination to remote anatomical sites [1]. Besides being the leading supplier of ATP, mitochondria could provide building blocks for the proliferation of malignant cells, they produce reactive oxygen species (ROS), and they are critical players in regulated cell death signaling [1].

Among the main mechanisms used by mitochondria for the malignant transformation of cells, first, there is the production of ROS, which favors the accumulation of potential oncogenic defects in DNA, and the activation of probable oncogenic signaling pathways [2]. Secondly, there is an abnormal accumulation of mitochondrial oncometabolite such as fumarate, succinate, and 2-hydroxyglutarate [3]. Thirdly, there are defects in the mitochondrial permeability transition (MPT), which allow the survival of malignant cells through the deregulation of regulated cell death processes [4]. Mitochondria influence the outcome of cancer cells to therapy through metabolic reprogramming between glycolysis and oxidative phosphorylation. The search for many anti-carcinogenic treatments is based on the identification of molecules that kill cancer cells or sensitize them to treatments by priming MPT [1].

Thus, the understanding of mitochondrial metabolism is fundamental in the development of new anti-cancer agents. Our research group is focused on the study of the Hypoxia Inducible Domain Family Member 2A, HIG2A, which is a small protein (106 amino acids) located in the inner membrane of the mitochondria. It has a hypoxia-induced-protein domain at the N-terminus [5]. HIG2A has a role in the respiratory supercomplexes assembly, a function that has been evidenced in the C2C12 mouse cell line, where the knockdown of *Higd2a* (nomenclature of mice gene) impaired supercomplex formation by the release of CIV [6,7]. Recently, we showed that the knockdown of *HIGD2A* (nomenclature of a human gene) decreases the activity of Complex I in the supercomplexes of HEK293 cells [8]. Noteworthy, in that study, the authors described the following results for the first time: the *Higd2a* gene exhibits differential expression in mice under basal physiological conditions that could be associated with different cell proliferation rates, and with differentiation and physiological oxygen levels in each tissue. Additionally, we also proved that physiological hypoxia induces *HIGD2A* (*Higd2a*) gene expression. Interestingly, the latter showed an increase during the cellular differentiation of C2C12 cells from myoblast to myotubes [8]. These results support a role for HIG2A in conditions of physiological stress, such as hypoxia in some tissues, and cell differentiation processes.

Further analysis of the *HIGD2A* gene promoter region in human chromosome 5 provided insights on how HIG2A could be related to cell cycle management. These studies evidenced several probable binding sites for different transcription factors related to cell cycle control, including E2F-1, E2F-2, E2F-3a, E2F-4, and E2F-5 [8]. These results agree with the evidence that under oxidative metabolism, E2F-1 directs cellular responses by acting as a regulatory switch from glycolytic to oxidative metabolism [9,10]. Moreover, we analyzed the effects of E2F-1 modulation on *HIGD2A* gene expression using roscovitine (inhibitor of CDKs), flavopiridol, and caffeic acid phenethyl ester (CAPE) (antiproliferative drugs) [8]. Roscovitine treatment significantly increased *HIGD2A* gene expression in the human embryonic kidney HEK293 cell line. Treatment with CAPE decreased *HIGD2A* gene expression in mouse myoblast C2C12 cells [8]. In the same work, the E2F-1 regulatory action in *HIGD2A* gene was studied, showing that the inhibition of cell proliferation treated with CAPE promotes E2F1 binding to the regulatory region of *HIGD2A*, thus setting a role for E2F-1 in the regulation of *HIGD2A* expression. Notably, analysis of *HIGD2A* genomic location showed a chromosome 5q35.2 section, a region where several chromosomal abnormalities are usually related to cancer [11–14].

Oncogenic mutations in the small GTPase Ras are highly prevalent in cancer. Depletion of *HIGD2A* selectively impairs the viability of colon adenocarcinoma cells (DLD1), which are Ras mutant cells, suggesting a role of HIG2A in cell cycle regulation and a potential target in cancer therapy [15]. Furthermore, the analysis of high definition expression profiles of *HIGD2A* with the Gene Expression Omnibus (GEO) repository [16,17] suggested a role for HIG2A in cancer biology. This analysis showed that *HIGD2A* expression is significantly increased in Methotrexate resistant colon cancer cell lines (HT29 resistant cells) (GDS3160) and Cisplatin-resistant non-small lung cancer cell lines (H460 resistant cells) (GDS5247). Additionally, when the estrogen receptor alpha is silenced in MCF7 breast cancer cells, a significant decrease of *HIGD2A* expression was evidenced (GDS4061). All the above data are suggesting a role of HIG2A in cell cycle regulation.

Accordingly, in light of the background mentioned above, the research objective was to perform a molecular biosystem analysis of *HIGD2A*, aiming to obtain insights on its implications in cancer biology.

2. Materials and Methods

2.1. Datasets

The Gene Expression Omnibus (GEO) [16] repository for gene expression profiles of DLBCL was screened, and datasets were analyzed with GEO2R [17]. The microarray Illumina Human HT-12 V4.0 expression bead chips were used in the study; "Role of hypoxia in Diffuse Large B-cell Lymphoma: Metabolic repression and selective translation of HK2 facilitates development of DLBCL". This study offers further conclusive proof of the contribution of HK2 in the development of B-cell lymphoma. It proposes that HK2 is a vital metabolic driver of DLBCL (Diffuse Large B-cell Lymphoma) phenotype. The authors contributed to the public dataset GSE104212 [18]. For this study, two human lymphoma cell lines, HLY-1 and SUDHL2, were cultured and assessed under hypoxic conditions ($n = 3$, biological replicates per cell line) or normoxia ($n = 3$, biological replicates per cell line), followed by a gene expression microarray analysis to examine the global gene expression differences under these conditions [18]. Another dataset analyzed was obtained with the Agilent-014850 Whole Human Genome Microarray 4×44K G4112F and were used in the study of gene-expression profiles in a series of non-Hodgkin lymphoma (NHL) patients (Dataset GSE32018). This study shows that PIM2 kinase inhibition is a logical process in DLBCL therapy and gives a new marker for patient stratification [19]. The gene-expression profiling from Dataset GSE32018 was conducted in a series of 114 B-cell non-Hodgkin lymphoma patients (DLBCL, Follicular Lymphoma (FL), Marginal Zone Lymphoma_Type (MALT), Mantle Cell Lymphoma (MCL), Chronic Lymphocytic Leukemia (CLL), and Nodal Marginal Zone Lymphoma (NMZL)). Seven freshly frozen lymph nodes and six freshly frozen reactive tonsils were used as controls [19]. The last Dataset GSE12453 obtained the expression profiling by array [HG-U133_Plus_2] Affymetrix Human Genome U133 Plus 2.0 Array was used in the study; origin and pathogenesis of lymphocyte-predominant Hodgkin lymphoma as revealed by global gene expression analysis. This study shows a relationship of microdissected lymphocytic and histiocytic (L&H) lymphoma cells to the origin from germinal center B cells at the transition to memory B cells. L&H cells are typified by abnormal ERK signaling and constitutive NF-κB activity [20]. The analysis of differential gene expression was performed in primary human lymphoma cells of Nodular Lymphocyte-Predominant Hodgkin Lymphoma (NLPHL) in comparison with primary lymphoma cells of classical Hodgkin lymphoma cells, and other B-non-Hodgkin Lymphoma (B-NHL) samples, and subsets of non-neoplastic B lymphocytes isolated from blood or tonsils [20].

2.2. In Silico Analysis

A homology modelling of HIG2A protein structure was generated with the SWISS-MODEL repository (https://swissmodel.expasy.org/repository/uniprot/Q9BW72?csm=205DE0AE39950053) [21,22]. Two crystal structures of backbone structure of human membrane protein HIGD1A and HIGD1B (protein data bank code: 2LON, 2LOM) were chosen as template for the construction of the three-dimensional HIG2A model (Model 1A and Model 1B). For validation, we used the PROCHECK program [23], which assesses the stereochemical quality of protein structures and the root mean square deviation (RMSD), superimposing the structures of proteins and calculating their deviation.

Additionally, we performed some in silico analysis for the prediction of nuclear localization signals (NLS) with the NLS Mapper software (nls-mapper.iab.keio.ac.jp) and DNA-binding residues in HIG2A protein with the DP-Bind software (lcg.rit.albany.edu/dp-bind), which is a web server for sequence-based prediction of DNA-binding residues in DNA-binding proteins. Moreover, we searched for post-translational modifications of HIG2A and with the GPS-SUMO prediction of SUMOylating sites and SUMOylating binding motifs (sumosp.biocuckoo.org).

DNA methylation and gene expression of *HIGD2A* in cancer was analyzed with MethHC, a database for human pan-cancer gene expression, methylation and microRNA expression [24] (http://methhc.mbc.nctu.edu.tw). The *HIGD2A* promoter was selected and the methylation level evaluation method was defined as maximum.

2.3. Immunofluorescence and Confocal Microscopy

The immunofluorescence analysis was performed according to the procedure previously reported [8] with brief addition for the inner nuclear membrane Lamin-B protein localization; anti-Lamin B antibody (Lamin B sc-6216 SANTA CRUZ BIOTECHNOLOGY, INC), the secondary antibody red signal-Alexa Fluor 546. Hoechst 33342 (Blue signal after DNA binding). Z-axis series were obtained using a Leica SP8 confocal microscopy.

2.4. Isolation of Mitochondria and Nucleus, and Western Blot

The isolation of mitochondria and nucleus and Western blot were performed according to the procedure previously reported [8].

2.5. Animals

The protocol of animal management was approved by the Bioethics Committee of the Vice-Rectory for Research and Postgraduate Studies of Universidad Andrés Bello, Approval Act 009/2010, of 8 July 2010. The animals were treated and handled according to the Chilean National Commission for Scientific and Technological Research-CONICYT requirements for the care and use of laboratory, in accordance with NIH guidelines (The Guide for the Care and Use of Laboratory Animals, 1996). Male C57BL/6 mice were housed in groups of nine mice per cage and maintained at 22 °C on a 12:12-h light–dark cycle, with food and water ad libitum before the procedures. Moreover, male C57BL/6 mice (12 months of age) were daily injected intraperitoneally (i.p) with either 50 mg/kg quercetin (Sigma-Aldrich, Cat # Q4951, Merck KGaA, Darmstadt, Germany) ($n = 9$), or vehicle (5% DMSO) plus PBS ($n = 9$) for 15 days, according to the protocol previously described [25].

2.6. Reverse Transcription and Quantitative Real-Time PCR (qRT-PCR)

Total RNA was extracted from mice tissues with TRIzol^{TM} Reagent (Invitrogen, Thermo Scientific, Waltham, MA, USA) according to the manufacturer's protocol. RNA quantification and quality assessment were determined using the spectrophotometer Infinite M200 Pro (TECAN AG, Zürich, Switzerland) and agarose electrophoresis. RNA (2 µg) was used for the reverse transcription with the RevertAid First Strand cDNA synthesis Kit (Thermo Scientific, Waltham, MA, USA). qPCR was performed using FastStart Essential DNA Green Master Kit (Roche, Risch-Rotkreuz, Zug, Switzerland) and the LightCycler® 96-Real time PCR system (Roche, Risch-Rotkreuz, Zug, Switzerland). Data are presented as relative mRNA levels of *HIGD2A* normalized to *PPIA* mRNA levels. The primers used were: *HIGD2A* Fw: 5′-GCCTTTTGATCCGTCCAAGC-3′, Rev: 5′-CTGAAACGGAGGGAGCAAGT-3′; *PPIA* Fw: 5′-GTGGTCTTTGGGAAGGTG-3′, Rev: 5′-GGTGATCTTCTTGCTGGTC-3′. The thermal conditions used were as follows: an initial three-step amplification (95 °C for 10 s, 60 °C for 10 s and 72 °C for 10 s), followed by a one-step melting (95 °C for 10 s, 65 °C for 60 s and 97 °C for 1 s) and finishing with a one-step cooling (37 °C for 30 s). All reactions were concluded with an integrated melting curve reaction to verify the specificity of the amplification. Two experimental replicates were analyzed in a "LightCycler" run, improving the precision within the test. In order to improve the variation between assays, four runs were carried out on four different days (biological replicates).

2.7. Statistical Analysis

All statistical analyses were performed with the Graphpad Prisma 6 software (San Diego, CA, USA). An unpaired Student's *t*-test followed by a Mann-Whitney test was used when comparing two average values. One way-ANOVA followed by a Dunnett´s multiple comparison test was also performed.

3. Results

3.1. Structural Features of HIG2A Protein

For the homology modeling of HIG2A protein, two crystal structures of backbone structure of human membrane protein HIGD1A and HIGD1B (protein data bank code: 2LON, 2LOM) were chosen as template for the construction of the three-dimensional HIG2A model (Model 1A and Model 1B) as it displayed a sequence identity of 36–36.14% and a similarity of 50.67–54.22%, see Figure 1. In the current study, the stereo-chemical evaluation of backbone psi and Phi dihedral angles of the HIG2A models showed that Model 1A and Model 1B residues were 70.3% and 70.4% in the most favorable region, and 0% and 14% in the additional allowed region, respectively (Table 1 and Figure 2). In general, a score close to 100% implies the good stereo-chemical quality of the model [26]. The total quality G-factor −0.29 and −0.23, for Model 1A and 1B, indicated a good quality model (acceptable values of the G-factor in PROCHECK are between 0 and −0.5, with the best models displaying values close to zero). The PROCHECK stereochemical analysis showed neither wrong contacts nor bad scores for main-chain or side-chain parameters. Therefore, these PROCHECK results suggest that the predicted model was of good quality.

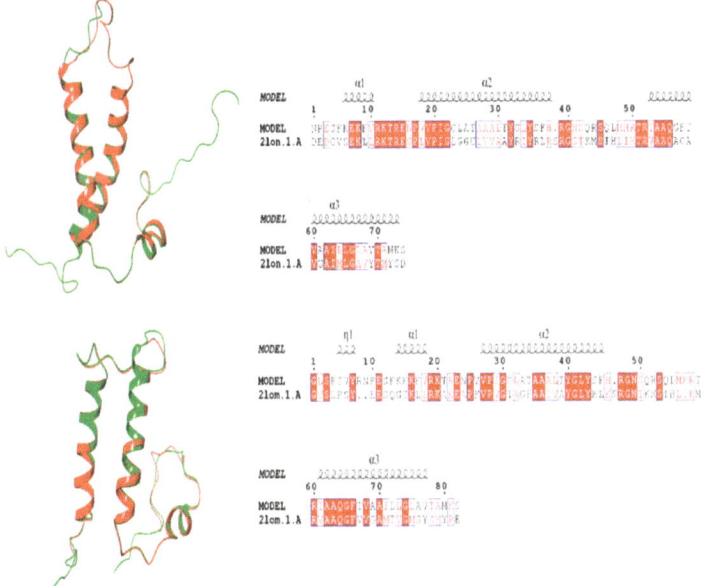

Figure 1. Images in the left side show superimposed template (green) on their respective model (red). Images in the right show alignment generated by the ESPript 3.0 webtool [27] of HIG2A protein with the PDBs: 2LON and 2LOM, accessions used to build the Models 1-A and 1-B.

Table 1. PROCHECK Summary.

	Ramachandran Plot Quality (%)				Goodness Factor		
	Most Favored	Additional Allowed	Generously Allowed	Dis-Allowed	Dihedral	Covalent	Overall
Model-1A	70.3	21.9	7.8	0.0	−0.30	−0.31	−0.29
Model-1B	70.4	23.9	4.2	1.4	−0.27	−0.22	−0.23

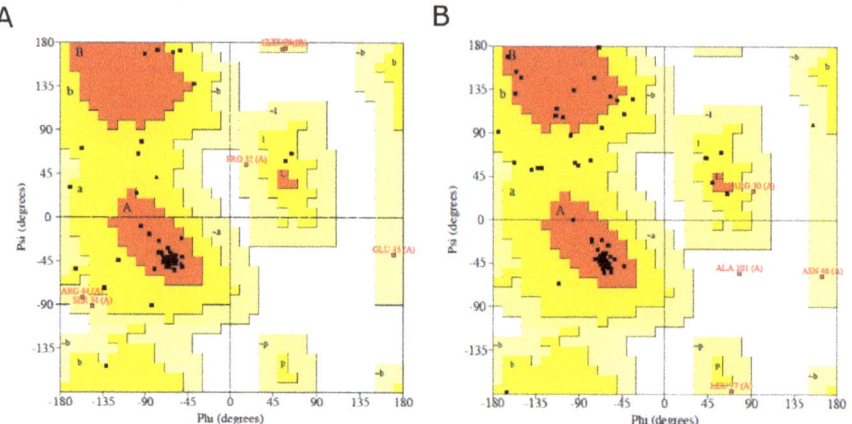

Figure 2. Ramachandran plots generated via PROCHECK for (**A**) HIG2A protein Model-1A and (**B**) HIG2A protein Model-1B. PROCHECK shows that the residues in most favored (red), additionally allowed (yellow), generously allowed (pale yellow) and disallowed regions (white color).

Our previous studies suggest that changes in oxygen concentration, cellular metabolism, and cell cycle regulate *HIGD2A* expression [8]. HIG2A protein might function as a regulator of respiratory supercomplexes assemblies in response to hypoxia, cellular metabolism, and cell cycle [8]. HIG2A could function as a hypoxia sensor in respiratory supercomplexes to activate signaling pathways of response to hypoxic stress. To explore the potential participation of HIG2A in cellular signaling pathways, we performed several analyses of the HIG2A protein sequence. With the nuclear localization signal, NLS Mapper software [28], for HIG2A, an importin α-dependent nuclear localization signal was predicted (Figure 3), which is a noncanonical NLSs recognized by importin α [29]. This NLS in HIG2A supports the participation of HIG2A in a cellular signaling pathway. HIG2A has a motif of DNA binding residues in the alpha-helix, which also supports the interaction of HIG2A with DNA (Figure 3).

Moreover, we looked at post-translational modifications for HIG2A that account for their participation in signaling pathways. In high throughput, proteomic screening was found acetylation in Ala 2- [30], phosphorylation in Thr 3 [31], and di-methylation in Arg 74 (PhosphoSitePlus®) in HIG2A (Figure 3). HIG2A protein localizes in the mitochondrial network and nucleus [8]. The immunofluorescence analysis of C2C12 cells by confocal microscopy allows observing the colocalization of HIG2A with the inner nuclear membrane protein, Lamin-B (Figure 4A). With the Western blot, an upper band of approximately 10 kDa higher than HIG2A was detected in the nucleus fraction with Anti-HIG2A antibody, suggesting that this upper band could be a post-translational modification of HIG2A (Figure 4B). For this reason, protein HIG2A was analyzed for SUMOylating; a probable SUMO interaction motif and a SUMOylating nonconsensus residue were identified (Figure 3). The sumoylation could regulate the nuclear localization of some proteins [32–35].

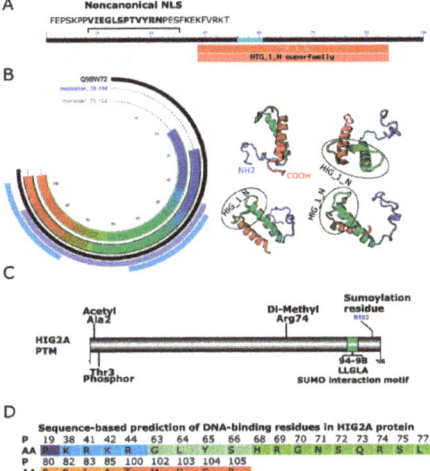

Figure 3. Structural features of HIG2A protein. (**A**) HIG2A noncanonical nuclear localization signals (NLS), (**B**) Q9BW72 (HIG2A_HUMAN) Homo sapiens (Human) from SWISS MODEL protein structure homology-modelling server, (**C**) post-translational modification of HIG2A, (**D**) sequence-based prediction of DNA-binding residues in HIG2A protein. P, position; AA, amino acid; No mitochondrial presequence; G 70 MPP cleavage site.

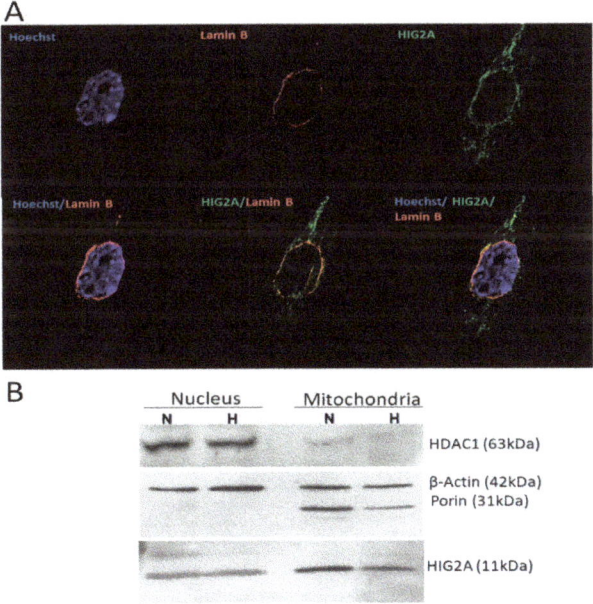

Figure 4. HIG2A protein localizes in mitochondria and nucleus. (**A**) Immunofluorescence image of an Anti-HIGD2A antibody stained C2C12 cells, the secondary antibody (Green signal, DyLight® 488). Lamin B (sc-6216) stained showing nuclear lamina localization, the secondary antibody red signal-Alexa Fluor 546. Hoechst 33342 (Blue signal after DNA binding). z-axis series were obtained using a Leica SP8 confocal microscopy. (**B**) Western blot of HIG2A in mitochondria and nucleus protein extract of HEK293 cells. Normoxia condition (N), Hypoxia condition (H).

3.2. Genetic Features of HIGD2A Gene in Cancer

The Catalogue of Somatic Mutations in Cancer (COSMIC) Cancer Gene Census (CGC) database indicates that the *HIGD2A* gene (COSG58129) has been reported as having mutations in 29 unique samples out of a total of 35183 samples; therefore, *HIGD2A* is not a known cancer-driving gene [36]. Moreover, mouse insertional mutagenesis experiments do not support the designation of *HIGD2A* as a cancer-causing gene [37]. On the other hand, DNA methylation is a vital epigenetic mechanism that stabilizes gene expression and cellular states; their alteration has a role in tumor initiation and evolution [38]. In the present study, we evaluated the correlation between DNA methylation and mRNA expression in the *HIGD2A* gene in cancer. For this purpose, we used the MethHC, a database of DNA methylation and gene expression in human cancer [24]. The comparison of average beta value in tumor samples, and matched normal samples, indicates significant alterations in DNA methylation and mRNA expression in the *HIGD2A* gene in diverse cancer: Breast Invasive Carcinoma (BRCA), Head and Neck Squamous Cell Carcinoma (HNSC), Kidney Renal Clear Cell Carcinoma (KIRC), Liver Hepatocellular Carcinoma (LIHC), Lung Adenocarcinoma (LUAD), Pancreatic Adenocarcinoma (PAAD), Prostate Adenocarcinoma (PRAD), and Rectum Adenocarcinoma (READ) (Figure 5). As shown in Figure 5, the correlation between DNA methylation and mRNA expression in the *HIGD2A* gene is significant for most of the cancers previously mentioned. The correlation and *p*-valued between DNA methylation and mRNA expression for each cancer are: BRCA (correlation: -0.023392995888958, *p*-value: $7.7715611723761E-16$); HNSC (correlation: -0.038296830523789, *p*-value: $8.8817841970013E-16$); KIRC (correlation: 0.026605097926286, *p*-value: $1.2061907028738E-9$); LIHC (correlation: 0.03121030048201, *p*-value: $3.5347748061909E-9$); LUAD (correlation: 0.00043286112981717, *p*-value: $2.246819973406E-7$); PAAD (correlation: 0.058019469632158, *p*-value: 0.40190361732643); PRAD (correlation: -0.19807571454707, *p*-value: 0.0002748122809052); and READ (correlation: 0.21585872962767, *p*-value: $7.0291561460323E-8$).

Moreover, we explored the microRNA-target interactions database (miRTarBase) analyzing microRNAs (miRNAs) for the *HIGD2A* gene [39]. These miRNAs are small non-coding RNAs that maintain cell homeostasis by negative regulation influencing each pathway practically from cell cycle checkpoint, cell proliferation to apoptosis [40]. Of the 17 miRNAs found, four miRNAs stand out as having experimental evidence and influence on different diseases related to cancer [39,41]. In Figure 6 the secondary structure of pre-miRNA; hsa-mir-181a-2, hsa-mir-181b-1, hsa-mir-181c, and hsa-mir-181d are presented. The word cloud of miRNA-disease information, for these miRNAs, are related to neoplasms, leukemia, carcinoma, lymphoma, among others. In Table 2, the significative clinical miRNA and gene expression profile (miRNA-Target expression profile) from The Cancer Genome Atlas (TCGA) is summarized. Briefly, the miRNA, hsa-mir-181a-2 prove a significant positive correlation for kidney chromophobe (KICH) and a negative correlation for PRAD. Besides, the miRNA, hsa-mir-181b-1, reveal a significant positive correlation for KICH and kidney renal papillary cell carcinoma (KIRP), and a negative correlation for HNSC, BRCA, and lung squamous cell carcinoma (LUSC). Moreover, the miRNA, hsa-mir-181c, indicates a significant positive correlation for KICH, liver hepatocellular carcinoma (LIHC), Cholangiocarcinoma (CHOL), and a negative correlation for BRCA and LUSC. Finally, the miRNA, hsa-mir-181d, demonstrate a significant positive correlation for LIHC and a negative correlation for BRCA and LUSC (Table 2).

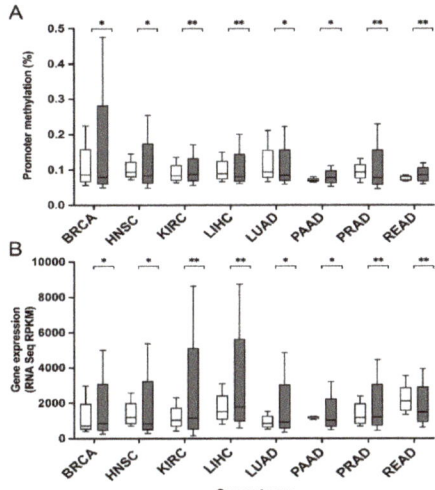

Figure 5. DNA Methylation (**A**) and mRNA Expression (**B**) in the *HIGD2A* gene in Cancer. The distinct methylation of *HIGD2A* in promoter region between cancer and normal tissues in GC patients (MethHC, a database of DNA methylation and gene expression in human cancer). The average beta value for the maximum methylation level evaluation method was used. Gene expression value was obtained from RNA Seq RPKM (Reads Per Kilobase per Million mapped reads) values in TCGA Data Portal by MethHC. Box plots in grey represent cancer samples and those in white represent normal samples. BRCA (*p*-value 0.020048563931465) cancer samples (*n* = 748), normal samples (*n* = 129); HNSC: Head and Neck Squamous Cell Carcinoma (*p*-value 0.0057123457160735), cancer samples (*n* = 517), normal samples (*n* = 67); KIRC: Kidney Renal Clear Cell Carcinoma (*p*-value 0.0010765698395251), cancer samples (*n* = 301), normal samples (*n* = 168); LIHC: Liver Hepatocellular Carcinoma (*p*-value 0.0014579663558734), cancer samples (*n* = 204), normal samples (*n* = 65); LUAD: Lung Adenocarcinoma (*p*-value 0.047325233745657), cancer samples (*n* = 452), normal samples (*n* = 48); PAAD: Pancreatic Adenocarcinoma (*p*-value 0.031511114364529), cancer samples (*n* = 91), normal samples (*n* = 16); PRAD: Prostate Adenocarcinoma (*p*-value 9.6625187628874E-7), cancer samples (*n* = 340), normal samples (*n* = 66); READ: Rectum Adenocarcinoma (*p*-value 0.002214301636065), cancer samples (*n* = 96), normal samples (*n* = 13). "*" indicates being statistically significant with $p < 0.05$. "**" indicates being statistically significant with $p < 0.005$.

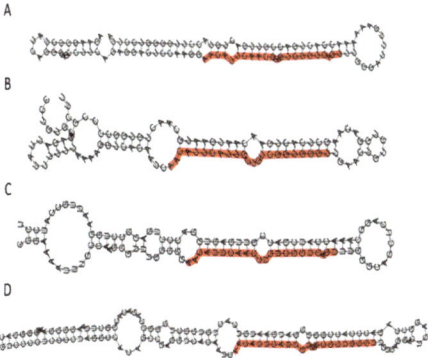

Figure 6. Secondary structure of pre-miRNA; hsa-mir-181a-2 (**A**), hsa-mir-181b-1 (**B**), hsa-mir-181c (**C**), and hsa-mir-181d (**D**) for *HIGD2A* target gene.

Table 2. Clinical microRNA (miRNA) and gene expression profile from TCGA (miRNA-Target expression profile).

miRNA. (Accession ID)	Mature miRNA Sequence	miRNA-Target Expression Profile (TCGA)		
		Tumor (n)	R (Pearson Correlation)	p-Value
hsa-mir-181a-2 (MIRT256742 [miRNA, hsa-miR-181a-5p :: HIGD2A, target gene])	39| AACAUUCAACGCUGUCGGUGAGU |61	KICH (25) PRAD (50)	0.346 −0.239	0.05 0.05
hsa-mir-181b-1 (MIRT256743 [miRNA, hsa-miR-181b-5p :: HIGD2A, target gene])	36| AACAUUCAUUGCUGUCGGUGGGU |58	HNSC (42) BRCA (84) KICH (25) LUSC (38) KIRP (32)	−0.409 −0.258 0.374 −0.276 0.296	3.6×10^{-3} 8.9×10^{-3} 0.03 0.05 0.05
hsa-mir-181c (MIRT256744 [miRNA, hsa-miR-181c-5p :: HIGD2A, target gene])	27| AACAUUCAACCUGUCGGUGAGU |48	BRCA (84) LIHC (49) CHOL (9) LUSC (38) KICH (25)	−0.312 0.283 0.642 −0.302 0.346	1.9×10^{-3} 0.02 0.03 0.03 0.05
hsa-miR-181d (MIRT256746 [miRNA, hsa-miR-181d-5p :: HIGD2A, target gene])	36| AACAUUCAUUGUUGUCGGUGGGU |58	BRCA (84) LUSC (38) LIHC (49)	−0.379 −0.389 0.236	1.9×10^{-4} 7.9×10^{-3} 0.05

3.3. Study of the Datasets of HIGD2A Expression in Diffuse Large B-cell Lymphoma by Profiling Arrays with Gene Expression Omnibus

Diffuse large B-cell lymphoma (DLBCL) is hematologic cancer and accounts for 35% to 40% of non-Hodgkin's lymphomas, the most common malignant lymphoid disease in adults [42,43]. Several classification schemes have been proposed for DLBCL, one of which was the molecular profiling of DLBCL revealing three subtypes: mitochondrial oxidative phosphorylation (OXPHOS), B-cell receptor/proliferation, and host response [44]. Another more widely accepted classification scheme was the cell-of-origin (COO), which presented two categories based on patterns of gene expression reminiscent of germinal center B cell (GCB group) and activated B cell (ABC group) [45]. However, the different subtypes of DLBCL are associated with different pathogenic mechanisms and outcomes [43]. OXPHOS-DLBCLs shows increased glutathione levels, enhanced mitochondrial energy transduction, and greater incorporation of nutrient-derived carbons into the tricarboxylic acid cycle [46]. The metabolic phenotypes of neoplastic lymphocytes, and adjacent stroma in DLBCL, indicate an OXPHOS phenotype in neoplastic lymphocytes while stromal cells in DLBCL samples display a glycolytic phenotype [47].

Bhalla et al. (2018) [18] studied the role of hypoxia in DLBCL using two human lymphoma cell lines, HLY-1 and SUDHL2, which were cultured under conditions of hypoxia or normoxia. In this study, a gene expression microarray analysis was employed to examine the global gene expression differences under these conditions. In this dataset, we analyzed the *HIGD2A* expression in DLBCL with GEO2R. Neither of the two cell lines displayed differential expression of the *HIGD2A* gene in response to hypoxia (Figure 7A). Bhalla et al. (2018) [18] suggested that the growth of lymphoma cell lines HLY-1 and SUDHL2 was resistant to hypoxic stress. Gómez-Abad et al., (2011) [19] also studied the gene-expression profile in a series of non-Hodgkin lymphoma patients, Follicular Lymphoma (FL), Marginal Zone Lymphoma_Type (MALT), Nodal Marginal Zone Lymphoma (NMZL), Diffuse Large B Cell Lymphoma (DLBCL), Mantle Cell Lymphoma (MCL), Chronic Lymphocytic Leukemia (CLL) and as controls, reactive tonsils, and lymph-node were used. In this dataset, we analyzed the *HIGD2A* expression, and the DLBCL indicated a *HIGD2A* expression significantly higher than the reactive tonsils (Figure 7B). The expression of *HIGD2A* in DLBCL is significantly higher than in NMZL (Figure 7B). Likewise, Brune et al., (2008) [20] studied the origin and pathogenesis of lymphocyte-predominant Hodgkin lymphoma, the analysis of differential gene expression in primary human lymphoma cells of nodular lymphocyte-predominant Hodgkin lymphoma in comparison with primary lymphoma cells of classical Hodgkin lymphoma cells and another B-non-Hodgkin lymphoma, including DLBCL.

Furthermore, our dataset analysis reveals a significant higher *HIGD2A* expression in DLBCL concerning all subsets of non- cancerous B lymphocytes isolated from blood or tonsils (naive B-cells, memory B-cells, centrocytes, centroblasts, and plasma cells) (Figure 7C). Lastly, the analysis of the GSE117556 dataset from the retrospective analysis of the whole transcriptome data for 928 DLBCL patients [48] proves no differences of *HIGD2A* expression between the molecular COO subtypes; GCB and ABC.

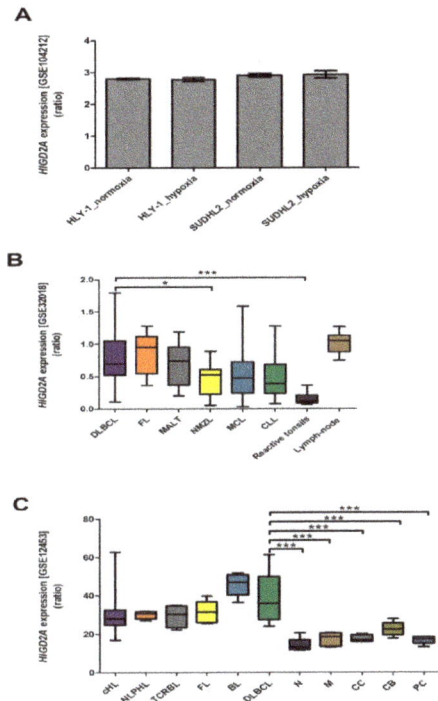

Figure 7. *HIGD2A* expression in DLBCL. (**A**) Dataset GSE104212, Role of hypoxia in Diffuse Large B-cell Lymphoma. Two human lymphoma cell lines, HLY-1 and SUDHL2, were cultured under conditions of hypoxia ($n = 3$) or normoxia ($n = 3$), hypoxia was induced at 1% oxygen in the presence of 5% CO2 for 24 to 48 h [18], and gene expression microarray analysis employed to examine the global gene expression differences under these conditions. (**B**) Dataset GSE32018, Gene-expression profile in a series of non-Hodgkin lymphoma (NHL) patients. FL, Follicular Lymphoma ($n = 23$); MALT, Marginal Zone Lymphoma_MALT type ($n = 15$); NMZL, Nodal Marginal Zone Lymphoma ($n = 13$); DLBCL, Diffuse Large B Cell Lymphoma ($n = 22$); MCL, Mantle Cell Lymphoma ($n = 24$); CLL, Chronic Lymphocytic Leukemia ($n = 16$); reactive tonsils ($n = 6$) and Lymph-node ($n = 7$) were used as controls. (**C**) Dataset GSE12453, Origin and pathogenesis of lymphocyte-predominant Hodgkin lymphoma as revealed by global gene expression analysis. cHL, classical Hodgkin lymphoma ($n = 12$); NLPHL, nodular lymphocyte-predominant Hodgkin lymphoma ($n = 5$); TCRBL, T-cell rich B-cell lymphoma ($n = 4$); FL, Follicular Lymphoma ($n = 5$); BL, Burkitt lymphoma ($n = 5$); DLBCL, Diffuse Large B Cell Lymphoma ($n = 11$); N, Naive B-cells ($n = 5$); M, Memory B-cells ($n = 5$); CC, Centrocytes ($n = 5$); CB, Centroblasts ($n = 5$); PC, Plasma cells ($n = 5$). * $p < 0.05$, *** $p < 0.001$.

The effect of *HIGD2A* high expression level on DLBCL patient survival illustrates a downward trend of survival probability in patients ($n = 11$) with high expression in relation with patients ($n = 36$) with low expression, $p = 0.85$ [49] (Figure 8). Other cancers with a high expression of *HIGD2A* present a downward trend survival of patients, being significant for Liver hepatocellular carcinoma (LIHC)

$p = 0.046$; Skin cutaneous melanoma (SKCM) $p = 0.024$; Uterine Corpus Endometrial Carcinoma (UCEC) $p \leq 0.0001$; and Uveal Melanoma (UVM) $p = 0.0055$ (Figure 8). Meanwhile, other cancers with high expression of *HIGD2A* present an upward trend in the survival of patients, being significant for Sarcoma (SARC) $p = 0.0087$ (Figure 8).

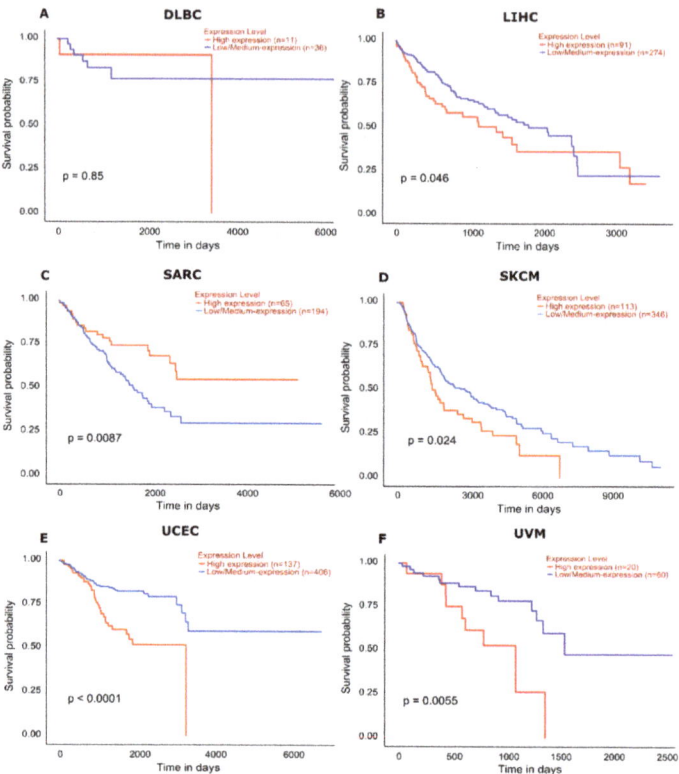

Figure 8. Effect of *HIGD2A* expression on cancer patient survival. The red lines represent a high expression level of *HIGD2A*, and blue lines represent a low/medium expression level of *HIGD2A*. (**A**) DLBCL $p = 0.85$; high expression ($n = 11$), Low/medium expression ($n = 36$). (**B**) LIHC (Liver hepatocellular carcinoma) $p = 0.046$; high expression ($n = 91$), Low/medium expression ($n = 274$). (**C**) SARC (Sarcoma) $p = 0.0087$; high expression ($n = 65$), Low/medium expression ($n = 194$). (**D**) SKCM (Skin cutaneous melanoma) $p = 0.024$; high expression ($n = 113$), Low/medium expression ($n = 346$). (**E**) UCEC (Uterine Corpus Endometrial Carcinoma) $p \leq 0.0001$; high expression ($n = 137$), Low/medium expression ($n = 406$). (**F**) UVM (Uveal Melanoma) $p = 0.0055$; high expression ($n = 20$), Low/medium expression ($n = 60$).

3.4. Effect of Quercetin on the Expression of Higd2a in Mouse Bone Marrow, Liver and Spleen

Quercetin is a natural polyphenolic flavonoid, abundant in the human diet, which has several properties: antioxidant, antihypertensive, antifibrotic, antidiabetic, anti-inflammatory, anticancer, and antibacterial [50]. Quercetin has a cancer cell-specific anti-proliferation effect; quercetin has been shown to prevent carcinogenesis in murine models. Quercetin induces anti-proliferation and arrests the G2/M phase in U937 cells; this was associated with a decrease in the E2F1 level [51]. Quercetin induced p21 CDK inhibitor with a related decrease of phosphorylation of pRb, which inhibits the G1/S cell cycle progression by blocking E2F1 [52]. The transcription factor E2F1 is related to the cell cycle. The inhibition of cell proliferation promotes E2F1 binding to the regulatory region of *HIGD2A*, thus setting a role for E2F-1 in the regulation of *HIGD2A* expression [8]. We wonder what would happen with the expression of *Higd2a* in an animal model treated with quercetin, where the cell cycle would present alterations due to quercetin. To this effect, different tissues involved in DLBCL were used: bone marrow, spleen, and liver, from C57BL/6 mice, injected with quercetin (50 mg/kg) and compared with control animals injected with the PBS/DMSO vehicle. The RT-qPCR technique analyzed the expression of the *Higd2a* gene. The relative quantification of the *Higd2a* gene showed tissue specific-differential expression, displaying higher expression in the bone marrow when compared with spleen and liver (Figure 9A). This result may be related to differences in tissues' proliferation rates. The latter is supported by the findings of Li et al., (2014) [53] who researched the downregulation of survival gene expression of an anti-cancerogenic treatment combined with quercetin. We wondered whether quercetin treatment modulated *Higd2a* expression in relevant tissues for DLBCL. Quercetin significantly increased the expression of *Higd2a* in spleen and bone marrow, while it decreased it in the liver (Figure 9B–D). Finally, the modulation by quercetin of the expression of *Higd2a* in liver, spleen, and bone marrow in adult mice might be related to the effect of quercetin on cellular proliferation.

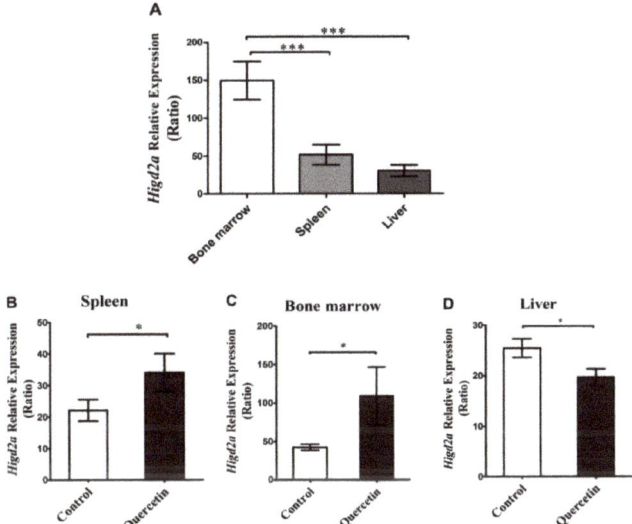

Figure 9. Effect of quercetin on mice *Higd2a* gene expression. Male adult C57BL/6 mice (12 months of age) were administered intraperitoneally daily (i.p.) with 50 mg/Kg quercetin (Cat # Q4951, Sigma-Aldrich) (*n* = 9) or with vehicle (5 % DMSO and PBS) for control animals (*n* = 9), for 15 days. The *Higd2a* gene expression was quantified by RT-qPCR with independent runs of the control spleen, control bone marrow and control liver (**A**). *Higd2a* quantification by Real-Time Quantitative Reverse Transcription Polymerase Chain Reaction (qRT-PCR) with independent runs of the spleen samples of control and quercetin treated; spleen (**B**); bone marrow (**C**) and liver (**D**). Each bar chart represents the mean ± SEM, analyzed by *t*-test ($p < 0.05$), followed by a Mann–Whitney test. * $p < 0.05$, *** $p < 0.001$.

4. Discussion

In this study, we report that the mitochondrial protein HIG2A might have a nuclear localization signal (NLS) and a potential sumoylation motif (Figure 3). The above structural features support the HIG2A nuclear localization, according to our observations made by confocal microscopy and detection of HIG2A in nuclear fractions [8] (Figure 4). HIG2A protein might function as a regulator of respiratory supercomplexes assemblies in response to hypoxia, cellular metabolism, and cell cycle [8]. HIG2A could function as a hypoxia sensor in respiratory supercomplexes to activate signaling pathways of response to hypoxic stress.

This study focuses on the molecular biosystem analysis of genetic features of the *HIGD2A* gene in cancer biology. We learned that the *HIGD2A* gene is not connected to cancer via mutation. However, DNA methylation and mRNA expression in the *HIGD2A* gene showed significant alterations in diverse cancer (Figure 5). Besides, four miRNAs for the *HIGD2A* gene have been reported as having an influence on cancer development [39,41], summarized in Figure 6 and Table 2. For instance, *HIGD2A* gene showed a significantly higher expression in Diffuse large B-cell lymphoma (DLBCL) (Figure 7). Intriguingly, the *HIGD2A* high expression level on DLBCL patients exhibited a downward trend of survival probability [49] (Figure 8). The correlation of *HIGD2A* high expression and poor patient survival is significant for liver hepatocellular carcinoma; cutaneous skin melanoma; uterine corpus endometrial carcinoma; and uveal melanoma (Figure 8).

In this study, we considerably evaluated the expression of the *Higd2a* gene in healthy bone marrow-liver-spleen tissues of mice after quercetin (50 mg/kg) treatment. The difference in the expression of the *Higd2a* gene in the bone marrow, liver, and spleen may be related to tissues' proliferation rates (Figure 9). Regardless of liver high metabolic rate, the liver is a quiescent organ (Phase G0 of the cell cycle) with a low rate of cellular proliferation with only 0.0012 to 0.01% of hepatocytes undergoing mitosis [54]. In contrast, the bone marrow is a tissue with a high rate of cellular proliferation of hematopoietic stem cells (HSCs) [55]. Bone marrow presents hypoxic niches [56] that might influence the expression of the *Higd2a* gene. Besides, the generation of red blood cells is stimulated when the blood oxygen levels decay [57].

Recently, a particular type of DLBCL called "bone marrow-liver-spleen" [58,59], which mainly deteriorates those tissues, [60] has been identified. The lymphoid tissues involved in DLBCL display low oxygen levels; bone marrow is hypoxic (pO2 1.3%) with extravascular oxygen tension ranging between pO2 0.6–4.2% [56], spleen also shows a hypoxic environment (pO2 0.5–4.5%) [61]. Meanwhile, the liver presents a higher pO2 of 3–12% [62]. Currently, the importance of hypoxia in this lymphoma has come into play. Hypoxia-Inducible Factor-1 alpha (HIF1α) is stabilized under hypoxic stress in DLBCL cell lines leading to global translational repression that is coupled with a decrease in mitochondrial function [18].

In most growing solid tumors, the vascular aspect is limiting and contains regions that experience hypoxia producing metabolic changes that support energy generation, anabolic processes, and the maintenance of redox potential, thus allowing cancer cells to survive and proliferate in a hostile tumor microenvironment [63,64]. In hypoxia, mitochondria work as an oxygen sensor to regulate cellular energetics, reactive oxygen species, and cell death [65].

In this work, we observed that quercetin modulated the expression of the *Higd2a* gene. In spleen and bone marrow, the expression was increased significantly, while in the liver, it decreased significantly (Figure 9). Modulation of *Higd2a* expression might be related to the effects of quercetin on cellular proliferation in promoting healthy bone marrow mesenchymal stem cell (BMSC) proliferation [66,67]. BMSCs cultured and treated with quercetin (0.1–5 µM and 1–10 µM for the isolation of mouse and rat tissues, respectively) significantly stimulated cells [66,67]. On the other hand, quercetin could have antiproliferative effects [68–71]. Quercetin at 2 µM shows antiproliferative activity against acute lymphoid leukemia and acute myeloid leukemia [70]. We previously reported that quercetin treatment also affected erythropoiesis. Immature erythroid populations showed a significant increase in the number of cells, while the iron-dependent cell populations of erythropoiesis for heme and hemoglobin biosynthesis significantly decreased in quercetin-treated mice [25].

Interestingly, quercetin at 50 µM has an antiproliferative effect on rat splenocytes. These cells have also shown a decrease in cell viability and apoptosis induction [71]. Moreover, human mesenchymal stem cell (MSC), isolated from bone marrow and cultured in the presence of two quercetin concentrations (0.1 and 10 µM), showed that quercetin (10 µM) inhibited cell proliferation of undifferentiated MSC [68]. Furthermore, primary rat hepatic stellate cells (HSCs) and Human LO2 hepatocytes were cultured and treated with quercetin 0.5–120 µM. Quercetin at 20 µM resulted in a significant inhibitory effect of HSC proliferation, and quercetin at concentrations higher than 80 µM significantly inhibited the proliferation of LO2 cells [69]. Besides, quercetin (1–10 µM) exerted inhibition of human breast carcinoma cells proliferation by cell cycle arrest in the G1 phase product of the induction of p21 and a decrease of phosphorylation of the retinoblastoma tumor suppressor protein (Rb) [52] (Figure 10). Remarkably, quercetin at 10 µM did not affect the proliferation of MCF-10A cells, which have the characteristics of normal breast epithelium [52]. All the above indicates that quercetin had selective inhibitory effects on cell proliferation at a specific dose range and suggests that quercetin has a cancer cell-specific anti-proliferation effect.

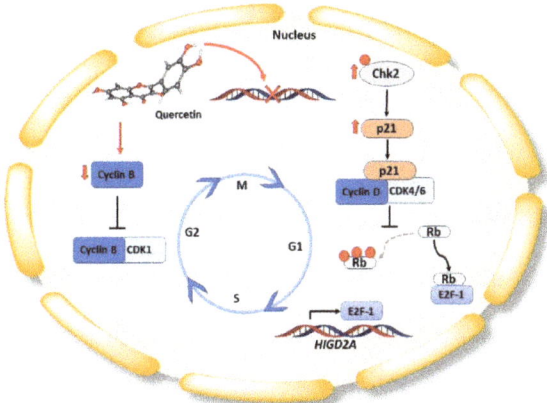

Figure 10. Quercetin can inhibit the progression of the cell cycle in cancer cells. Quercetin induces the arrest of the cell cycle in the G0/G1 phase; Low doses of Quercetin, induces slight damage in the DNA causing the activation Chk2, a primary transcriptional regulator of p21. The p21 protein is a kinase-dependent cyclin inhibitor (CDK), p21 binds to the cyclin/CDK complex in the G1 phase, causing the decrease in the phosphorylation of the retinoblastoma protein (pRb). When pRb is in its hypophosphorylated state, it is bound to the transcription factor E2F1, inhibiting the cell cycle progression in G1 / S, due to the capture of E2F1 by pRb. The transcription factor E2F1 is involved in the regulation of *HIGD2A* gene expression. Quercetin decreases the expression of the cyclin B1 protein by arresting the cell cycle progression in the G2/M phase; Quercetin inhibits the recruitment of the transcription factor NF-Y to the promoter region of the cyclin B1 gene, decreasing its transcriptional expression. Cyclin B1 is an essential component for the function of CDK1 and the progression of the cell cycle in the G2/M phase.

The transcription factor E2F1 is involved in the regulation of *HIGD2A* gene expression [8] (Figure 10). E2F1 plays a role in energy homeostasis, acting as a metabolic switch from oxidative to glycolytic metabolism under stressful conditions [9,10]. Roscovitine is an inhibitor of CDK that suppresses the proliferation of mammalian cells lines, and roscovitine induced a significant increase in *HIGD2A* gene expression in the human embryonic kidney HEK293 cell line. However, in a mouse myoblast C2C12 cell line, the treatment with Caffeic acid phenethyl ester and Flavopiridol, both antiproliferative agents, decreased *HIGD2A* gene expression [8]. While inhibition of cell proliferation in HEK293 was associated with increased expression of *HIGD2A*, in C2C12 it was associated with *HIGD2A* decreased expression. Therefore, *HIGD2A* expression is not an indicator of cell proliferation.

5. Conclusions

DNA methylation and mRNA expression of *HIGD2A* gene present significant alterations in several types of cancer.

Four miRNAs for *HIGD2A* gene show significant gene expression profile related to neoplasms, leukemia, carcinoma, and lymphoma.

HIGD2A gene expression is upregulated in DLBCL.

HIGD2A gene expression was higher in DLBLC than in Nodal Marginal Zone Lymphoma (NMZL). Although this is not specific for DLBLC, it is a more generalized aspect of cancer cells.

The effect of *HIGD2A* high expression level on DLBCL shows a downward trend of survival probability in patients.

The correlation of *HIGD2A* high expression and poor patient survival is significant for liver hepatocellular carcinoma, skin cutaneous melanoma, uterine corpus endometrial carcinoma, and uveal melanoma.

Quercetin induced the expression of *Higd2a* gene in bone marrow and spleen of healthy mice, while it was reduced in the liver.

It is worth further exploring the role of HIG2A in cancer biology.

Author Contributions: Conceptualization, N.C. and L.M.R.; Methodology, C.S., O.Y., W.T., and L.M.R.; Software, O.Y. and W.T.; Validation, C.S., O.Y., and L.M.R.; Formal analysis, C.S., O.Y., and L.M.R.; Investigation, C.S., O.Y., and L.M.R.; Resources, A.A.E., O.G.-B., W.T. and L.M.R.; Data curation, C.S., O.Y., and L.M.R.; Writing—original draft preparation, C.S., and L.M.R.; Writing—review and editing, O.Y., N.C., A.A.E., O.G.-B., W.T., and L.M.R.; Visualization, C.S.; Supervision, L.M.R. and A.A.E.; Project administration, L.M.R.; Funding acquisition, L.R., W.T., O.G.-B., and A.A.E. All authors have read and agreed to the published version of the manuscript.

Funding: This research was funded by FONDECYT 11130192 (LR), FONDECYT 1181165 (W.T.) and FONDECYT 1180983 (AE). Millennium Institute on Immunology and Immunotherapy P09-016-F (AE).

Conflicts of Interest: The authors declare no conflict of interest. The funders had no role in the design of the study; in the collection, analyses, or interpretation of data; in the writing of the manuscript, or in the decision to publish the results.

References

1. Porporato, P.E.; Filigheddu, N.; Pedro, J.M.B.-S.; Kroemer, G.; Galluzzi, L. Mitochondrial metabolism and cancer. *Cell Res.* **2018**, *28*, 265–280. [CrossRef] [PubMed]
2. Sabharwal, S.S.; Schumacker, P.T. Mitochondrial ROS in cancer: Initiators, amplifiers or an Achilles' heel? *Nat. Rev. Cancer* **2014**, *14*, 709–721. [CrossRef] [PubMed]
3. Gaude, E.; Frezza, C. Defects in mitochondrial metabolism and cancer. *Cancer Metab.* **2014**, *2*, 10. [CrossRef] [PubMed]
4. Czabotar, P.E.; Lessene, G.; Strasser, A.; Adams, J.M. Control of apoptosis by the BCL-2 protein family: Implications for physiology and therapy. *Nat. Rev. Mol. Cell Biol.* **2014**, *15*, 49–63. [CrossRef]
5. Gracey, A.Y.; Troll, J.V.; Somero, G.N. Hypoxia-induced gene expression profiling in the euryoxic fish Gillichthys mirabilis. *Proc. Natl. Acad. Sci. USA* **2001**, *98*, 1993–1998. [CrossRef]
6. Chen, Y.-C.; Taylor, E.B.; Dephoure, N.; Heo, J.-M.; Tonhato, A.; Papandreou, L.; Nath, N.; Denko, N.C.; Gygi, S.P.; Rutter, J. Identification of a Protein Mediating Respiratory Supercomplex Stability. *Cell Metab.* **2012**, *15*, 348–360. [CrossRef]
7. Rieger, B.; Shalaeva, D.N.; Söhnel, A.-C.; Kohl, W.; Duwe, P.; Mulkidjanian, A.Y.; Busch, K.B. Lifetime imaging of GFP at CoxVIIIa reports respiratory supercomplex assembly in live cells. *Sci. Rep.* **2017**, *7*, 46055. [CrossRef]
8. Salazar, C.; Elorza, A.A.; Cofre, G.; Ruiz-Hincapie, P.; Shirihai, O.; Ruiz, L.M. The OXPHOS supercomplex assembly factor HIG2A responds to changes in energetic metabolism and cell cycle. *J. Cell. Physiol.* **2019**, *234*, 17405–17419. [CrossRef]
9. Blanchet, E.; Annicotte, J.-S.; Lagarrigue, S.; Aguilar, V.; Clape, C.; Chavey, C.; Fritz, V.; Casas, F.; Apparailly, F.; Auwerx, J.; et al. E2F transcription factor-1 regulates oxidative metabolism. *Nat. Cell Biol.* **2011**, *13*, 1146–1152. [CrossRef]
10. Fajas, L.; Landsberg, R.L.; Huss-Garcia, Y.; Sardet, C.; Lees, J.A.; Auwerx, J. E2Fs regulate adipocyte differentiation. *Dev. Cell* **2002**, *3*, 39–49. [CrossRef]

11. Johannsdottir, H.K.; Jonsson, G.; Johannesdottir, G.; Agnarsson, B.A.; Eerola, H.; Arason, A.; Heikkila, P.; Egilsson, V.; Olsson, H.; Johannsson, O.T.; et al. Chromosome 5 imbalance mapping in breast tumors from BRCA1 and BRCA2 mutation carriers and sporadic breast tumors. *Int. J. Cancer* **2006**, *119*, 1052–1060. [CrossRef] [PubMed]
12. Kram, A.; Li, L.; Zhang, R.D.; Yoon, D.S.; Ro, J.Y.; Johnston, D.; Grossman, H.B.; Scherer, S.; Czerniak, B. Mapping and Genome Sequence Analysis of Chromosome 5 Regions Involved in Bladder Cancer Progression. *Lab. Investig.* **2001**, *81*, 1039. [CrossRef] [PubMed]
13. Westbrook, C.A.; Keinänen, M.J. Myeloid malignancies and chromosome 5 deletions. *Baillière's Clin. Haematol.* **1992**, *5*, 931–942. [CrossRef]
14. Wu, X.; Zhao, Y.; Kemp, B.L.; Amos, C.I.; Siciliano, M.J.; Spitz, M.R. Chromosome 5 aberrations and genetic predisposition to lung cancer. *Int. J. Cancer* **1998**, *79*, 490–493. [CrossRef]
15. Luo, J.; Emanuele, M.J.; Li, D.; Creighton, C.J.; Schlabach, M.R.; Westbrook, T.F.; Wong, K.-K.; Elledge, S.J. A Genome-wide RNAi Screen Identifies Multiple Synthetic Lethal Interactions with the Ras Oncogene. *Cell* **2009**, *137*, 835–848. [CrossRef]
16. Edgar, R.; Domrachev, M.; Lash, A.E. Gene Expression Omnibus: NCBI gene expression and hybridization array data repository. *Nucleic Acids Res.* **2002**, *30*, 207–210. [CrossRef]
17. Gene Expression Omnibus (GEO) Repository. Available online: http://www.ncbi.nlm.nih.gov/geoprofiles/ (accessed on 14 April 2019).
18. Bhalla, K.; Jaber, S.; Nahid, M.N.; Underwood, K.; Beheshti, A.; Landon, A.; Bhandary, B.; Bastian, P.; Evens, A.M.; Haley, J.; et al. Role of hypoxia in Diffuse Large B-cell Lymphoma: Metabolic repression and selective translation of HK2 facilitates development of DLBCL. *Sci. Rep.* **2018**, *8*, 1–15. [CrossRef]
19. Gómez-Abad, C.; Pisonero, H.; Blanco-Aparicio, C.; Roncador, G.; González-Menchén, A.; Martinez-Climent, J.A.; Mata, E.; Rodríguez, M.E.; Muñoz-González, G.; Sánchez-Beato, M.; et al. PIM2 inhibition as a rational therapeutic approach in B-cell lymphoma. *Blood* **2011**, *118*, 5517. [CrossRef]
20. Brune, V.; Tiacci, E.; Pfeil, I.; Döring, C.; Eckerle, S.; van Noesel, C.J.M.; Klapper, W.; Falini, B.; von Heydebreck, A.; Metzler, D.; et al. Origin and pathogenesis of nodular lymphocyte-predominant Hodgkin lymphoma as revealed by global gene expression analysis. *J. Exp. Med.* **2008**, *205*, 2251–2268. [CrossRef]
21. Waterhouse, A.; Bertoni, M.; Bienert, S.; Studer, G.; Tauriello, G.; Gumienny, R.; Heer, F.T.; de Beer, T.A.P.; Rempfer, C.; Bordoli, L.; et al. SWISS-MODEL: Homology modelling of protein structures and complexes. *Nucleic Acids Res.* **2018**, *46*, W296–W303. [CrossRef]
22. Bienert, S.; Waterhouse, A.; de Beer, T.A.P.; Tauriello, G.; Studer, G.; Bordoli, L.; Schwede, T. The SWISS-MODEL Repository-new features and functionality. *Nucleic Acids Res.* **2017**, *45*, D313–D319. [CrossRef] [PubMed]
23. Laskowski, R.A.; MacArthur, M.W.; Moss, D.S.; Thornton, J.M. PROCHECK: A program to check the stereochemical quality of protein structures. *J. Appl. Crystallogr.* **1993**, *26*, 283–291. [CrossRef]
24. Huang, W.-Y.; Hsu, S.-D.; Huang, H.-Y.; Sun, Y.-M.; Chou, C.-H.; Weng, S.-L.; Huang, H.-D. MethHC: A database of DNA methylation and gene expression in human cancer. *Nucleic Acids Res.* **2015**, *43*, D856–D861. [CrossRef] [PubMed]
25. Ruiz, L.M.; Salazar, C.; Jensen, E.; Ruiz, P.A.; Tiznado, W.; Quintanilla, R.A.; Barreto, M.; Elorza, A.A. Quercetin Affects Erythropoiesis and Heart Mitochondrial Function in Mice. *Oxidative Med. Cell. Longev.* **2015**, *2015*, 836301. [CrossRef]
26. Reddy, C.S.; Vijayasarathy, K.; Srinivas, E.; Sastry, G.M.; Sastry, G.N. Homology modeling of membrane proteins: A critical assessment. *Comput. Biol. Chem.* **2006**, *30*, 120–126. [CrossRef]
27. Robert, X.; Gouet, P. Deciphering key features in protein structures with the new ENDscript server. *Nucleic Acids Res.* **2014**, *42*, W320–W324. [CrossRef]
28. Kosugi, S.; Hasebe, M.; Tomita, M.; Yanagawa, H. cNLS Mapper: Prediction of Importin α-Dependent Nuclear Localization Signals. Available online: http://nls-mapper.iab.keio.ac.jp/cgi-bin/NLS_Mapper_form.cgi (accessed on 15 May 2019).
29. Kosugi, S.; Hasebe, M.; Tomita, M.; Yanagawa, H. Systematic identification of cell cycle-dependent yeast nucleocytoplasmic shuttling proteins by prediction of composite motifs. *Proc. Natl. Acad. Sci. USA* **2009**, *106*, 10171. [CrossRef]

30. Vaca Jacome, A.S.; Rabilloud, T.; Schaeffer-Reiss, C.; Rompais, M.; Ayoub, D.; Lane, L.; Bairoch, A.; Van Dorsselaer, A.; Carapito, C. N-terminome analysis of the human mitochondrial proteome. *Proteomics* **2015**, *15*, 2519–2524. [CrossRef]
31. Sui, S.; Wang, J.; Yang, B.; Song, L.; Zhang, J.; Chen, M.; Liu, J.; Lu, Z.; Cai, Y.; Chen, S.; et al. Phosphoproteome analysis of the human Chang liver cells using SCX and a complementary mass spectrometric strategy. *Proteomics* **2008**, *8*, 2024–2034. [CrossRef]
32. Chen, L.; Ma, Y.; Qian, L.; Wang, J. Sumoylation regulates nuclear localization and function of zinc finger transcription factor ZIC3. *Biochim. Biophys. Acta (BBA) Mol. Cell Res.* **2013**, *1833*, 2725–2733. [CrossRef]
33. Du, J.X.; Bialkowska, A.B.; McConnell, B.B.; Yang, V.W. SUMOylation regulates nuclear localization of Krüppel-like factor 5. *J. Biol. Chem.* **2008**, *283*, 31991–32002. [CrossRef] [PubMed]
34. Palczewska, M.; Casafont, I.; Ghimire, K.; Rojas, A.M.; Valencia, A.; Lafarga, M.; Mellström, B.; Naranjo, J.R. Sumoylation regulates nuclear localization of repressor DREAM. *Biochim. Biophys. Acta (BBA) Mol. Cell Res.* **2011**, *1813*, 1050–1058. [CrossRef] [PubMed]
35. Sun, X.; Li, J.; Dong, F.N.; Dong, J.-T. Characterization of nuclear localization and SUMOylation of the ATBF1 transcription factor in epithelial cells. *PLoS ONE* **2014**, *9*, e92746. [CrossRef] [PubMed]
36. Sondka, Z.; Bamford, S.; Cole, C.G.; Ward, S.A.; Dunham, I.; Forbes, S.A. The COSMIC Cancer Gene Census: Describing genetic dysfunction across all human cancers. *Nat. Rev. Cancer* **2018**, *18*, 696–705. [CrossRef] [PubMed]
37. Abbott, K.L.; Nyre, E.T.; Abrahante, J.; Ho, Y.-Y.; Isaksson Vogel, R.; Starr, T.K. The Candidate Cancer Gene Database: A database of cancer driver genes from forward genetic screens in mice. *Nucleic Acids Res.* **2014**, *43*, D844–D848. [CrossRef]
38. Flavahan, W.A.; Gaskell, E.; Bernstein, B.E. Epigenetic plasticity and the hallmarks of cancer. *Science* **2017**, *357*, eaal2380. [CrossRef]
39. Chou, C.-H.; Shrestha, S.; Yang, C.-D.; Chang, N.-W.; Lin, Y.-L.; Liao, K.-W.; Huang, W.-C.; Sun, T.-H.; Tu, S.-J.; Lee, W.-H.; et al. miRTarBase update 2018: A resource for experimentally validated microRNA-target interactions. *Nucleic Acids Res.* **2018**, *46*, D296–D302. [CrossRef]
40. Mishra, S.; Yadav, T.; Rani, V. Exploring miRNA based approaches in cancer diagnostics and therapeutics. *Crit. Rev. Oncol./Hematol.* **2016**, *98*, 12–23. [CrossRef]
41. Riley, K.J.; Rabinowitz, G.S.; Yario, T.A.; Luna, J.M.; Darnell, R.B.; Steitz, J.A. EBV and human microRNAs co-target oncogenic and apoptotic viral and human genes during latency. *EMBO J.* **2012**, *31*, 2207–2221. [CrossRef]
42. Coiffier, B. Rituximab therapy in malignant lymphoma. *Oncogene* **2007**, *26*, 3603. [CrossRef]
43. Chapuy, B.; Stewart, C.; Dunford, A.J.; Kim, J.; Kamburov, A.; Redd, R.A.; Lawrence, M.S.; Roemer, M.G.M.; Li, A.J.; Ziepert, M.; et al. Molecular subtypes of diffuse large B cell lymphoma are associated with distinct pathogenic mechanisms and outcomes. *Nat. Med.* **2018**, *24*, 679–690. [CrossRef] [PubMed]
44. Monti, S.; Savage, K.J.; Kutok, J.L.; Feuerhake, F.; Kurtin, P.; Mihm, M.; Wu, B.; Pasqualucci, L.; Neuberg, D.; Aguiar, R.C.T.; et al. Molecular profiling of diffuse large B-cell lymphoma identifies robust subtypes including one characterized by host inflammatory response. *Blood* **2005**, *105*, 1851. [CrossRef] [PubMed]
45. Alizadeh, A.A.; Eisen, M.B.; Davis, R.E.; Ma, C.; Lossos, I.S.; Rosenwald, A.; Boldrick, J.C.; Sabet, H.; Tran, T.; Yu, X.; et al. Distinct types of diffuse large B-cell lymphoma identified by gene expression profiling. *Nature* **2000**, *403*, 503–511. [CrossRef] [PubMed]
46. Caro, P.; Kishan, A.U.; Norberg, E.; Stanley, I.A.; Chapuy, B.; Ficarro, S.B.; Polak, K.; Tondera, D.; Gounarides, J.; Yin, H.; et al. Metabolic signatures uncover distinct targets in molecular subsets of diffuse large B cell lymphoma. *Cancer Cell* **2012**, *22*, 547–560. [CrossRef]
47. Gooptu, M.; Whitaker-Menezes, D.; Sprandio, J.; Domingo-Vidal, M.; Lin, Z.; Uppal, G.; Gong, J.; Fratamico, R.; Leiby, B.; Dulau-Florea, A.; et al. Mitochondrial and glycolytic metabolic compartmentalization in diffuse large B-cell lymphoma. *Semin. Oncol.* **2017**, *44*, 204–217. [CrossRef]
48. Sha, C.; Barrans, S.; Cucco, F.; Bentley, M.A.; Care, M.A.; Cummin, T.; Kennedy, H.; Thompson, J.S.; Uddin, R.; Worrillow, L.; et al. Molecular High-Grade B-Cell Lymphoma: Defining a Poor-Risk Group That Requires Different Approaches to Therapy. *J. Clin. Oncol.* **2018**, *37*, 202–212. [CrossRef]
49. Chandrashekar, D.S.; Bashel, B.; Balasubramanya, S.A.H.; Creighton, C.J.; Ponce-Rodriguez, I.; Chakravarthi, B.V.S.K.; Varambally, S. UALCAN: A Portal for Facilitating Tumor Subgroup Gene Expression and Survival Analyses. *Neoplasia* **2017**, *19*, 649–658. [CrossRef]

50. Baccan, M.M.; Chiarelli-Neto, O.; Pereira, R.M.S.; Espósito, B.P. Quercetin as a shuttle for labile iron. *J. Inorg. Biochem.* **2012**, *107*, 34–39. [CrossRef]
51. Lee, T.-J.; Kim, O.H.; Kim, Y.H.; Lim, J.H.; Kim, S.; Park, J.-W.; Kwon, T.K. Quercetin arrests G2/M phase and induces caspase-dependent cell death in U937 cells. *Cancer Lett.* **2006**, *240*, 234–242. [CrossRef]
52. Jeong, J.H.; An, J.Y.; Kwon, Y.T.; Rhee, J.G.; Lee, Y.J. Effects of low dose quercetin: Cancer cell-specific inhibition of cell cycle progression. *J. Cell. Biochem.* **2009**, *106*, 73–82. [CrossRef]
53. Li, X.; Wang, X.; Zhang, M.; Li, A.; Sun, Z.; Yu, Q. Quercetin potentiates the antitumor activity of rituximab in diffuse large B-cell lymphoma by inhibiting STAT3 pathway. *Cell Biochem. Biophys.* **2014**, *70*, 1357–1362. [CrossRef]
54. Mangnall, D.; Bird, N.C.; Majeed, A.W. The molecular physiology of liver regeneration following partial hepatectomy. *Liver Int.* **2003**, *23*, 124–138. [CrossRef]
55. Khurana, S. The effects of proliferation and DNA damage on hematopoietic stem cell function determine aging. *Dev. Dyn.* **2016**, *245*, 739–750. [CrossRef] [PubMed]
56. Spencer, J.A.; Ferraro, F.; Roussakis, E.; Klein, A.; Wu, J.; Runnels, J.M.; Zaher, W.; Mortensen, L.J.; Alt, C.; Turcotte, R.; et al. Direct measurement of local oxygen concentration in the bone marrow of live animals. *Nature* **2014**, *508*, 269–273. [CrossRef] [PubMed]
57. Haase, V.H. Hypoxic regulation of erythropoiesis and iron metabolism. *Am. J. Physiol. Ren. Physiol.* **2010**, *299*, F1–F13. [CrossRef] [PubMed]
58. Lyapichev, K.A.; Chapman, J.R.; Iakymenko, O.; Ikpatt, O.F.; Teomete, U.; Sanchez, S.P.; Vega, F. Bone Marrow-Liver-Spleen Type of Large B-Cell Lymphoma Associated with Hemophagocytic Syndrome: A Rare Aggressive Extranodal Lymphoma. *Case Rep. Hematol.* **2017**, *2017*, 8496978. [CrossRef] [PubMed]
59. Yeh, Y.-M.; Chang, K.-C.; Chen, Y.-P.; Kao, L.-Y.; Tsai, H.-P.; Ho, C.-L.; Wang, J.-R.; Jones, D.; Chen, T.-Y. Large B cell lymphoma presenting initially in bone marrow, liver and spleen: An aggressive entity associated frequently with haemophagocytic syndrome. *Histopathology* **2010**, *57*, 785–795. [CrossRef]
60. Knutson, M.D. Iron transport proteins: Gateways of cellular and systemic iron homeostasis. *J. Biol. Chem.* **2017**, *292*, 12735–12743. [CrossRef]
61. Caldwell, C.C.; Kojima, H.; Lukashev, D.; Armstrong, J.; Farber, M.; Apasov, S.G.; Sitkovsky, M.V. Differential Effects of Physiologically Relevant Hypoxic Conditions on T Lymphocyte Development and Effector Functions. *J. Immunol.* **2001**, *167*, 6140. [CrossRef]
62. Godoy, P.; Hewitt, N.J.; Albrecht, U.; Andersen, M.E.; Ansari, N.; Bhattacharya, S.; Bode, J.G.; Bolleyn, J.; Borner, C.; Böttger, J.; et al. Recent advances in 2D and 3D in vitro systems using primary hepatocytes, alternative hepatocyte sources and non-parenchymal liver cells and their use in investigating mechanisms of hepatotoxicity, cell signaling and ADME. *Arch. Toxicol.* **2013**, *87*, 1315–1530. [CrossRef]
63. Bensaad, K.; Harris, A.L. Hypoxia and Metabolism in Cancer. In *Tumor Microenvironment and Cellular Stress. Advances in Experimental Medicine and Biology*; Koumenis, C., Hammond, E., Giaccia, A., Eds.; Springer: New York, NY, USA, 2014; Volume 772, pp. 1–39.
64. Hanahan, D.; Weinberg, R.A. Hallmarks of Cancer: The Next Generation. *Cell* **2011**, *144*, 646–674. [CrossRef]
65. Snyder, C.M.; Chandel, N.S. Mitochondrial regulation of cell survival and death during low-oxygen conditions. *Antioxid. Redox Signal.* **2009**, *11*, 2673–2683. [CrossRef]
66. Pang, X.-G.; Cong, Y.; Bao, N.-R.; Li, Y.-G.; Zhao, J.-N. Quercetin Stimulates Bone Marrow Mesenchymal Stem Cell Differentiation through an Estrogen Receptor-Mediated Pathway. *BioMed. Res. Int.* **2018**, *2018*, 4178021. [CrossRef] [PubMed]
67. Zhou, Y.; Wu, Y.; Jiang, X.; Zhang, X.; Xia, L.; Lin, K.; Xu, Y. The Effect of Quercetin on the Osteogenesic Differentiation and Angiogenic Factor Expression of Bone Marrow-Derived Mesenchymal Stem Cells. *PLoS ONE* **2015**, *10*, e0129605. [CrossRef] [PubMed]
68. Casado-Díaz, A.; Anter, J.; Dorado, G.; Quesada-Gómez, J.M. Effects of quercetin, a natural phenolic compound, in the differentiation of human mesenchymal stem cells (MSC) into adipocytes and osteoblasts. *J. Nutr. Biochem.* **2016**, *32*, 151–162. [CrossRef] [PubMed]
69. He, L.; Hou, X.; Fan, F.; Wu, H. Quercetin stimulates mitochondrial apoptosis dependent on activation of endoplasmic reticulum stress in hepatic stellate cells. *Pharm. Biol.* **2016**, *54*, 3237–3243. [CrossRef] [PubMed]

70. Larocca, L.M.; Teofili, L.; Leone, G.; Sica, S.; Pierelli, L.; Menichella, G.; Scambia, G.; Benedetti Panici, P.; Ricci, R.; Piantelli, M.; et al. Antiproliferative activity of quercetin on normal bone marrow and leukaemic progenitors. *Br. J. Haematol.* **1991**, *79*, 562–566. [CrossRef] [PubMed]
71. López-Posadas, R.; Ballester, I.; Abadía-Molina, A.C.; Suárez, M.D.; Zarzuelo, A.; Martínez-Augustin, O.; Sánchez de Medina, F. Effect of flavonoids on rat splenocytes, a structure–activity relationship study. *Biochem. Pharmacol.* **2008**, *76*, 495–506. [CrossRef] [PubMed]

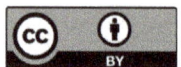
© 2020 by the authors. Licensee MDPI, Basel, Switzerland. This article is an open access article distributed under the terms and conditions of the Creative Commons Attribution (CC BY) license (http://creativecommons.org/licenses/by/4.0/).

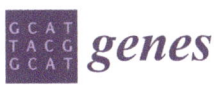

Article

iMethyl-Deep: N6 Methyladenosine Identification of Yeast Genome with Automatic Feature Extraction Technique by Using Deep Learning Algorithm

Omid Mahmoudi [1,†], Abdul Wahab [1,†] and Kil To Chong [2,*]

1. Department of Electronics and Information Engineering, Jeonbuk National University, Jeonju 54896, Korea; omidmahmoudi75@jbnu.ac.kr (O.M.); me.wahabqayyum@gmail.com (A.W.)
2. Advanced Electronics and Information Research Center, Jeonbuk National University, Jeonju 54896, Korea
* Correspondence: kitchong@jbnu.ac.kr
† These authors contributed equally to this work.

Received: 8 April 2020; Accepted: 5 May 2020; Published: 9 May 2020

Abstract: One of the most common and well studied post-transcription modifications in RNAs is N6-methyladenosine (m6A) which has been involved with a wide range of biological processes. Over the past decades, N6-methyladenosine produced some positive consequences through the high-throughput laboratory techniques but still, these lab processes are time consuming and costly. Diverse computational methods have been proposed to identify m6A sites accurately. In this paper, we proposed a computational model named iMethyl-deep to identify m6A *Saccharomyces Cerevisiae* on two benchmark datasets M6A2614 and M6A6540 by using single nucleotide resolution to convert RNA sequence into a high quality feature representation. The iMethyl-deep obtained 89.19% and 87.44% of accuracy on M6A2614 and M6A6540 respectively which show that our proposed method outperforms the state-of-the-art predictors, at least 8.44%, 8.96%, 8.69% and 0.173 on M6A2614 and 15.47%, 28.52%, 25.54 and 0.5 on M6A6540 higher in terms of four metrics Sp, Sn, ACC and MCC respectively. Meanwhile, M6A6540 dataset never used to train a model.

Keywords: RNA N6-methyladenosine site; yeast genome; methylation; computational biology; deep learning; bioinformatics

1. Introduction

Presently, many possibilities of methylation as an additional post-transcriptional modification of RNA have been found in sequence RNAs particularly mRNA [1]. The first internal of the mRNA modification discovery is N6-methyladenosine (m6A) modification which plays a fundamental regulatory role in different biological processes, such as brain development abnormalities [2], mRNA stability and splicing [3], RNA localization and degradation [4] and microRNA biogenesis [5]. It was reported that m6A modification associated with lots of diseases such as thyroid tumor [6], prostate cancer [7], breast cancer [8–10], pancreatic cancer [11,12], leukemia [13] and etc. Undoubtedly, the identification of m6A sites would be a great benefit for cell biology and disease mechanism research.

The high-throughput laboratory techniques such as two-dimensional thin layer chromatography [14], high performance liquid chromatography [15] and next-generation sequencing techniques (e.g., m6A-seq [16] and MeRIP-Seq [2]) have been developed to identify m6A sites but all of these are time consuming and costly. Because of these restrictions of experimental methods, finding an accurate and fast computational method for m6A sites identification is a significant task.

To date, some computational methods [17–19] have been proposed to build a predictive model for detecting transcriptome and m6A sites in different species of RNAs such as *Saccharomyces cerevisiae*, *Homo sapiens*, *Mus musculus* and *Arabidopsis thaliana*. *S. cerevisiae* is one of the most widely utilized organisms in biotechnology over the globe. The first computational method was proposed by Schwartz et al., for identifying of m6A sites [20], where they used machine learning technique logistic regression and inputted handcrafted features.

Chen et al., developed two sequence based predictors for the detection of m6A sites in S. cerevisiae called iRNA-Methyl [17] and RAM-ESVM [18] by using the support vector machine through pseudo nucleotide composition and pseudo dinucleotide composition respectively. iRNA-Methyl and RAM-ESVM have an ability to predict with the accuracy of 65.59% and 78.35% respectively. Xing et al., also contributed to improve the efficiency for the identification of m6A sites by introduced RAM-NPPS [19] model in which they used position-specific condition propensity as feature representation by using support vector machine. Their contribution increased the accuracy of 79.59%. Last but not least, another model was built by the Leyi et al., called DeepM6APred [21] with the handcrafted features by using different machine learning and neural network techniques. Until now DeepM6APred is competing all the predictors by the accuracy of 80.50%. All of these methods were trained and tested by using Chen et al. dataset [17]. They used handcrafted features for the feature representation and machine learning algorithms for constructing the models. For the fair assessment of the performance, each model used 10 fold and jackknife cross-validation.

In this study, we aimed to construct a deep learning model on M6A2614 and M6A6540 datasets which were based on the pioneering work of Chen et al. [17] and Xiaolei Zhu et al. [20] respectively. The proposed predictor which is called iMethyl-deep has a novel and powerful method to identify m6A S. Cerevisiae sites by using single nucleotide resolution to convert RNA sequence into high-quality feature representation in the robust deep learning technique convolution neural network (CNN). It extracts the important features automatically from the inputted RNA samples. This idea purely implemented for multiple extents of features for which deep learning is more robust. The proposed model outperforms in comparison with the state-of-the-art methods and successfully achieves ACC of 89.19% and 87.44% on M6A2614 and M6A6540 benchmark datasets respectively.

2. Materials and Methods

2.1. Benchmark Datasets

Two benchmark datasets for the S. cerevisiae genome were used in this work. The first dataset, named M6A2614, was proposed by Schwartz et al. [22], contains 1307 positive RNA sequences as methylated sites and 1307 negative RNA sequences as non-methylated sites. Several state-of-the-art computational identifiers used the M6A2614 dataset for their predictors [17–19,21]. The second dataset is called as M6A6540 dataset which was introduced by Xiaolei Zhu et al.'s [20] contains 3270 positive RNA sequences regarded as methylated sites and 3270 negative RNA sequences regarded as non-methylated sites, all steps for preparing the dataset was mentioned in their work. Both M6A2614 and M6A6540 benchmark datasets are mutually exclusive and to avoid the redundancy both datasets used CD-HIT-EST software [23]. The length of each sequence is 51 bp in both benchmark datasets. A depiction of the datasets is shown in Table 1.

Table 1. Benchmark datasets demonstration.

Datasets	Positive	Negative	Total
M6A2614	1307	1307	2614
M6A6540	3270	3270	6540

As per the literature, the datasets are divided into training and testing set. The training dataset is characteristically used for the learning of the model, whereas the testing dataset is worked to evaluate the model. The most effective way for testing is the k-fold cross-validation test [24], which we got the combinations of different independent test datasets.

2.2. Formulation and Representation of RNA Samples

It is important to make data in the form of deep learning recognition because all algorithms take input as a vector or discrete, so we formulated RNA sequences into vector form. It also needs to consider the loss of pattern sequence information while converting into vector form, mostly it happens in the discrete model. There are many introduced techniques to avoid it, for example, PseAAC [25], which is widely used in proteomics. There is some vigorous software regarding PseAAC known as PseAAC-Builder [26], Propy [27], and PseAAC-General [28] was developed as an open source. Another approach, Pseudo K-tuple nucleotide composition (PseKNC), was introduced to provoke different feature vectors for RNA and DNA sequences, which used widely in many research works [29–32]. The sequence of RNA in the benchmark datasets is represented as $R = \{N1, N2, N3, N4\ldots, Ni\}$, where $N1$ denoted as the first single nucleotide in a sequence, $N2$ the second nucleotide and so on until the end of the sequence. In each sequence, there are four nucleotides A, C, G, U represented as a string form with different combinations like $AGCUAUAG\ldots UGACAU$.

We started with a suitable format of deep learning to convert an RNA sequence into vector form for the formulation of the sequence instead of manually crafted features such as chemical properties and nucleotide frequency. One-hot encoding is used for this purpose, which maps the categorical variables into a binary representation. The four unique nucleotides A, C, G, and U mapped as (1, 0, 0, 0), (0, 1, 0, 0), (0, 0, 1, 0), (0, 0, 0, 1) respectively. Several deep learning models used one-hot encoding for the representation of the sequences such as [33,34]. Each sequence in both datasets is 51 bp long and after one-hot encoding, it transformed into a matrix. The matrix is represented as 4 columns and 51 rows, each column signifies an RNA base of sequence and the rows signify mapped representations of unique nucleotides.

3. The Proposed Model

We presented a model based on a CNN instead of handcrafted features extraction models as a classifier such as support-vector machine (SVM) [17,35–37]. CNN has been used in deep learning techniques and the area of bioinformatics extensively [33,34,38–40] and also in other fields [41,42]. It has the ability to gather all the worthwhile features automatically from the RNA m6A sequences during the training process. The input of the iMethyl-deep is one-hot encoded RNA sequences, each one has a length of 51 bp and four channels. CNN is processed with various layers and functions such as the convolution layer, pooling layer, activation function, and dropout to get exceptional results. We implemented a grid search algorithm while the learning process of the model with different hyper-parameters tuning. The fine-tuning parameters consist of convolution layers, filters, filter size, pool-size, stride length, and dropout values. The range of hyper-parameters is illustrated in Table 2.

The best resultant optimized parameters were chosen while considering the minimum validation loss to evade the overfitting and underfitting. In the proposed model, we implemented two 1-D (one-dimensional) convolution layers, which are represented as Conv1D. Each layer of Conv1D has 16 filters, with a filter-size of five. However, the convolution layer has the most pivot functionality on CNN. It extracts the features from the RNA positive and negative samples of m6A sites. We used the L2 regularization and bias regularization as a parameter in the convolution layer to avoid the overfitting problem with the value of 0.001 for both Conv1D. The exponential linear unit (ELU) is used as an activation function. A group normalization layer (GN) was used after both convolution layers, which helped to decrease the outcomes of convolution layers produced by each filter of Conv1D. Group normalization distributes the outcomes of convolution layers into groups and performs the normalization in each group. The group size is set as four. After each GN layer, a max-pooling layer was implemented to reduce the redundancy of the features from preceding layers. We set the pool-size of 4 and stride of two in both layers. The dropout layer was used after the second max-pooling layer with a rate of 0.35, which prevents overfitting and enhances the authenticity of the model. The dropout layer works as a strainer to discard some intermediary features while the training period, by arbitrarily shutting down some neurons and setting zero value for them. We used flatten function to unstack all multidimensional tensors of previous layers into a 1D tensor and fed to the fully connected (FC) layer. FC layer has 32 hidden units and also uses the L2 regularization parameter for the weights and bias with the value of 0.0001. We used the ELU activation function for the FC layer. In the end, a fully connected layer was implemented with the sigmoid function for binary classification. Sigmoid function squeezes the output values between 0 and 1.

Table 2. Range of Hyper-parameters.

Parameters	Range
Convolution layers	[1, 2, 3, 4]
Filters in convolution Layer	[6, 8, 16, 24, 32, 44, 64]
Filter size	[2, 4, 5, 7, 8, 10, 13]
Pool-size in Maxpooling	[2, 4]
Stride length in Maxpooling	[2, 4]
Dropout values	[0.3, 0.35, 0.4, 0.45, 0.5]

The architecture of the proposed model is described in Table 3, where Conv1D (f, k, s) is a convolution layer as one-dimensional, parameter f is the number of filters, k is the kernel-size, and s represents the stride. ELU signifies as an activation function. The GroupNormalization (g) is a normalization layer, where g is a number of groups. The Maxpooling1D (l, r) is a max-pooling layer with two parameters, l is used as pool-size and r for the stride. The Dropout (d) denotes as a dropout layer with the value of d and the Dense (e) is a FC layer with the number of e nodes. At the last, the Sigmoid () function as an activation function makes it possible that the range of output should be between 0 and 1. Figure 1 demonstrates the comprehensive graphical architecture of the proposed model.

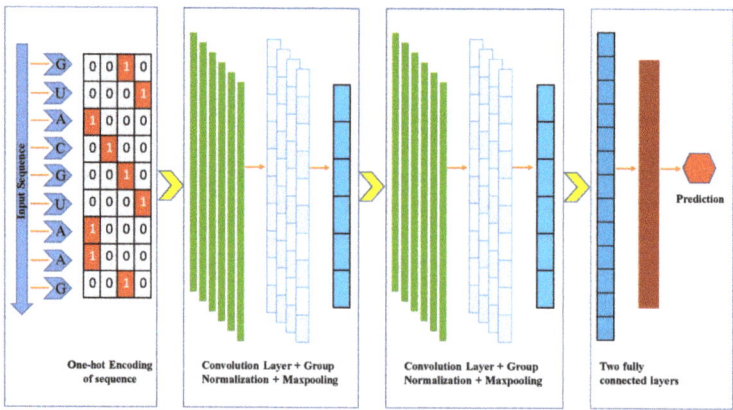

Figure 1. A graphical illustration of iMethyl-deep. Inputted RNA sequence converted into one-hot encoded, then fed into the Convolution Neural Network (CNN) layers for training the datasets.

Table 3. The architecture of the proposed model.

Layer	Output Shape
Input	(51, 4)
Conv1D(16, 5, 1)	(47, 16)
ELU	(47, 16)
GroupNormalization(4)	(47, 16)
MaxPool1D (4, 2)	(22, 16)
Conv1D(16, 5, 1)	(18, 16)
ELU	(18, 16)
GroupNormalization(4)	(18, 16)
MaxPool1D(4,2)	(8, 16)
Flatten	(128)
Dropout(0.35)	(128)
Dense(32)	(32)
Dense(1)	1
Sigmoid	1

In iMethyl-deep, we used stochastic gradient descent (SGD) optimizer with the momentum of 0.95 and binary cross-entropy as a loss function [43], Learning rate for SGD is set as 0.003. The epoch and batch sizes are set to 100 and 32 respectively. The callbacks function is used to handle the checkpoint for saving the models and their best weights which have high accuracy. The early stopping is also used to stop the prediction accuracy when the validation stops improving, the value for the patience level is set to 30. The iMethyl-deep is implemented on the Keras framework [44].

4. Performance Evaluation

To calculate the performance of the prediction system, we used 10 folds cross-validation. Choosing a precise cross-validation method is a foremost part of investigating a prediction achievement. The k-fold cross validation method is a resampling method that provides a more accurate estimate of algorithm performance. It does this by first shuffling whole data and splitting them into k groups. Then the algorithm is trained and evaluated k times and the performance summarized by taking the mean performance score. Each unique group holds out as eight folds for training, one fold for validation, and the last one for testing. Each model was fitted on the training set and will be saved which one gives the highest accuracy on the validation fold. The performance of the model was evaluated on test fold, keeping the evaluated scores and abandoning the model. The Average scores of 10 repetitions were calculated and used as the performance evaluation of the proposed model. Four standard evaluation metrics were used in many research publication [45,46], which consist of overall accuracy (ACC), Mathew's correlation coefficient (MCC), specificity (Sp), and sensitivity (Sn). The following are the mathematical formulation of four metrics [47–50].

$$ACC = \frac{TP + TN}{TP + TN + FP + FN} \qquad (1)$$

$$SN = \frac{TP}{TP + FN} \tag{2}$$

$$SP = \frac{TN}{TN + FP} \tag{3}$$

$$MCC = \frac{TP \times TN - FP \times FN}{\sqrt{(TP + FP) \times (TP + FN) \times (TN + FP) \times (TN + FN)}} \tag{4}$$

where TP indicates a true positive which means a positive number of sequences predicted correctly and TN indicates as a true negative which can be described as a negative number of sequences predicted correctly. Meanwhile, FP designates as false positive which can be explained as a negative number of sequences identified falsely as positive and FN represents a false negative which means a positive number of sequences predicted falsely as negative. The receiver operating characteristics curve (ROC) and area under the ROC curve (AUC) are also used to evaluate the performance of the proposed model.

5. Results and Discussion

We evaluated the identification performance of our model, iMethyl-deep, on two RNA m6A benchmark datasets M6A2146 [22] and M6A6540 [20] for the *S. cerevisiae* genome. The results of the proposed model on the benchmark datasets show better performance in terms of all evaluation metrics. We used the same proposed model for both datasets.

5.1. The Performance of iMethyl-Deep on M6A2146 Benchmark Dataset

After validating the effectiveness of the proposed method, by comparing its performance with four state-of-the-art methods iRNA-Methyl [17], RAM-ESVM [18], RAM-NPPS [19], and DeepM6APred [21] which used the same benchmark dataset, we obtained 89.92%, 88.46%, 89.19% and 0.783 for Sp, Sn, ACC and MCC respectively. Comparing with Deepm6Apred method, which is the best among the other existing methods, the performance of the proposed predictor is 8.96%, 8.44%, 8.69% and 0.173 higher in terms of four metrics respectively. We observed the proposed method is capable to distinguish m6A sites from non-m6A sites more accurately as compared to the other state-of-the-art predictors. Additionally, the less false positives are achieved by the highest Sp, which we reached. Table 4 shows the detail results of the iMethyl-deep model and Figure 2 represents the graphical illustration of results. We achieved 0.931 of AUC to prove the successful performance of the iMethyl-deep as depicted in Figure 3. The visualization representation of the confusion matrix is also shown in Figure 4.

Table 4. Performance comparison of iMethyl-deep with other four state-of-the-art methods on M6A2614 dataset. Overall accuracy (ACC), Mathew's correlation coefficient (MCC), specificity (Sp), and sensitivity (Sn).

Model	Sp (%)	Sn (%)	ACC (%)	MCC
iRNA-Methyl	60.63	70.55	65.59	0.29
RAM-ESVM	77.78	78.93	78.35	0.57
RAM-NPPS	80.87	78.42	79.65	0.59
DeepM6APred	81.48	79.50	80.50	0.61
iMethyl-deep	89.92	88.46	89.19	0.78

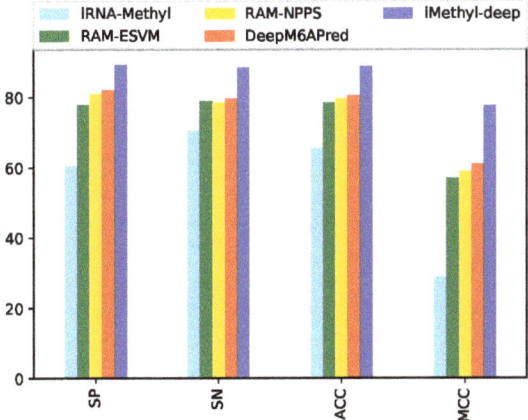

Figure 2. Performance evaluation illustration of iMethyl-deep on M6A2146 dataset.

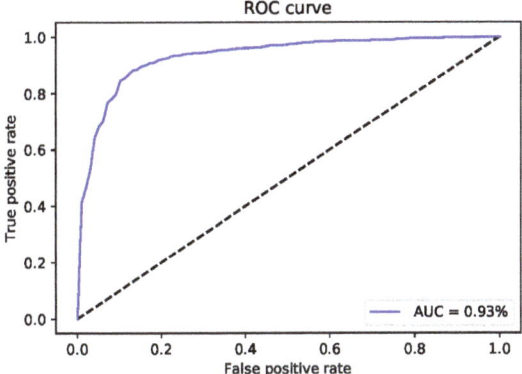

Figure 3. The receiver operating characteristics (ROC) curve of iMethyl-deep on M6A2614 dataset.

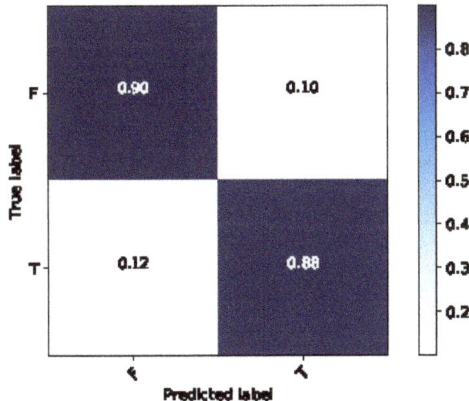

Figure 4. Graphical illustration of confusion matrix of iMethyl-deep on M6A2614 dataset.

5.2. The Performance of iMethyl-Deep on M6A6540 Benchmark Dataset

In this section, the results of iMethyl-deep on benchmark dataset M6A6540 which were introduced by Zhu et al. [20] are shown. We should mentioned the DeepM6APred was just trained and tested on M6A2614 and not considered on M6A6540 dataset. Meanwhile, The M6A6540 never used to train in the other mentioned models. As shown in Table 5 and Figure 5, we obtained 86.54% of specificity, 88.34% of sensitivity, 87.44% of accuracy, and 0.749 of MCC. It is clear that our proposed model can outperform all four metrics in comparison with three state-of-the-art model RAM-NPPS [19], iRNA-Methyl [17] and RAM-ESVM [18] which had the maximum value for Sp, Sn, ACC and MCC repectively. Moreover, same M6A2146 dataset we reached to 0.931 of AUC for M6A6540 dataset. The AUC curve and the visualization representation of the confusion matrix are depicted in Figures 6 and 7 respectively.

Table 5. The results of iMethyl-deep on benckmark M6A6540 dataset.

Model	Sp (%)	Sn (%)	ACC (%)	MCC
RAM-NPPS	71.07	34.59	52.83	0.06
iRNA-Methyl	61.68	59.82	60.75	0.22
RAM-ESVM	64.53	59.27	61.90	0.24
iMethyl-deep	86.54	88.34	87.44	0.74

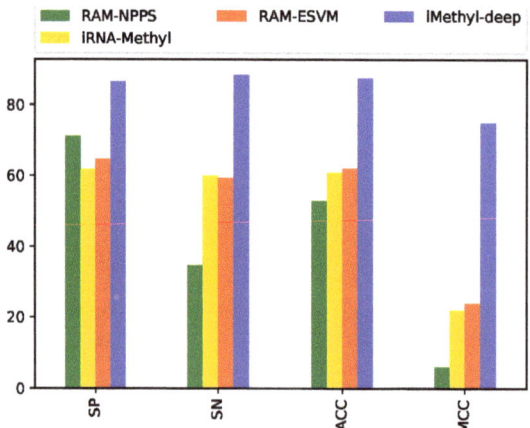

Figure 5. Performance evaluation illustration of iMethyl-deep on M6A6540 dataset.

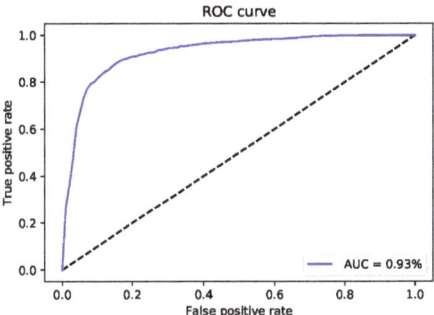

Figure 6. The receiver operating characteristics (ROC) curve of iMethyl-deep on M6A6540 dataset.

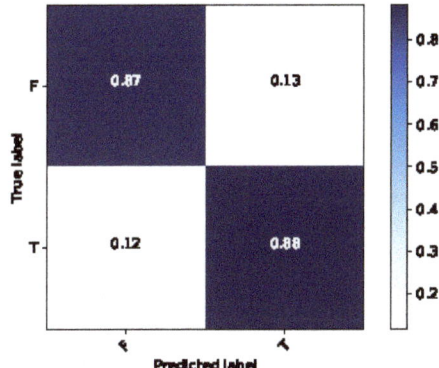

Figure 7. Graphical illustration of confusion matrix of iMethyl-deep on M6A6540 dataset.

6. Conclusions

In this study, we proposed iMethyl-deep as a new computational predictor to identify N6-methyladenosine sites from RNA sequences. Two different benchmark datasets M6A2146 and M6A6540 were compiled to evaluate the performance of the proposed model. We used a one-hot encoding method to input RNA sequence and fed into a CNN. The simulated results show that iMethyl-deep can significantly and robustly improve the performance of deep learning to identify m6A sites. To access the effectiveness of the proposed predictor, we compared its performance with four state-of-the-art models. It predicts all evaluation metrics Sp, Sn, ACC, MCC and AUC better than the others. Potentially, the method proposed in this paper can be extended to be effective in brain development abnormalities, mRNA stability and splicing. In the future, we will further study in other kinds of modifications. The datasets and model is available at https://github.com/abdul-bioinfo/iMethyl-deep.

Author Contributions: conceptualization, O.M., A.W. and K.T.C.; methodology, O.M. and A.W.; software, O.M. and A.W.; validation, O.M., A.W. and K.T.C.; investigation, O.M., A.W. and K.T.C.; writing—original draft preparation: O.M., A.W.; writing, review and editing, O.M., A.W. and K.T.C.; supervision, K.T.C. All authors have read and agreed to the published version of the manuscript.

Funding: This research was supported by the Brain Research Program of the National Research Foundation (NRF) funded by the Korean government (MSIT) (No. NRF-2017M3C7A1044815).

Conflicts of Interest: The authors declare no conflict of interest. The funders had no role in the design of the study; in the collection, analyses, or interpretation of data; in the writing of the manuscript, or in the decision to publish the results.

References

1. Desrosiers, R.; Friderici, K.; Rottman, F. Identification of methylated nucleosides in messenger RNA from Novikoff hepatoma cells. *Proc. Natl. Acad. Sci. USA* **1974**, *71*, 3971–3975. [CrossRef]
2. Meyer, K.D.; Saletore, Y.; Zumbo, P.; Elemento, O.; Mason, C.E.; Jaffrey, S.R. Comprehensive analysis of mRNA methylation reveals enrichment in 3 UTRs and near stop codons. *Cell* **2012**, *149*, 1635–1646. [CrossRef] [PubMed]
3. Nilsen, T.W. Internal mRNA methylation finally finds functions. *Science* **2014**, *343*, 1207–1208. [CrossRef] [PubMed]
4. Meyer, K.D.; Jaffrey, S.R. The dynamic epitranscriptome: N 6-methyladenosine and gene expression control. *Nat. Rev. Mol. Cell Biol.* **2014**, *15*, 313–326. [CrossRef] [PubMed]
5. Alarcón, C.R.; Lee, H.; Goodarzi, H.; Halberg, N.; Tavazoie, S.F. N 6-methyladenosine marks primary microRNAs for processing. *Nature* **2015**, *519*, 482–485. [CrossRef]
6. Heiliger, K.J.; Hess, J.; Vitagliano, D.; Salerno, P.; Braselmann, H.; Salvatore, G.; Ugolini, C.; Summerer, I.; Bogdanova, T.; Unger, K.; et al. Novel candidate genes of thyroid tumourigenesis identified in Trk-T1 transgenic mice. *Endocr. Relat. Cancer* **2012**, *19*, 409. [CrossRef]
7. Machiela, M.J.; Lindström, S.; Allen, N.E.; Haiman, C.A.; Albanes, D.; Barricarte, A.; Berndt, S.I.; Bueno-de Mesquita, H.B.; Chanock, S.; Gaziano, J.M.; et al. Association of type 2 diabetes susceptibility variants with advanced prostate cancer risk in the Breast and Prostate Cancer Cohort Consortium. *Am. J. Epidemiol.* **2012**, *176*, 1121–1129. [CrossRef]
8. Akilzhanova, A.; Nurkina, Z.; Momynaliev, K.; Ramanculov, E.; Zhumadilov, Z.; Rakhypbekov, T.; Hayashida, N.; Nakashima, M.; Takamura, N. Genetic profile and determinants of homocysteine levels in Kazakhstan patients with breast cancer. *Anticancer Res.* **2013**, *33*, 4049–4059.
9. Reddy, S.; Sadim, M.; Li, J.; Yi, N.; Agarwal, S.; Mantzoros, C.; Kaklamani, V. Clinical and genetic predictors of weight gain in patients diagnosed with breast cancer. *Br. J. Cancer* **2013**, *109*, 872–881. [CrossRef]
10. Long, J.; Zhang, B.; Signorello, L.B.; Cai, Q.; Deming-Halverson, S.; Shrubsole, M.J.; Sanderson, M.; Dennis, J.; Michailiou, K.; Easton, D.F.; et al. Evaluating genome-wide association study-identified breast cancer risk variants in African-American women. *PLoS ONE* **2013**, *8*. [CrossRef]
11. Lin, Y.; Ueda, J.; Yagyu, K.; Ishii, H.; Ueno, M.; Egawa, N.; Nakao, H.; Mori, M.; Matsuo, K.; Kikuchi, S. Association between variations in the fat mass and obesity-associated gene and pancreatic cancer risk: A case–control study in Japan. *BMC Cancer* **2013**, *13*, 337. [CrossRef] [PubMed]
12. Pierce, B.L.; Austin, M.A.; Ahsan, H. Association study of type 2 diabetes genetic susceptibility variants and risk of pancreatic cancer: An analysis of PanScan-I data. *Cancer Causes Control* **2011**, *22*, 877–883. [CrossRef] [PubMed]
13. Casalegno-Garduno, R.; Schmitt, A.; Wang, X.; Xu, X.; Schmitt, M. *Wilms' Tumor 1 as A Novel Target for Immunotherapy of Leukemia*; Transplantation Proceedings; Elsevier: Amsterdam, The Netherlands, 2010; Volume 42, pp. 3309–3311.
14. Keith, G. Mobilities of modified ribonucleotides on two-dimensional cellulose thin-layer chromatography. *Biochimie* **1995**, *77*, 142–144. [CrossRef]
15. Zheng, G.; Dahl, J.A.; Niu, Y.; Fedorcsak, P.; Huang, C.M.; Li, C.J.; Vågbø, C.B.; Shi, Y.; Wang, W.L.; Song, S.H.; et al. ALKBH5 is a mammalian RNA demethylase that impacts RNA metabolism and mouse fertility. *Mol. Cell* **2013**, *49*, 18–29. [CrossRef]
16. Dominissini, D.; Moshitch-Moshkovitz, S.; Schwartz, S.; Salmon-Divon, M.; Ungar, L.; Osenberg, S.; Cesarkas, K.; Jacob-Hirsch, J.; Amariglio, N.; Kupiec, M.; et al. Topology of the human and mouse m6A RNA methylomes revealed by m 6 A-seq. *Nature* **2012**, *485*, 201–206. [CrossRef] [PubMed]
17. Chen, W.; Feng, P.; Ding, H.; Lin, H.; Chou, K.C. iRNA-Methyl: Identifying N6-methyladenosine sites using pseudo nucleotide composition. *Anal. Biochem.* **2015**, *490*, 26–33. [CrossRef] [PubMed]
18. Chen, W.; Xing, P.; Zou, Q. Detecting N 6-methyladenosine sites from RNA transcriptomes using ensemble Support Vector Machines. *Sci. Rep.* **2017**, *7*, 1–8. [CrossRef]
19. Xing, P.; Su, R.; Guo, F.; Wei, L. Identifying N 6-methyladenosine sites using multi-interval nucleotide pair position specificity and support vector machine. *Sci. Rep.* **2017**, *7*, 46757. [CrossRef]

20. Zhu, X.; He, J.; Zhao, S.; Tao, W.; Xiong, Y.; Bi, S. A comprehensive comparison and analysis of computational predictors for RNA N6-methyladenosine sites of *Saccharomyces cerevisiae*. *Briefings Funct. Genomics* **2019**, *18*, 367–376.
21. Wei, L.; Su, R.; Wang, B.; Li, X.; Zou, Q.; Gao, X. Integration of deep feature representations and handcrafted features to improve the prediction of N6-methyladenosine sites. *Neurocomputing* **2019**, *324*, 3–9. [CrossRef]
22. Schwartz, S.; Agarwala, S.D.; Mumbach, M.R.; Jovanovic, M.; Mertins, P.; Shishkin, A.; Tabach, Y.; Mikkelsen, T.S.; Satija, R.; Ruvkun, G.; et al. High-resolution mapping reveals a conserved, widespread, dynamic mRNA methylation program in yeast meiosis. *Cell* **2013**, *155*, 1409–1421. [CrossRef]
23. Fu, L.; Niu, B.; Zhu, Z.; Wu, S.; Li, W. CD-HIT: Accelerated for clustering the next-generation sequencing data. *Bioinformatics* **2012**, *28*, 3150–3152. [CrossRef]
24. Chou, K.C.; Zhang, C.T. Prediction of protein structural classes. *Crit. Rev. Biochem. Mol. Biol.* **1995**, *30*, 275–349. [CrossRef]
25. Chou, K.C. Using amphiphilic pseudo amino acid composition to predict enzyme subfamily classes. *Bioinformatics* **2005**, *21*, 10–19. [CrossRef]
26. Du, P.; Wang, X.; Xu, C.; Gao, Y. PseAAC-Builder: A cross-platform stand-alone program for generating various special Chou's pseudo-amino acid compositions. *Anal. Biochem.* **2012**, *425*, 117–119. [CrossRef]
27. Cao, D.S.; Xu, Q.S.; Liang, Y.Z. propy: A tool to generate various modes of Chou's PseAAC. *Bioinformatics* **2013**, *29*, 960–962. [CrossRef]
28. Du, P.; Gu, S.; Jiao, Y. PseAAC-General: Fast building various modes of general form of Chou's pseudo-amino acid composition for large-scale protein datasets. *Int. J. Mol. Sci.* **2014**, *15*, 3495–3506. [CrossRef]
29. Chen, W.; Lei, T.Y.; Jin, D.C.; Lin, H.; Chou, K.C. PseKNC: A flexible web server for generating pseudo K-tuple nucleotide composition. *Anal. Biochem.* **2014**, *456*, 53–60. [CrossRef]
30. Chen, W.; Lin, H.; Chou, K.C. Pseudo nucleotide composition or PseKNC: An effective formulation for analyzing genomic sequences. *Mol. BioSystems* **2015**, *11*, 2620–2634. [CrossRef]
31. Chen, W.; Tang, H.; Ye, J.; Lin, H.; Chou, K.C. iRNA-PseU: Identifying RNA pseudouridine sites. *Mol. Ther. Nucleic Acids* **2016**, *5*, e332.
32. Liu, B.; Fang, L.; Long, R.; Lan, X.; Chou, K.C. iEnhancer-2L: A two-layer predictor for identifying enhancers and their strength by pseudo k-tuple nucleotide composition. *Bioinformatics* **2016**, *32*, 362–369. [CrossRef] [PubMed]
33. Wahab, A.; Ali, S.D.; Tayara, H.; Chong, K.T. iIM-CNN: Intelligent identifier of 6mA sites on different species by using convolution neural network. *IEEE Access* **2019**, *7*, 178577–178583. [CrossRef]
34. Yu, H.; Dai, Z. SNNRice6mA: A deep learning method for predicting DNA N6-methyladenine sites in rice genome. *Front. Genet.* **2019**, *10*, 1071. [CrossRef] [PubMed]
35. Chen, W.; Ding, H.; Zhou, X.; Lin, H.; Chou, K.C. iRNA (m6A)-PseDNC: Identifying N6-methyladenosine sites using pseudo dinucleotide composition. *Anal. Biochem.* **2018**, *561*, 59–65. [CrossRef]
36. Zhou, Y.; Zeng, P.; Li, Y.H.; Zhang, Z.; Cui, Q. SRAMP: Prediction of mammalian N6-methyladenosine (m6A) sites based on sequence-derived features. *Nucleic Acids Res.* **2016**, *44*, e91. [CrossRef]
37. Chen, W.; Feng, P.M.; Lin, H.; Chou, K.C. iRSpot-PseDNC: Identify recombination spots with pseudo dinucleotide composition. *Nucleic Acids Res.* **2013**, *41*, e68. [CrossRef]
38. Tahir, M.; Tayara, H.; Chong, K.T. iDNA6mA (5-step rule): Identification of DNA N6-methyladenine sites in the rice genome by intelligent computational model via Chou's 5-step rule. *Chemom. Intell. Lab. Syst.* **2019**, *189*, 96–101. [CrossRef]
39. Tahir, M.; Tayara, H.; Chong, K.T. iRNA-PseKNC (2methyl): Identify RNA 2'-O-methylation sites by convolution neural network and Chou's pseudo components. *J. Theor. Biol.* **2019**, *465*, 1–6. [CrossRef]
40. Akbar, S.; Hayat, M.; Iqbal, M.; Tahir, M. iRNA-PseTNC: Identification of RNA 5-methylcytosine sites using hybrid vector space of pseudo nucleotide composition. *Front. Comput. Sci.* **2020**, *14*, 451–460. [CrossRef]
41. Ilyas, T.; Khan, A.; Umraiz, M.; Kim, H. SEEK: A Framework of Superpixel Learning with CNN Features for Unsupervised Segmentation. *Electronics* **2020**, *9*, 383. [CrossRef]
42. Zhang, K.; Zuo, W.; Zhang, L. FFDNet: Toward a fast and flexible solution for CNN-based image denoising. *IEEE Trans. Image Process.* **2018**, *27*, 4608–4622. [CrossRef] [PubMed]
43. De Boer, P.T.; Kroese, D.P.; Mannor, S.; Rubinstein, R.Y. A tutorial on the cross-entropy method. *Ann. Oper. Res.* **2005**, *134*, 19–67. [CrossRef]

44. Chollet, F. Keras: Deep Learning Library for Theano and Tensorflow. Available online: https://keras.Io/ (accessed on 8 May 2020).
45. Manavalan, B.; Basith, S.; Shin, T.H.; Lee, D.Y.; Wei, L.; Lee, G. 4mCpred-EL: An ensemble learning framework for identification of DNA N4-Methylcytosine sites in the mouse genome. *Cells* **2019**, *8*, 1332. [CrossRef]
46. Liu, Z.; Xiao, X.; Yu, D.J.; Jia, J.; Qiu, W.R.; Chou, K.C. pRNAm-PC: Predicting N6-methyladenosine sites in RNA sequences via physical–chemical properties. *Anal. Biochem.* **2016**, *497*, 60–67. [CrossRef] [PubMed]
47. Chen, J.; Liu, H.; Yang, J.; Chou, K.C. Prediction of linear B-cell epitopes using amino acid pair antigenicity scale. *Amino Acids* **2007**, *33*, 423–428. [CrossRef] [PubMed]
48. Chou, K.C. Using subsite coupling to predict signal peptides. *Protein Eng.* **2001**, *14*, 75–79. [CrossRef] [PubMed]
49. Chou, K.C. Prediction of signal peptides using scaled window. *Peptides* **2001**, *22*, 1973–1979. [CrossRef]
50. Zeng, F.; Fang, G.; Yao, L. A deep neural network for identifying DNA N4-methylcytosine sites. *Front. Genet.* **2020**, *11*, 209. [CrossRef]

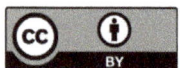

© 2020 by the authors. Licensee MDPI, Basel, Switzerland. This article is an open access article distributed under the terms and conditions of the Creative Commons Attribution (CC BY) license (http://creativecommons.org/licenses/by/4.0/).

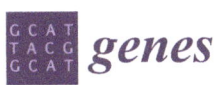

Article

Classification of Microarray Gene Expression Data Using an Infiltration Tactics Optimization (ITO) Algorithm

Javed Zahoor * and Kashif Zafar

Department of Computer Science, National University of Computer and Emerging Sciences (NUCES), Lahore 54000, Pakistan; kashif.zafar@nu.edu.pk
* Correspondence: javed.zahoor@gmail.com; Tel.: +92-321-462-5747

Received: 20 May 2020; Accepted: 9 July 2020; Published: 18 July 2020

Abstract: A number of different feature selection and classification techniques have been proposed in literature including parameter-free and parameter-based algorithms. The former are quick but may result in local maxima while the latter use dataset-specific parameter-tuning for higher accuracy. However, higher accuracy may not necessarily mean higher reliability of the model. Thus, generalized optimization is still a challenge open for further research. This paper presents a warzone inspired "infiltration tactics" based optimization algorithm (ITO)—not to be confused with the ITO algorithm based on the Itō Process in the field of Stochastic calculus. The proposed ITO algorithm combines parameter-free and parameter-based classifiers to produce a high-accuracy-high-reliability (HAHR) binary classifier. The algorithm produces results in two phases: (i) Lightweight Infantry Group (LIG) converges quickly to find non-local maxima and produces comparable results (i.e., 70 to 88% accuracy) (ii) Followup Team (FT) uses advanced tuning to enhance the baseline performance (i.e., 75 to 99%). Every soldier of the ITO army is a base model with its own independently chosen Subset selection method, pre-processing, and validation methods and classifier. The successful soldiers are combined through heterogeneous ensembles for optimal results. The proposed approach addresses a data scarcity problem, is flexible to the choice of heterogeneous base classifiers, and is able to produce HAHR models comparable to the established MAQC-II results.

Keywords: infiltration tactics optimization algorithm; classification; clustering; cancer; microarray; ensembles; machine learning; infiltration; computational intelligence

1. Introduction

Microarray experiments produce a huge amount of gene-expression data from a single sample. The ratio of number of genes (features) to the number of patients (samples) is very skewed which results in the well-known curse-of-dimensionality problem [1]. This further imposes two self-inflicting limitations on any proposed model: (i) processing all the data is not always feasible; and (ii) processing only a subset of data may result in loss of information, overfitting, and local maxima. These two limitations directly impact the accuracy and reliability of any machine learning model. To address the curse-of-dimensionality, a lot of research has been done in the past to identify the most impactful feature subset [2–5]. Both evolutionary as well as statistical methods have been proposed in the literature for this purpose. Feature Subset Selection (FSS) techniques like Minimum Redundancy Maximum Relevance (mRMR), Joint Mutual Information (JMI), and Joint Mutual Information Maximization (JMIM) are amongst the most prominent statistical methods [6–8] while advanced approaches like Particle Swarm Optimization (PSO), Genetic Algorithm (GA), Deep Neural Networks (DNN), Transfer Learning, mining techniques, etc. have also been shown in the literature to produce highly accurate results [9–11]. The microarray data classification process is typically carried out in two major phases: (i) Feature Selection: this phase focuses on selecting the most relevant features from otherwise a huge dataset to reduce noise, computational overheads, and overfitting. (ii) Classifier Training: this phase builds a model from the selected features to classify a given microarray sample accurately and reliably [12]. Advanced techniques like Deep Neural Network (DNN), Convolutional Neural Network (CNN), Transfer learning, Image processing, ANT Miner, and other exploratory approaches have been proposed in the literature [13–21]. While the advanced approaches for both FSS and Classifier training are capable of producing high accuracies, they need to be tuned according to the underlying dataset in a controlled setup to achieve these good results. However, in practice, there are a number of factors that can impact the accuracy and reliability of a model. These include the different cancer types that need analysis of different tissues, the differences in microarray toolkits/hardware e.g., data ranges and durabilities, experimental setups, number of samples, number of features used, type of preprocessing methods applied, validation method used, etc. Due to these variations and No Free Lunch (NFL) theorem, many of the existing methods can not be generalized across datasets. Thus, it is still a challenging problem for researchers to develop a generalized approach that can enhance both the reliability and accuracy of the model across datasets and variations. The algorithm proposed in this paper puts these variations at an advantage by using ensembles for the classification of microarray gene expression data. The Infiltration Tactics Optimization (ITO) algorithm proposed in this paper is inspired by classic war-zone tactics [22]—not to be confused with the ITO algorithm based on the Itō Process in the field of Stochastic calculus [23,24]. It is comprised of four phases: Find, Fix, Flank/Fight, and Finish i.e., the so called Four F's of the basic war strategy. A small light-infantry group (LIG) penetrates into the enemy areas to setup a quick command and control center while the follow-up troops (FT) launch a detailed offensive with heavier and sophisticated weapons to gain finer control and victory over the enemy. Both the LIG and FT members independently identify enemy weak-points and choose their own routes, targets, movements, and methods of attack. The "successful" LIG members are then combined to form a heterogeneous group that can become operational in a short time-interval. This LIG group is joined by the "successful" survivors from the FT to gain full control. The following text describes the four Fs (i.e., Find, Fix, Flank/Fight and Finish stages):

1. **Find:** In this stage, the LIG members analyze the field position to make a strategy and find the most appropriate target to attack.
2. **Fix:** In this stage, the LIG members use different light-weight weapons to infiltrate into enemy areas.
3. **Flank/Fight:** In this stage, LIG members keep the enemy pinned down so they could not reorganize their forces while the FT performs a detailed offensive in the area independently.
4. **Finish:** In this stage, the FT members apply heavier weapons to cleanup the area and gain full control over the enemy.

The proposed ITO algorithm is inspired by the Super Learner algorithm [25] but works in two phases to build the overall model. In the first phase, ITO builds a heterogeneous ensemble of parameter-free classifiers which can produce comparable results in a very short time-span. This sets a bar for the minimum accuracy and reliability of the overall ensemble which is further refined when fully tuned parameterized classifiers are available. The final model is guaranteed to meet this bar for accuracy and reliability at the minimum. Parameter tuning is generally very time-consuming and mostly it produces the most optimal results.

The microarray technology produces thousands of gene expressions in a single experiment. However, the number of samples/patients is much smaller (upto few hundreds) as compared to the number of features (several thousands). The small number of samples (training data) are not sufficient to build an efficient model from the available data. This is known as data scarcity in the field of machine learning. The ITO algorithm overcomes the data scarcity problem by building multiple heterogeneous base classifiers. ITO does not restrict the use of any base classifiers as LIG and/or FT members. It is possible to use the most performant classifiers from literature with this algorithm.

The LIG and FT use exploration to learn about the different configurations and gain knowledge about rewards while the ensembling phase exploits the best performers from both LIG and FT to build an optimal model. The ITO algorithm achieves generalization and reliability by addressing data scarcity problems and producing HAHR models.

The rest of the paper is organized as follows; Section 2 provides a background of microarray-based cancer classification domain and literature review, Section 3 presents the proposed algorithm, Section 4 describes the experimental setup. Section 5 discusses the results and analysis and Section 9 presents the conclusions and future directions.

2. Background and Literature Review

Microarray gene expression data processing is a multidisciplinary area of computer science spanning graph analysis, machine learning, clustering, and classification [13]. Microarray technology allows measuring several thousand gene expressions in a single experiment. Gene expression levels help determine correlated genes and disease progression, which in turn helps in early diagnosis and prognosis of different types of cancers.

2.1. Phases of Microarray Gene Expression Data

2.1.1. Phase 1: Pre-Processing

First of all, the gene expression data are discretized for noise reduction, missing values are imputed, and the data are normalized [13].

2.1.2. Phase 2: Feature Subset Selection

Feature subset selection (FSS) helps in reducing the width of dataset which is skewed due to a very high features-to-samples ratio. A feature subset is selected such as to reduce feature redundancy without loss of information. There are generally three approaches for feature subset selection: i.e., filtering, wrapper based, or hybrid. Filtering approaches include minimum Redundancy and Maximum Relevance (mRMR), Mutual Information (MI), Joint Mutual Information (JMI), Joint Mutual Information Maximization (JMIM), etc. [4,5,8]. They perform feature selection without any information about the downstream classifier to be used. Thus, the feature selection is independent of classification. Wrapper-based approaches result in higher accuracy but are computationally expensive because they use an embedded classifier to gauge their performance [4,5]. A hybrid approach makes use of a combination of both filtering and wrappers [4,5], but the classifier used during feature selection may be different from the downstream classifier used for actual classification.

2.1.3. Phase 3: Learning and Classification

In this phase, generally supervised classifiers are used with a subset of feature to train the model. Different techniques are used for two-class and multi-class classification. State of the art includes advanced techniques like transfer-learning, deep learning, convolutional neural networks, etc. or swarm optimization techniques like Ant Colony Optimization (ACO), Bat algorithm (BA), etc. However, overfitting (due to few training samples) and no-free-lunch theorem (NFL) (due to variations in underlying Microarray technology, cancer subtypes and different cancers resulting in different expressive genes, etc.) still remain two major challenges for most of the machine learning based techniques [9,26]. This research covers two-class problem only and uses ensemble of heterogeneous base classifiers to overcome overfitting and data scarcity.

2.2. Literature Review

2.2.1. Microarray Quality Control (MAQC)

MAQC was a series of studies to monitor and standardize the common practices for development and validation of microarray based predictive models. The first phase of this project focused on addressing inter and intra-platform inconsistencies of results produced by different alternatives and methods. The aim was to setup guidelines for reproducible results in different setups using different hardware [27–29]. MAQC-II was the second phase of this project which aimed to establish a baseline for microarray gene expression data analysis practices. The purpose of establishing this baseline was to assess the reliability of clinical and pre-clinical predictions made through different models. For this purpose, 36 independent teams analyzed six microarray datasets with respect to 13 end points indicative of lung or liver toxicity in rodents or of breast cancer, multiple myeloma or neuroblastoma in humans. More than 30,000 different models were produced by these teams using different alternatives of analysis methods. MAQC-II used Matthews Correlation Coefficient (MCC) as the primary metric to evaluate the models [12]. MCC is used as a measure of quality for two-class classification. It ranges between $[-1, 1]$ interval with MCC = 1 representing perfect prediction, MCC = 0 representing random predictions and MCC = -1 representing completely $-$ve correlation between the predictions and actual classes. MCC works better than other measures such as F-Score for microarray data with unbalanced class distribution [30]. The subsequent phase of MAQC (SEQC/MAQC-III) was focused on quality control for RNA Sequencing technologies rather than Microarray technology [31]. The MAQC-II established baseline results are thus taken up in this study to compare our results against using MCC as a primary metric. However, very limited research have reported results in the form of MCC.

2.2.2. Feature Selection Algorithms

In 2005, Ding et al. proposed the famous minimum Redundancy and Maximum Relevance (mRMR) technique which made it possible to identify most relevant genes that can be used to reduce computational cost while maintaining high accuracy [6]. It uses mutual information with the target classes to determine relevant of a feature and dissimilarity of a selected feature with the already selected features. Since it computes both relevance and dependency independently, it is very likely that it may miss out a feature that individually looks irrelevant but when used in combination with other features may become significant i.e., it may miss out on interdependence of the features.

In 2014, Nguyen et al. analyzed the Mutual Information (MI) based approaches and contended that most of them are greedy in nature, thus are prone to sub-optimal results. They proposed that the performance can be improved by utilizing MI systematically to attain global optimization. They also reviewed the Quadratic Programming Feature Selection (QPFS) in detail and pointed out several discrepancies in QPFS regarding self-redundancy. They proposed spectral relaxation and semi-definite programming to solve this global optimization problem for mutual information-based feature selection. Their experiments show that spectral relaxation approach returns a solution identical to semi-definite programming approach but at a much lesser cost [32]. In addition, the spectral relaxation reduced the computation time to $O(n^2)$ equivalent to mRMR. They also demonstrated empirically that their proposed method was much more scalable as compared to other methods in terms of computational time needed and working memory requirements. However, the computational time for mRMR with careful optimization was much better than their proposed global method.

In 2019, Potharaju et al. introduced a novel distributed feature selection method to remedy the curse-of-dimensionality of microarray data [33]. Their technique is inspired by an academic method of forming final year project groups. They used Symmetrical Uncertainty, Information Gain, and Entropy to build multiple balanced feature clusters. Each cluster is used to train a multi-layer perceptrons (MLP) and the most performant cluster is chosen for further processing. The MLP training and tuning itself is a very time-consuming task. Training multiple such clusters makes it even more resource hungry. However, the use of MLP makes it possible to stop the process prematurely and pick up the cluster with the highest accuracy and lowest root mean square for further processing. This approach may not scale well for a very large number of features because of computational and working memory requirements. It will further require a way to strike a balance between the cluster size and number of clustered required for such large datasets.

2.2.3. Ensemble Based Approaches

In 2006, Wang et al. used Neuro-Fuzzy Ensemble (NFE) approach to utilize many inputs by dividing them into small (not necessarily disjoint) subsets that were used as input to individual Neuro-fuzzy units to learn a model. The outputs of these units were then used in an ensemble to jointly estimate the class of a sample. This approach made the biological interpretation of the selected features more sensible [34]. However, this approach requires encoding of prior knowledge from different sources, interpretation of the complete ensemble is still very complex, and it does not suggest how to balance between accuracy and use of existing knowledge for interpretability. These problems also make it hard to scale.

In 2009, Chen et al. proposed and showed that Artificial Neural Network (ANN) Ensemble with Sample Filtering is more accurate and stable than single neural network. This method also outperformed Bagging, Filtering, SVM, and Back Propagation [35]. However, the homogeneous ensemble of ANN requires a lot of computational time and resources to train each of the base ANN, thus it is not scalable for datasets with a very large number of features.

In 2013, Bosio used biological knowledge e.g., gene activation from Gene Ontology databases and statistical methods to generate meta-genes. Each meta-gene represented the common attributes of the contributing genes, thus replacing a number of genes with a representative meta-gene that yields better accuracy. He used Improved Sequential Floating Forward Selection (IFFS) and meta-genes to consistently out perform other models from literature [36]. However, this approach is mostly brute-force i.e., it needs to compute all pairwise correlations to generate meta genes which are also treated as genes/features for further processing. Although the IFFS algorithm eventually generates very small feature subset comprising of both meta-genes and raw genes where meta-genes represent cluster/tree-let of genes; however, based on the iterative nature of IFFS algorithm at each step, it chooses the best gene from amongst all genes and checks if adding increases the model performance; if not, then it checks if any existing genes should be removed or replaced with some other genes to make the feature subset the most optimal one. This makes the overall feature selection step very time consuming. Thus, scaling this approach for larger datasets will be a challenge.

2.2.4. Heterogeneous Ensemble Classifiers

In 2008, Gashler et al. showed that a heterogeneous ensemble of different tree algorithms performs better than homogeneous forest algorithms when the data contain noise or redundant attributes [37]. This is particularly suitable for microarray data which contains a huge number of features, some of which could be a mere noise and other noise introduced during data digitization from the microarray chip. They use Entropy reducing Decision Trees and a novel Mean Margin Decision Trees (MMDT) to build the heterogeneous ensemble. Their work also showed that a small heterogeneous ensemble performs better than relatively larger homogeneous ensemble of trees. They used a diverse datasets comprising of many diseases, cars, wines, etc. to show how a heterogeneous ensemble can potentially address the NFL constrains. However, their work does not include MAQC-II Datasets and hence is not comparable with that benchmark.

In 2018, Yujue Wu proposed a Multi-label Super Leaner based on Heterogeneous ensembles to improve the classification accuracy of multi-class Super Learner [38]. A multi-label classification is a problem where each sample can represent more than one class labels simultaneously e.g., a picture may be assigned sea and beach or sea and mountains simultaneously depending upon the objects it contains. This work was not in the bio-informatics domain as such, but it was shown to outperform all other methods for music sentiment analysis, birds acoustics, and scenery datasets. Again, the diversity of problems it addresses shows the potential of heterogeneous ensemble to overcome NFL constrains.

In 2019, Yu et al. proposed a novel method using medical imaging, advanced machine learning algorithms, and Heterogeneous Ensembles to accurately predict diagnostically complex cases of cancer patients. They also used this system to explain what imaging features make them difficult to diagnose even with typical Computer-Aided Diagnosis (CAD) programs [39]. Their work takes lung images as input, performs segmentation of the image, and extracts features from them. These features are used to train the heterogeneous base classifiers and build an ensemble of trained classifiers. Their work improved the overall prediction accuracy to 88.90% as opposed to the highest accuracy reported in literature as 81.17%.

2.2.5. Bio-Inspired Algorithms

In 2011, a very detailed overview summarizing the overall research carried out in the literature was compiled by Elloumi et al. covering the challenges, solutions, and future directions for Bio-Inspired algorithms [40].

In 2014, Selvaraj et al. compiled a list of applications of modern bio-inspired algorithms. Some of these algorithms have been applied to cancer detection already. These algorithms can be applied to microarray gene expression data to resolve the complex optimization problems posed by this data [14].

In 2016, Mohapatra et al. used modified Cat Swarm Optimization algorithm for feature selection along with Kernel Ridge Regression (KRR) for classification. They demonstrated that KRR outperforms wavelet kernel ridge regression (WKRR) and radial basis kernel ridge regression (RKRR), irrespective of the dataset used. Their technique performs relatively better on two-class datasets as opposed to multi-class datasets [41].

2.2.6. Deep Learning Based Approaches

In 2013, Rasool et al. used Deep Learning based unsupervised feature learning technique and microarray data to detect cancer. PCA was used for dimensionality reduction. PCA along with a random subset of features (to ensure that nonlinear relations amongst the features are not completely lost due to PCA) are fed to auto-encoders to learn the gene-expression profiles. These gene-expression profiles are compared with healthy tissues' profiles to detect the disease. This approach generalizes the feature subsets across different cancer subtypes. Their proposed method combines data from different tissues (cancer types and subtypes) to train the classifier for type-agnostic cancer detection. Thus, addressing data scarcity problem as well [9]. However, they did not use MAQC-II datasets in their study. They claim their approach to be scalable across cancer types and bigger datasets. However, because of missing time complexity analysis, missing parameter details of DNN, and very high level description of steps, this claim can not be validated.

In 2016, Chen et al. proposed a deep learning based model code-named D-GEX to infer the gene expression-levels of correlated genes based on the "landmark" genes. The idea of landmark genes suggests that carefully selected 1000 genes can help infer 80% of the genome-wide gene expression levels [10]. They trained their system using Microarray Omnibus dataset (not used MAQC-II datasets) This idea can be used as a pre-processing step to impute missing values for microarray data. The proposed model in this paper was compared with Linear Regression based current model and KNN based models and shown to outperform both of the. However, the interpretation of the learned hidden layers was found to be extremely difficult due to the complex way DNNs work i.e., lots of weights and nodes representing learned hidden structures from data. In addition, their implementation used random splitting of genes into smaller clusters due to hardware limitations. In its current state, this model is not scalable. However, as proposed in the paper, with the help of gene expression profiles, related genes could be clustered together and dimensionality reduction could be applied at a cluster level before processing them with DNN. This can greatly simplify the hidden structure that the DNN needs to learn and hence reduce computational needs for DNN.

In 2019, Liao et al. presented a novel Multi-task Deep Learning (MTDL) method that can reliably predict rare cancer types by exploiting cross cancer gene-expression profiling [21]. They used different datasets one for each type of cancer and common hidden layers that are extracted from these datasets to train the model. The trained model's learning is then transferred as additional input to the prediction model. Their work showed significant improvement in correct diagnosis when there is inadequate data available. The performance improvements were evident in all but the Leukemia database where multi-class data are used. The proposed model learns common features from 12 different types of cancers to effectively exploit the right features for a given cancer type. Their work also showed the way to generalize a model across cancer-type and across datasets. The simplified approach of combining single task learners through a DNN and use of Transfer learning makes it a scalable model for two-class problems. For multi-class problems, further improvement will need to be done.

2.2.7. Image Based Cancer Classification

In 2016, Huynh et al. extracted tumor information from mammograms to train their SVM classifier for cancer detection. They showed that the image-features learnt from mammograms performed comparable to the analytical feature selection methods [17]. A separate study by Spanhol et al. in 2016 used patches of histopathological breast images from BreaKHis database with CNN to classify samples for breast cancer. They used simple fusion rules to improve the recognition rates. Their final results outperformed the other results reported in the literature [18]. In another study in the same year, L'evy et al. used pre-segmented mammograms with Convolutional Neural Networks to measure breast-mass for binary cancer classification. Their method surpassed the expert human performance [20].

In 2017, Han et al. used histopathological breast images in conjunction with Deep Convolution Neural Networks (DCNN) to achieve automated cancer multi-class classification (subtype detection). Their proposed method achieved over 93% accuracy over a large-scale dataset BreaKHis. Employing Class-Structure aware approach (hence the name CSDCNN), they used oversampling over the training dataset to balance the class distributions amongst unbalanced classes. They also showed that the performance of their proposed method was significantly better with transfer learning (from an Imagenet dataset fine-tuned on the BreaKHis dataset) than learning the model from scratch directly on BreaKHis. Their work was the first attempt at Image based classification of Breast Cancers [19].

In 2020, Duncan et al. compiled a set of the ten most recent contributions in the fields of Big-Data, Machine Learning, and Image analysis in the Biomedical field and set the stage for upcoming cross-cutting concerns in these three areas [15].

2.2.8. Cancer Detection Using Transfer Learning

In 2016, Huynh et al. used transfer learning from a deep CNN to learn tumor information (features) from the mammograms. These features were used with SVM to classify cancerous samples. They showed that this approach produced comparable results to the conventional FSS techniques. Furthermore, they formed an ensemble to achieve an accuracy higher than these two methods [17].

In 2017, Ravishankar et al. studied the process of transferring a CNN trained on ImageNet for general image classification to kidney detection problem in ultrasound images. They proved that transfer learning can outperform any state-of-the-art feature selection pipeline [42]. They further proved that a hybrid approach can increase the accuracy by 20%.

In 2018, transfer learning with Deep Neural Networks was used on unsupervised data from other tumor types to learn the salient features of a certain type of cancer. They tested their approach on 36 binary benchmark datasets from GEMLeR repository to prove that their approach outperformed many of the general cancer classification approaches [11].

The use of datasets for other cancer types and use of Transfer Learning makes these approaches scalable and worthy for further investigation. The effectiveness of their approach should be tested on MAQC-II benchmark datasets to gauge their reliability.

2.2.9. Summary of Literature Review

Based on the advanced techniques presented in literature review, most of the studies have reported comparable results in terms of accuracy and reliability. However, not all of the studies are based on MAQC-II datasets and they use different scoring metrics like T-test, chi-test, MCC, error rate, confusion matrix, etc. Therefore, they cannot be benchmarked uniformly and compared on a common ground.

3. Proposed Algorithm

The proposed algorithm is inspired by warzone tactics. It is comprised of the Four Fs (Find, Fix, Flank/Fight, and Finish) of basic war strategy for infiltration into enemy areas i.e., small light-infantry group (LIG) backed by follow-up troops (FT) are used to conquer the area.

In our case, the LIG members are parameter-free classifiers that can be trained quickly to classify a sample with reasonable accuracy and reliability. The LIG members independently choose to identify enemy weak-points and choose their own routes, targets, movements, and methods of attack. While the overall approach does not restrict the user to use any particular classifiers and any set of parameter-free classifiers can be used; for this research, Decision Tree Classifier (DTC) [43], Adaptive Boosting (AdaBoost) [13,44–46] and Extra Tree Classifier (also known as Extremely Randomized Trees) [47] were used as LIG members with default settings.

The "successful" LIG members are then combined to form a heterogeneous ensemble which can reliably classify a given unseen sample. In parallel, the FT applies heavier and sophisticated techniques (i.e., parameter tuning) to find a better model. Random Forest [48], Deep Neural Network (DNN) a.k.a. Multi-layer Perceptron (MLP) [16,49] and Support Vector Machine (SVM) [50–52] were used as FT members with Grid Search and Random Grid Search for parameter tuning for binary classification. The "successful" FT members are used to update the overall ensemble for enhanced accuracy and reliability.

In the following text, we map the Four Fs (i.e., Find, Fix, Flank/Fight, and Finish stages) onto the proposed algorithm:

1. **Find:** In this stage, a random grid search is applied on the 4-dimensional search space comprising of pre-processing methods, FSS methods, Subset sizes, and Validation methods to generate "attack vectors" (tuples of length 4 each from the search space with different combinations) for LIG and FT members e.g., (Quantile method, mRMR, 50 features, 10 Fold CV) is one such tuple. Details of the options used for each of these dimensions are given below.
2. **Fix:** In this stage, each of the LIG members use one of the attack vectors to construct individual models. An efficiency index ρ is calculated using Matthews Correlation Coefficient (MCC) and average classification accuracy (score) as:

$$\rho_{LIG(i)} = MCC_{LIG(i)} \times score_{LIG(i)}, \qquad (1)$$

where LIG(i) is the i-th member of LIG. Similar to MAQC-II benchmarks, MCC and accuracy are used to compute ρ_{LIG}. In addition, our analysis from earlier experimentation showed that, in the case of overfitting, though the average accuracy/score of the model seemingly improves but simultaneously the MCC of the model decreases. Hence, these two measures were used to decide the trade-off between accuracy and MCC at the time of base classifier selection. The value of MCC ranges between -1 and $+1$, but, for our experimentation, we used only (0, 1] or MCC > 0 i.e., anything better than random guess. The accuracy ranges between [0, 1] range. Both measures are equally important, thus we use product as a statistical conjunction function. It helps balance the trade-offs between MCC and Accuracy. In our experiments, we observed that ρ_{LIG} helped in improving both the MCC and accuracy in some cases and helped achieve a good trade-off between MCC and accuracy in other cases. A fitness threshold ϵ_{LIG} is used to filter in "successful" members from the whole LIG i.e.,

$$\rho_{LIG(i)} > \epsilon_{LIG}, 1 > \epsilon_{LIG} > 0 \qquad (2)$$

The value of ϵ_{LIG} is chosen such that it filters at least the top 33% of the LIG members for $LIG_{Ensemble}$. Once the ensemble is formed, the value of ϵ can be adjusted to tune the ensemble for maximum $\rho_{LIG-Ensemble}$ yield as explained below.

3. **Flank/Fight**: In this stage, a heterogeneous ensemble of a subset of "successful" LIG members (MCC > 0) is formed such that:

$$\rho_{LIG-Ensemble} \geq \forall \rho_{LIG(i)} \qquad (3)$$

The ensemble is formed iteratively using a majority-vote method. In each iteration, the top LIG(i) is added to the $LIG_{Ensemble}$ and $\rho_{LIG-Ensemble}$ is computed to ensure that the newly added LIG(i) did not deteriorate the ensemble performance. If an LIG(i) causes decline in the $\rho_{LIG-Ensemble}$, it is discarded.

The $LIG_{Ensemble}$ takes relatively very short time to build while each FT(i) may take several hours to days to train (depending upon the parameter-space), thus, for the time-sensitive cases e.g., in the domain of pandemic diseases where an early prediction may be required, $LIG_{Ensemble}$ can be used until FT(i) are being trained. When the FT(i) are trained and the ensemble updated for improved performance, a follow-up prediction could be done which will either strengthen the confidence in prediction if both $LIG_{Ensemble}$ and $Final_{Ensemble}$ agree on the prediction Or $Final_{Ensemble}$ could be used to over-ride the earlier prediction.

4. **Finish**: In this stage, the FT members apply advanced classifiers such as Deep Neural Networks, SVM, etc. to build fine-tuned models. The "successful" FT members are filtered in using:

$$\rho_{FT(i)} = MCC_{FT(i)} \times score_{FT(i)} \qquad (4)$$

where FT(i) is the ith member of FT. A fitness threshold is used to filter in "successful" FT members i.e.,

$$\rho_{FT(i)} > \epsilon_{FT}, 1 > \epsilon_{FT} > 0 \qquad (5)$$

Then, $FT_{Ensemble}$ is computed from FT subsets such that:

$$\rho_{FT-Ensemble} \geq \forall \rho_{FT(i)} \qquad (6)$$

Finally, a $Ensemble_{Final}$ is formed using filtered-in LIG(i) and filtered-in FT(i). The following different approaches can be used to build the $Ensemble_{Final}$:

(a) simply combine all the LIG and FT members from $LIG_{Ensemble}$ & $FT_{Ensemble}$, respectively. However, through empirical analysis, it was found that this approach actually causes a decline in MCC and/or average accuracy of the model.

(b) start with one of $LIG_{Ensemble}$ or $FT_{Ensemble}$ and call it $Ensemble_{Final}$. Choose base classifiers from the other ensemble with $\rho \geq \rho_{Final-Ensemble}$ and add to $Ensemble_{Final}$. However, starting with an ensemble with higher ρ would cause all of them to fail on $\rho \geq \rho_{Final-Ensemble}$, thus resulting in no further improvement. In addition, our experiments showed that, starting with an ensemble with lower ρ, the optimization gain was not as good as the next approach because the condition $\rho \geq \rho_{Final-Ensemble}$ filtered out many classifiers which still could help with reducing misclassifications of ensembles hence improve both the accuracy and MCC.

(c) rebuild the $Ensemble_{Final}$ from scratch using LIG(i) ∪ FT(i) ordered by ρ. This approach was found effective to further enhance the performance.

While the proposed algorithm is flexible to allow the choice of any classifiers, the pre-processing method, validation method, subset size, and FSS methods, etc., the following configurations were used in this study for LIG and FT members to carry out the Four Fs.

The imputer method [51] was used for data normalization. During feature exclusion, the features with any missing values were completely removed from the dataset because (i) the number of features are in abundance already and, (ii) due to missing values, these features do not represent the sample space sufficiently. For scaling of the data Quantile method, Robust method, and Standard method were used [51].

While, in the most recent studies [53,54], multi-objective feature selection methods have been shown to outperform the single-objective methods; however, their implementations are not widely available for public use. Thus, for feature subset selection (FSS), also known as Variable Selection, three publicly available single-objective methods, namely Joint Mutual Information (JMI), Joint Mutual Information Maximization (JMIM), and minimum Redundancy Maximum Relevance (mRMR) were used [6–8,51]. The minimum number of features that should be chosen, largely depends upon the dataset being used. For the basic techniques like JMI and JMIM the produced subset may contain some level of redundancy whereas mRMR ensures that the chosen features in a subset have minimum redundancy and maximum relevance to the class label [6,8]. These are brute-force techniques and all the features are considered to compute a ranked list of features based on statistical relevance and hence it is a computationally expensive step [8]. The selection of these algorithms was done due to their out-of-the-box availability for Python, not requiring an implementation from scratch.

For validation, 10-Fold Cross Validation (CV) and Leave-one-out CV (LOOCV) were considered, both of which have been proven in the literature to be amongst the best validation techniques [36].

Pseudo Code

The ITO Algorithm (Algorithm 1) computes $LIG_{Ensemble}$ using Algorithm 2. This produces an initial baseline result which is either the best of LIG members or an improved output from the ensemble. The Grid G on line 2 of Algorithm 1 has 4-tuples i.e., four elements wide and the length of G will be |preps| × |searchRadius| × |searchStrategy| × |successEvaluation| to hold all possible combinations of these four sets. The variables t_{LIG} and t_{LIG} (also 4-tuples) are subsets of G, for our experiments, we used half the size of G. The Compute$Ensemble_{Final}$ (Algorithm 3) conditionally updates this ensemble using a ranked list of FT(i) if they improve the overall results.

Algorithm 1: ITO Algorithm

input :
    T: t × f matrix - training dataset with t samples and f features;
    V: v × f matrix - validation dataset - with v samples and f features;
    preps={Imputer, Robust, Quantile, Standard, ...} - set of preprocessing methods;
    searchRadius={10, 50, 100, 150, 200, 250, ...} - set of FSS sizes;
    searchStrategy={JMI, JMIM, mRMR ...} - set of FSS methods;
    successEvaluation={10 Fold CV, LOOCV, ...} - set of validation methods;
    LIG$_{Options}$={DT, AdaBoost, Extra Tree, ...} - set of parameter-free classifiers;
    FT$_{Options}$={DNN, SVM, Random Forest, ...} - set of parameterized classifiers

output: $Ensemble_{Final}$

BEGIN
G ← GenerateOptionsGrid(searchRadius, searchStrategy, successEvaluation, preps);
Choose $t_{LIG} \subset G$ using Randomized Grid Search;
$LIG_{Ensemble}$ ← ComputeLIG$_{Ensemble}$ (T, V, LIG$_{Options}$, t_{LIG}) //Algorithm 2;
Choose $t_{FT} \subset G$ using Randomized Grid Search;
$Ensemble_{Final}$ ← ComputeEnsemble$_{Final}$ (T, V, FT$_{Options}$, t_{FT}) //Algorithm 3;
return $Ensemble_{Final}$;
END

Algorithm 2: ComputeLIG$_{Ensemble}$

input :
    T: t × f matrix - training dataset with t samples and f features;
    V: v × f matrix - validation dataset with v samples and f features;
    t_{LIG}: subset of configuration tuples each representing a combination with a preprocessing method, FSS size, FSS method, validation method;
    LIG$_{Options}$={DT, AdaBoost, Extra Tree, ...} - set of parameter-free classifiers

output: $LIG_{Ensemble}$

BEGIN
$LIG_{Ensemble}$ ← {};
Train $\forall LIG(i)$ as LIG $\in LIG_{Options}$ using every tuple from t_{LIG};
Compute $\forall \rho_{LIG}$ using Equation (1);
Sort descending on ρ_{LIG};
Pickup top (50 OR 33%, which ever is bigger size) LIG members;
if $\rho_{LIG} > \epsilon_{LIG}$ **then**
    | //i.e., Equation (2);
    | $LIG_{Filtered}$ ← $LIG_{Filtered} \cup LIG(i)$;
    | Update $LIG_{Ensemble}$ such that $\rho_{LIG_{Ensemble}} \geq \rho_{LIG(i)}$ using Equation (3);
return $LIG_{Ensemble}$;
END

Algorithm 3: ComputeEnsemble$_{Final}$

input :
    T: t × f matrix - training dataset with t samples and f features;
    V: v × f matrix - validation dataset with v samples and f features;
    t_{FT}: subset of configuration tuples each representing a combination with a preprocessing method, FSS size, FSS method, validation method;
    $FT_{Options}$={DNN, SVM, Random Forest, ...} - set of parameterized classifiers;
    $LIG_{Ensemble}$: the LIG ensemble computed by Algorithm 2;
    $LIG_{Filtered}$: The top 33% filtered LIG(i) based on ρLIG

output: Ensemble$_{Final}$

BEGIN
$FT_{Ensemble} \leftarrow \{\}$;
Train $\forall$ FT(i) as FT $\in FT_{Options}$ using every tuple from t_{FT};
Compute $\forall \rho_{FT}$ using Equation (4);
Sort descending on ρ_{FT};
Pickup top (50 OR 33%, which ever is bigger size) FT members;
if $\rho_{FT} > \epsilon_{FT}$ **then**
    //i.e., Equation (5);
    $FT_{Filtered} \leftarrow FT_{Filtered} \cup FT(i)$;
    Update $FT_{Ensemble}$ such that $\rho_{FT_{Ensemble}} \geq \rho_{FT(i)}$ using Equation (6);
$All_{Filtered} \leftarrow LIG_{Filtered} \cup FT_{Filtered}$;
//Iteratively build Ensemble$_{Final}$ from $All_{Filtered}$ such that
$\rho_{Final} \geq argmax(\rho_{LIG_{(i)}}, \rho_{FT_{(i)}}, \rho_{LIG_{Ensemble}}, \rho_{FT_{Ensemble}})$
Sort $All_{Filtered}$ on ρ;
Ensemble$_{Final}$ = {};
for *each classifier* $clf \in All_{Filtered}$ **do**
    $Temp_{EnsembleFinal} \leftarrow clf \cup Ensemble_{Final}$;
    if $\rho_{Temp_{EnsembleFinal}} > \rho_{Ensemble_{Final}}$ **then**
        $Ensemble_{Final} \leftarrow Ensemble_{Final} \cup clf$;
    else
        //else ignore clf and continue with next element
end
return Ensemble$_{Final}$;
END

4. Experimental Setup

The ITO Algorithm was run on each of the Datasets A, B, and C to Compute Ensemble$_{Final}$ for each of the datasets, respectively.

4.1. Benchmark Datasets

There are a number of publicly available datasets that have been used in different research papers [13,40,55]. However, this research uses datasets A (Hamner), B (Iconix), and C (NIEHS) from Microarray Quality Control Study—Phase II (MAQC-II) [12] as listed in Table 1.

Table 1. MAQC-II datasets available at https://www.ncbi.nlm.nih.gov/geo/query/acc.cgi.

Dataset	Endpoint	Accession Code	Features	Training Samples			Validation Samples		
				+ve	−ve	Total	+ve	−ve	Total
Dataset A	Hamner	GSE24061	1004004	26	44	70	28	60	88
Dataset B	Iconix	GSE24417	0010560	73	143	216	57	144	201
Dataset C	NIEHS	GSE24363	0695556	79	135	214	78	126	204

4.2. Description of Datasets Used

Dataset A (Hamner), Dataset B (Iconix), and Dataset C (NIEHS) from the MAQC II study have been used in this research. MAQC was a series of studies conducted by American Health Association (AHA) to establish a baseline for a reliable model for data classification Microarray data.

Dataset A (accession code GSE24061) was obtained from mice while conducting Lung tumorigen vs. non-tumorigen study using an Affymetrix Mouse 430 2.0 platform [12]. The training and validation datasets have 1,004,004 features (using raw .CEL files). The training dataset contains 26 positive samples and 44 negative samples (70 samples in total), while the validation dataset is comprised of 28 positive and 60 negative samples (88 samples).

Dataset B (accession code GSE24417) was data obtained for mice while conducting non-genotoxic liver carcinogens vs. non-carcinogens study. The separation of the training and validation set was based on the time when the microarray data were collected; i.e., microarrays processed earlier in the study were used as training and those processed later were used for validation. This study was conducted on an Amersham Uniset Rat 1 Bioarray platform. The training and validation datasets have 10,560 features (using GSE24417_Training_DataMatrix.txt.gz file). The training dataset contains 216 samples with 73 positive and 173 negative samples, while the validation dataset contains 57 positive and 144 negative samples (total 201 samples).

Dataset C (accession code GSE24363) was obtained from rat-liver while conducting liver necrosis prediction. The data was collected from 418 rats using an Affymetrix Rat 230 2.0 microarray. The training and validation datasets have 695,556 features (using raw .CEL files). The training dataset contains 214 total samples with 79 positive and 135 negative samples. The validation dataset contains 204 samples with 78 positive and 126 negative samples.

The experimental data used to support the findings of this study are available at https://github.com/JavedZahoor/phd-thesis-iv.

4.3. FT Parameter Setting

The objective of this research was not to find the most optimal parameters for the individual FT members but to demonstrate the effectiveness of the proposed algorithm over whatever base classifiers are used; hence, the best parameters found for FT members during these experiments are not guaranteed to be the most optimal ones. In addition, since, in the final run, 199 FT(i) were filtered-in for Dataset A based on ρ, 12 for Dataset B and 108 FT(i) for dataset C, thus, for the sake of brevity, the list of those 312 optimal parameters is skipped from the paper. However, for the interested readers, some details are provided here. The grid search was used on a small set of choices to find the best available setting for individual FT members. For DNN/MLP, the following parameter grid was used:

1. learning_rate: ["constant", "invscaling", "adaptive"]
2. alpha: [1, 0.1, 0.001, 0.0001, 0.00001, 0.000001, 0.0000001, 0.00000001]
3. activation: ["logistic", "relu", "tanh"]
4. hidden_layer_sizes: [(100,1), (100,2), (100,3)]

For SVM, the following parameter grid was used:

1. C = [0.001, 0.01, 0.1, 1, 10]

2. gamma = [0.001, 0.01, 0.1, 1]
3. kernels = ['rbf','linear']

For the Random Forest, the following parameter grid was used:

1. estimators: [100, 300, 500, 800, 1000]
2. criterion: ['gini', 'entropy']
3. bootstrap: [True, False]

4.4. ITO Parameter Setting

The ϵ_{LIG} and ϵ_{FT} are used to control the number of classifiers that will be considered for $Ensemble_{LIG}$ and $Ensemble_{FT}$, respectively. These ϵ_{LIG} and ϵ_{FT} are set to control the number of LIG and FT members that are considered "successful". This helps in preventing overcrowded ensembles. For this study, we numerically computed ϵ_{LIG} and ϵ_{FT} to ensure that the top 33% members for Datasets A & C are included for which hundreds of LIG and FT members produced MCC > 0. However, for Dataset B, where only few (less than 20) produced MCC > 0, we set the value of ϵ_{LIG} and ϵ_{FT} very low to allow all of them to be included. Table 2 summarizes the settings for ϵ_{LIG} and ϵ_{FT} that were used:

Table 2. ϵ Thresholds.

Dataset	ϵ_{LIG}	ϵ_{FT}
A	0.639793072	0.4923244337
B	0.1025047719	0.09680510363
C	0.6312148229	0.6648090879

5. Results and Analysis

The ITO algorithm optimizes the overall model in two phases, LIG optimization and FT optimization.

5.1. LIG Optimizations

Figure 1a–c show the filtered LIG(i) of Datasets A, B, and C respectively sorted on their efficiency index (ρ). As it can be seen from Figure 1, selection of LIG members can not be done based on the MCC values or average accuracy alone, since they exhibit different and unrelated behavior for different LIG members. Thus, the efficiency index (ρ) is used as a fitness measure to rank LIG(i) from most efficient to least efficient. As a heuristic, only the top 33% of the successful (i.e., ($\rho > 0$) LIG(i) were filtered-in for further processing.

For Dataset A, $LIG_{Filtered}$ is comprised of 98 members. The $LIG_{Filtered}$ had MCC ranging in an 0.84–0.95 interval (avg 0.89) and the accuracy ranging in a 70–81% interval (avg 75%). For Dataset B, smaller subset sizes produced a high accuracy but poor MCC value hence the size of LIG group was only 7 members. The average accuracy of LIG(i) was found to be 63–75% (an average of 69%), whereas $LIG_{Ensemble}$ improved the average accuracy to 72%. However, due to poor MCC values in the range 0.14–0.21, the ensemble contained only one LIG member i.e., the highest performing member. For Dataset C, the chosen LIG group comprised of 80 LIG members and the LIG(i) average accuracy is 88% (in the range of 85–91%) with average MCC of 0.76 (in the range of 0.72–0.82).

An $LIG_{Ensemble}$ was formed for each of the datasets using a majority-voting ensembling method to even out the individual biases of LIG(i). Figure 2a–c shows the efficiency index for $LIG_{Ensemble}$ (shown at i = 0 in the graph) for Datasets A, B, and C, respectively. For Dataset A, the $LIG_{Ensemble}$ resulted in a higher accuracy (95%) and MCC (0.90) as compared to the individual LIG(i) as shown in Figure 2a. For Dataset B, the accuracy improved to 72% with an improved MCC value of 0.21 as shown in Figure 2b. For Dataset C, the accuracy improved to 90% with an improved MCC of 0.82 as shown in Figure 2c. Table 3 summarizes the performance improvements through $LIG_{Ensemble}$:

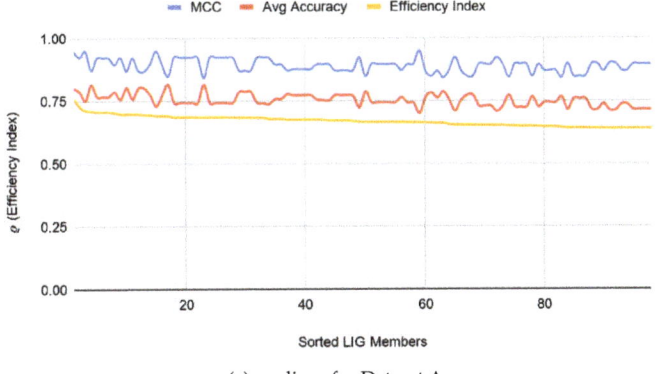

(a) readings for Dataset A

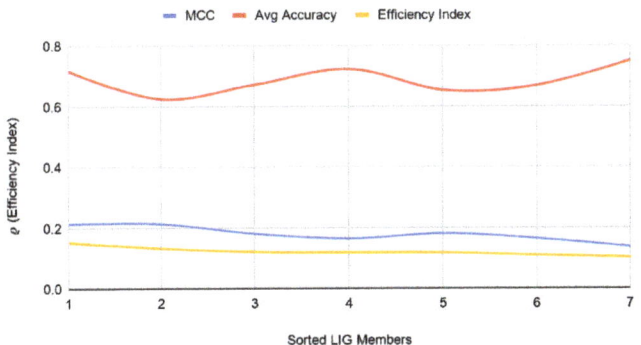

(b) readings for Dataset B

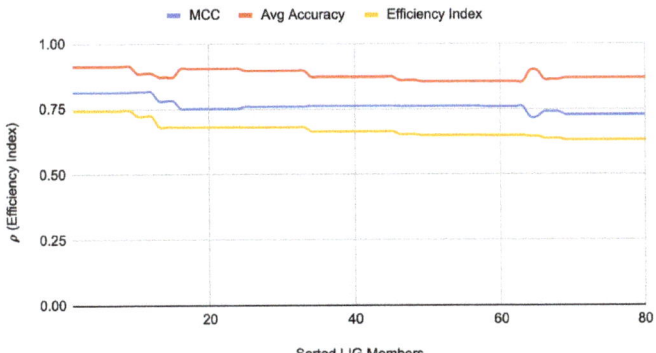

(c) readings for Dataset C

Figure 1. LIG(i) filtered-in accuracy, MCC, and ρ.

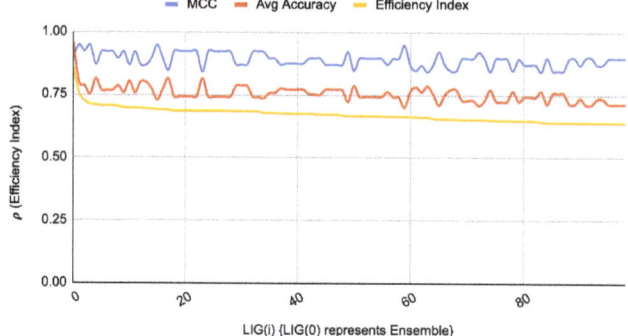

(a) readings for Dataset A

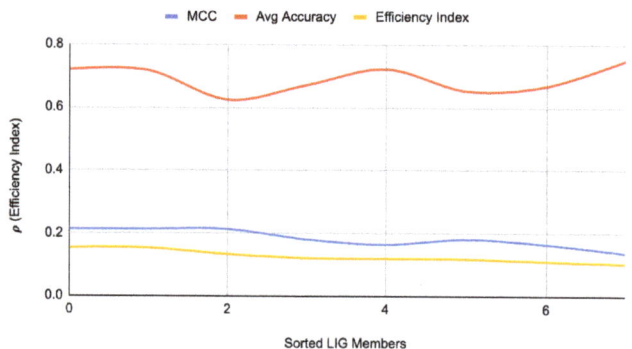

(b) readings for Dataset B

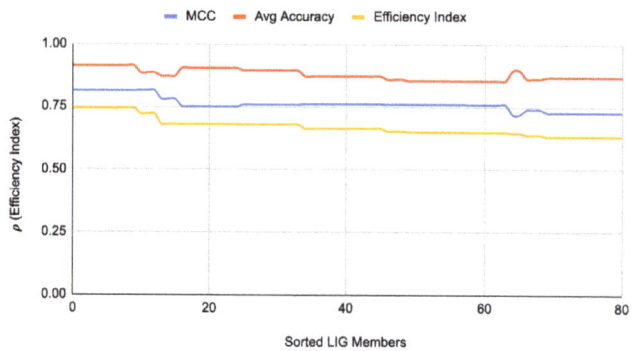

(c) readings for Dataset C

Figure 2. $LIG_{Ensemble}$ vs LIG(i) filtered-in accuracy, MCC, and ρ.

Table 3. Improvements by $LIG_{Ensemble}$.

		LIG(i)		$LIG_{Ensemble}$	
Dataset	|LIG|	Accuracy	MCC	Accuracy	MCC
A	98	75%	0.89	95%	0.90
B	07	69%	0.18	72%	0.21
C	80	88%	0.76	90%	0.82

Note that the value of ρ (Equation (1)) will always fall below the accuracy and MCC, but, due to its relative nature, the max value of ρ will always indicate the best LIG(i) (or FT(i)).

5.2. FT Optimizations

As a next step, the FTs were trained on each dataset under the same configuration options except the set of classifiers, which, in this case, were parameterized classifiers, each requiring its own parameter tuning. Figure 3 shows filtered-in FT(i) and their ρ. For Dataset A, top 75 FT(i) were filtered-in based on their ρ. Similar to LIG(i) selection, as a heuristic, top 33% of "successful" FT(i) were chosen to construct the $FT_{Ensemble}$ which achieved an accuracy 97% as compared to average accuracy of 70% (ranging from 58–79%) and MCC to 0.92 as compared to average MCC of 0.82 (0.65–0.90). For Dataset C, the $FT_{Ensemble}$ improved the average accuracy to 91%, average MCC to 0.84 as shown in Figure 3c. For Dataset B, like before, only 12 members were chosen from FTs due to poor MCC values for all other members. The accuracies, MCC, and $\rho_{FT-Ensemble}$ of FT(i) can be seen in Figure 3b. Dataset B is a hard dataset to model [12], and it might be possible to get better individual results through the use of advanced base-classifiers such as CNN or PSO based implementations, etc. The limited choice of LIG and FT models used in this study (due to their out of box availability) did not produce higher MCC. Table 4 summarizes the performance improvements through $FT_{Ensemble}$:

ITO works independent of these choices, hence any better models can be used as a member for both LIG and FT. The proposed optimization method was still able to produce comparable overall accuracy and enhance the MCC value through optimization as shown in Figure 3c. Table 4 shows that, for dataset B, the ITO algorithm produced a HAHR model with comparable reliability and accuracy.

Table 4. Improvements by $FT_{Ensemble}$.

		FT(i)		$FT_{Ensemble}$	
Dataset	|FT|	Accuracy	MCC	Accuracy	MCC
A	199	70%	0.82	97%	0.92
B	12	68%	0.16	72%	0.08
C	108	90%	0.81	91%	0.84

From raw results, it was interesting to note that a noticeable majority of successful FT(i) were using RandomForest, followed by a relatively small number of FT(i) using SVM. $FT_{Ensemble}$ constructed from FT(i) resulted in a relatively very high efficiency index as shown in Figure 4a. It is interesting to note that, except for the first few LIG(i) and FT(i), the MCC values and average accuracies of the individual LIG(i) or FT(i) seemed to be inversely proportional to each other i.e., the higher accuracy, the lower reliability, and vice versa. This is a clear indication of over/under fitting of individual LIG(i) or FT(i).

Finally, Figure 5 shows that the proposed algorithm produced an overall best result. It is interesting to note that, instead of choosing only $\rho_{FT(i)} > \rho_{LIG-Ensemble}$, updating the $LIG_{Ensemble}$ with top FT(i) without this constraint improved the $\rho_{LIG-Ensemble}$ i.e., $\rho_{overall-Ensemble} \geq argmax(_{LIG-Ensemble}, \rho_{FT-Ensemble}, \rho_{LIG(i)}, \rho_{FT(i)})$. Tables 5 and 6 show the values-of and %age improvement in MCC, Accuracy and ρ between ITO Tuned Ensemble against LIG(i), FT(i), $LIG_{Ensemble}$, $LIG_{Ensemble}$, and Combined Ensemble (i.e., an ensemble of all LIG(i) and FT(i)), respectively. Tables 7 and 8 show that, for datasets A & C respectively, the ITO algorithm produced a HAHR model with significantly higher reliability and accuracy, whereas, for dataset B (Table 9, however, the accuracy increased, but the MCC decreased a bit.

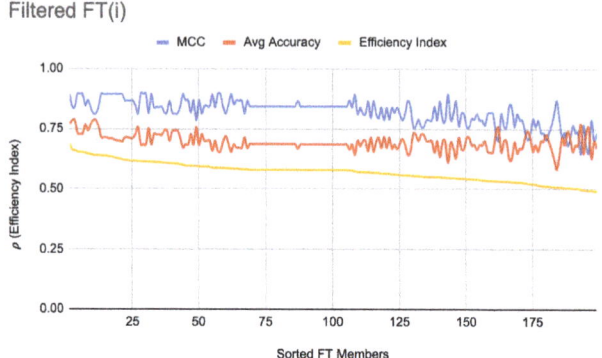

(a) readings for Dataset A

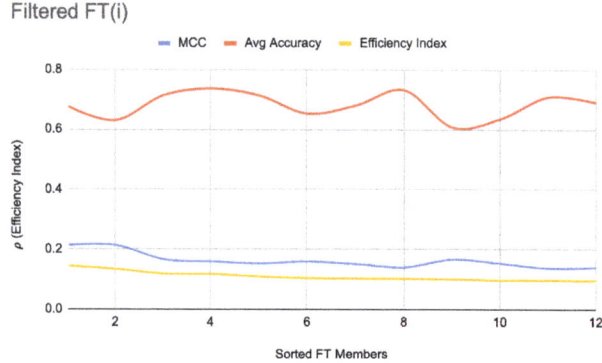

(b) readings for Dataset B

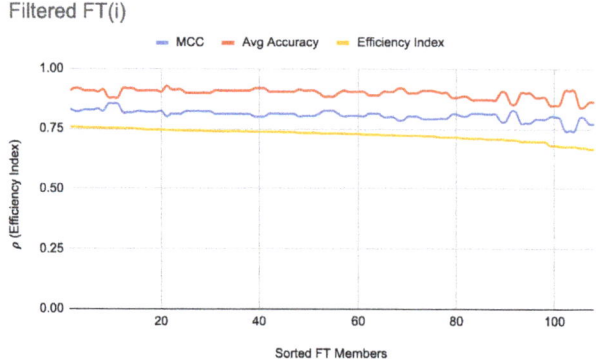

(c) readings for Dataset C

Figure 3. FT(i) filtered-in accuracy, MCC, and ρ.

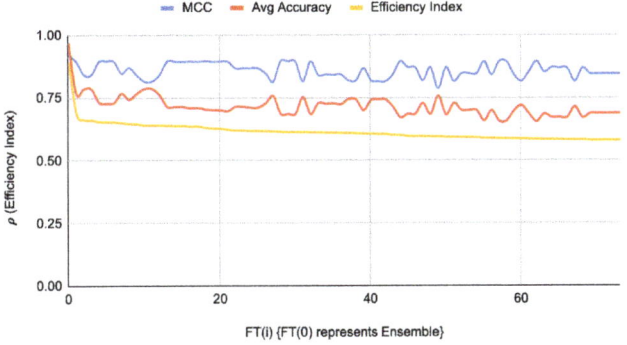

(a) readings for Dataset A

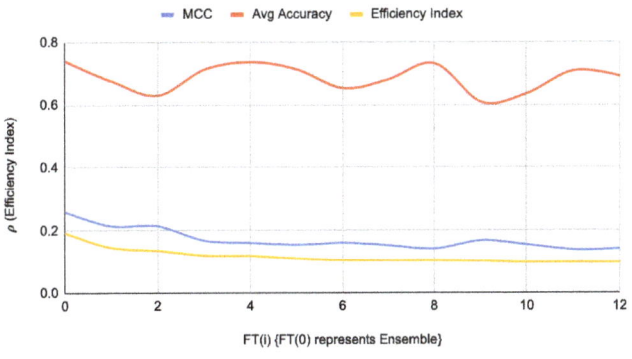

(b) readings for Dataset B

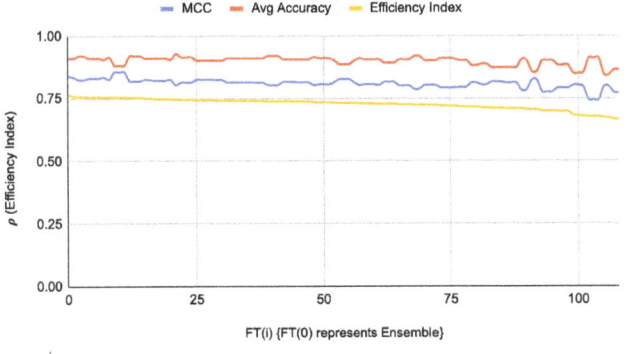

(c) readings for Dataset C

Figure 4. $FT_{Ensemble}$ vs. FT(i) filtered-in accuracy, MCC, and ρ.

Table 5. All Datasets—Accuracy, MCC, and ρ.

Dataset	Measure	Ensembles					
		LIG(i) (X1)	FT(i) (X2)	LIG (X3)	FT (X4)	LIG & FT Combined (X5)	ITO Tuned (X6)
A	Accuracy	0.75	0.70	0.95	0.97	0.98	**0.99**
	MCC	0.89	0.82	0.90	0.92	0.95	**0.97**
	Efficiency (ρ)	0.76	0.69	0.86	0.89	0.93	**0.96**
B	Accuracy	0.69	0.68	0.71	0.72	0.71	**0.75**
	MCC	0.18	0.16	0.06	0.08	0.00	**0.33**
	Efficiency (ρ)	0.15	0.14	0.05	0.06	0.00	**0.24**
C	Accuracy	0.88	0.90	0.90	0.91	0.90	**0.92**
	MCC	0.76	0.81	0.82	0.84	0.83	**0.87**
	Efficiency (ρ)	0.74	0.76	0.74	0.76	0.75	**0.80**

Table 6. All Datasets—ITO Improvement %age over LIG(i), FT(i), LIG Ensemble, FT Ensemble, and Combined Ensemble.

Dataset	Measure	ITO Improvement % Age Over				
		LIG (X6−X1)/X6%	FT (X6−X2)/X6%	LIG Ensemble (X6−X3)/X6%	FT Ensemble (X6−X4)/X6%	LIG & FT Combined Ensemble (X6−X5)/X6%
A	Accuracy	24.24%	29.29%	04.04%	02.02%	01.01%
	MCC	08.25%	15.46%	07.22%	05.15%	02.06%
	Efficiency (ρ)	20.83%	28.12%	10.42%	07.29%	03.12%
B	Accuracy	08.00%	09.33%	05.33%	04.00%	05.33%
	MCC	45.45%	51.52%	81.82%	75.76%	100%
	Efficiency (ρ)	37.50%	41.66%	79.17%	75.00%	100%
C	Accuracy	04.35%	02.17%	02.17%	01.07%	02.17%
	MCC	12.64%	06.90%	05.75%	03.45%	04.60%
	Efficiency (ρ)	07.50%	05.00%	07.50%	05.00%	06.25%

Table 7. Comparison with Results reported in Literature for an MAQC-II Dataset A.

Method	MCC	Accuracy
MAQC-II [12]	0.210	-
AID [56]	0.293	-
Kun [56]	0.407	-
Kun$_{tie}$ [56]	0.303	-
Kun$_{genes}$ [56]	0.346	-
EJLR [57]	0.57	-
Monte Carlo simulation as reported in [36]	0.270	67.3%
ITO algorithm	**0.950**	**98%**

Table 8. Comparison with Results reported in Literature for MAQC-II Dataset C.

Method	MCC	Accuracy
MAQC-II [12]	0.830	-
AID [56]	0.793	-
Kun [56]	0.812	-
Kun$_{tie}$ [56]	0.804	-
Kun$_{genes}$ [56]	0.781	-
Kun$_{all}$ [56]	0.792	-
t-test with KNN (Mean Centering) [57]	0.80	-
Monte Carlo simulation as reported in [58]	0.795	90.25%
ITO algorithm	**0.870**	**92%**

Table 9. Comparison with Results reported in Literature for MAQC-II Dataset B.

Method	MCC	Accuracy
MAQC-II [12]	0.42	-
Ratio-G [57]	**0.50**	-
ITO algorithm	0.33	75%

Figure 5 and Tables 5 and 6 show that ITO was able to enhance both the accuracy as well as MCC (and hence ρ) for all the datasets regardless of the base LIG and FT classifiers.

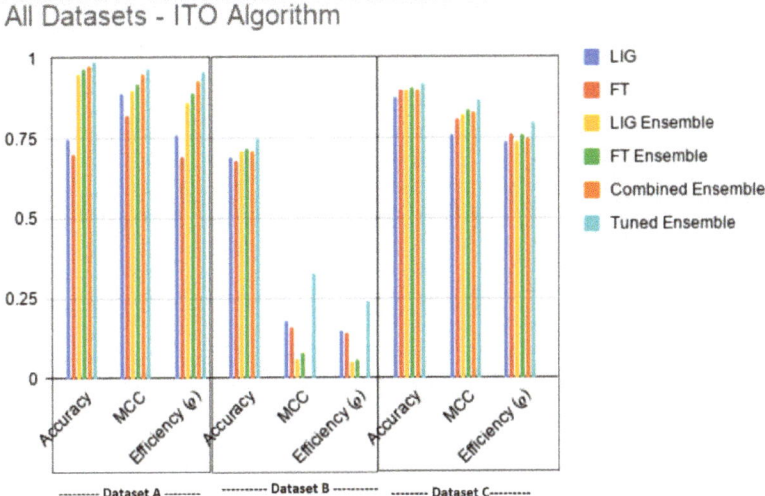

Figure 5. Overall improved results produced by ITO Algorithm on all datasets.

6. Machine Specifications

The experiments were performed on a shared machine with 64-bit ASUS GPU, 32 GB RAM, Quad-core 64-bit Intel i7-4790K CPU, with 800MHz-4.4 GHz speed.

7. Time Complexity

The overall time complexity of the algorithm depends on:

1. number of samples (t)
2. number of features (f)
3. number of different preprocessing methods (P) and maximum execution time for preprocessing (t_{prep}) of dataset of size txf
4. number of FSS methods (FM) and maximum execution time for feature selection (t_{fss}) from f features. This is one of the most time-consuming steps of the algorithm because the underlying methods need to calculate pair-wise mutual information for feature ranking, which is eventually used to pick the top features.
5. Subset sizes (S)
6. Validation methods (V)
7. number of parameterized classifiers (C_p) and maximum time to train a parameterized classifier (t_p) This is the second most time-consuming step of the algorithm. Parameter tuning for the classifiers requires trying different combinations of parameter values and find the most effective one.

8. number of non-parameterized (parameter-free) classifiers (C_n) and maximum time to train a parameter-free classifier (t_f).
9. Ensemble construction time (E_{FT}=FT Ensemble, E_{LIG}=LIG Ensemble, E_{ITO}=Overall Ensemble).

The time complexity of ITO algorithm would be as given in Equation (7).

$$(P \times t_{prep}) \times (FM \times t_{fss}) \times S \times V \times (C_p \times t_p + C_n \times t_f) + E_{LIG} + E_{FT} + E_{ITO} \qquad (7)$$

8. Execution Times

FSS was a very time-consuming step because, for the chosen methods, all pairwise correlations are computed between features to rank the most relevant features for final selection. To stay focused on the generalization problem, the FSS method was chosen solely considering the availability of out-of-the-box implementation or library for Python. Table 10 shows the minimum and maximum times it took to generate FSS for datasets A, B, and C.

Table 10. Min and Max times for FSS Generation for Datasets A, B, and C

Data set	Number of Features	Min Time for FSS (Size 10)	Max Time for FSS (Size 250)
A	1,004,004	26 h	>72 h
B	10,560	50 min	2.6 h
C	695,556	24 h	72 h

LIG training and filtering: As can be seen from Figures: 6–8, the training time for the filtered-in LIG(i) was under 15 s each.

LIG ensemble formation: In this phase, an ensemble is formed iteratively using the majority-voting method. The execution time for this step was under 500 s.

FT training and filtering: The training times for the filtered-in FT(i) are relatively much larger than LIG(i) as shown in Figures 9–11. However, the total execution times for ITO included training and parameter-tuning for SVM and DNN as well which may have been filtered-out for Datasets A and B. For example, for Dataset C, SVM training times fell around 3000 s to 4000 s (1.1 h each) while DNN training times fell around 30,000 s to 35,000 s (8.3–9.7 each).

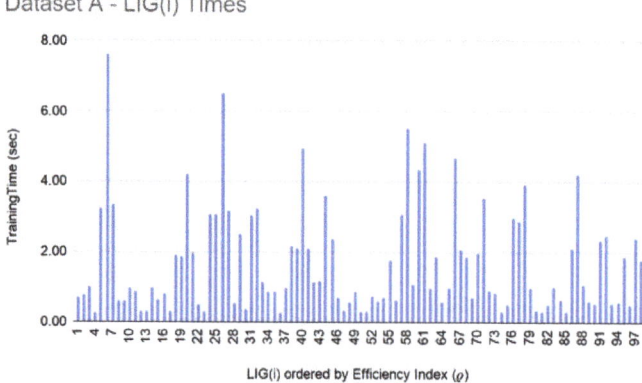

Figure 6. Dataset A—LIG(i) filtered-in training times.

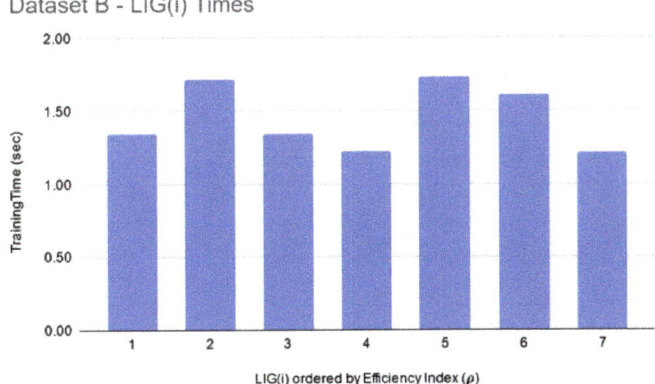

Figure 7. Dataset B—LIG(i) filtered-in training times.

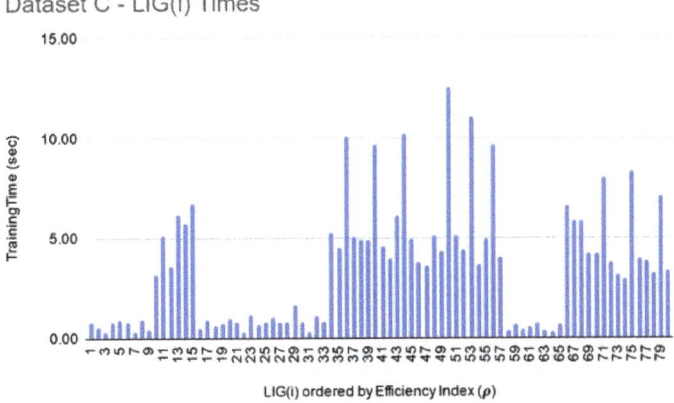

Figure 8. Dataset C—LIG(i) filtered-in training times.

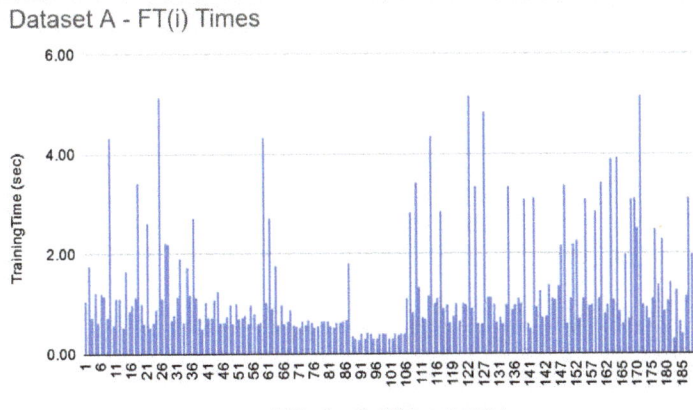

Figure 9. Dataset A—FT(i) filtered-in training times.

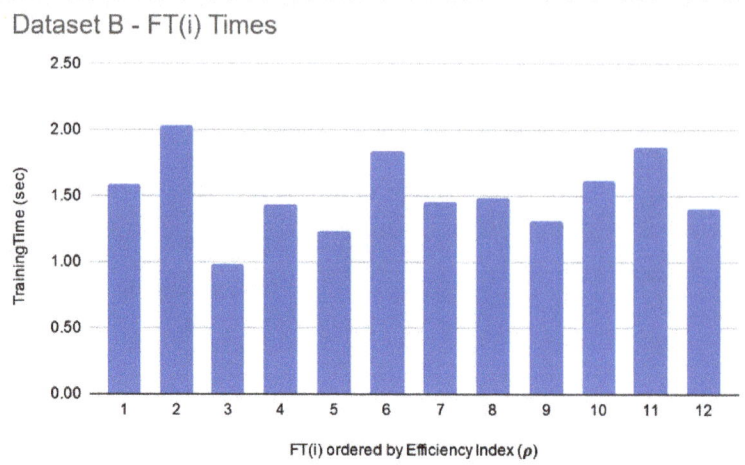

Figure 10. Dataset B—FT(i) filtered-in training times.

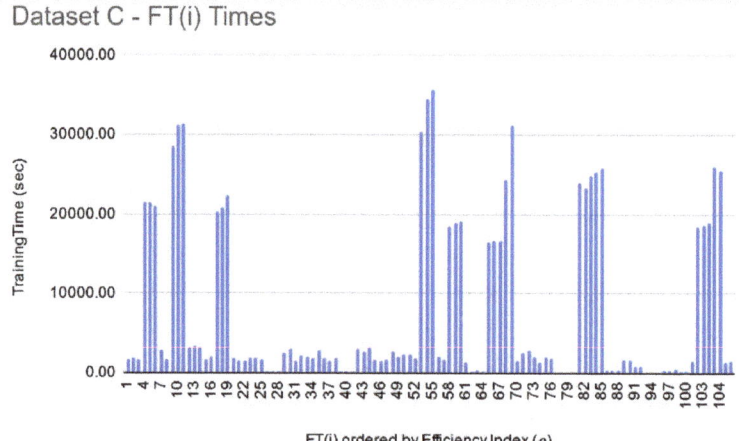

Figure 11. Dataset C—FT(i) filtered-in training times.

9. Conclusions and Future Directions

The scarcity of samples, digitization errors, and curse-of-dimensionality of microarray data makes it hard to reliably and accurately classify cancerous cells and avoid overfitting. A number of FSS and classification techniques have been applied to this domain to produce higher accuracies; however, there is still room for more improvement on reliability and generalization of these techniques. The curse of dimensionality and data scarcity can be addressed through the use of heterogeneous models built from subsets of data.

This paper showed that, regardless of the dataset, the accuracy and reliability of a model is inversely proportional (Figure 3a–c and Figure 1a–c) and hence both these factors should be considered when evaluating a model. A notion of efficiency index ρ is introduced which can be used as a single, more dependable factor to choose the best model amongst the available choices. The ITO algorithm introduced in this paper enhances the efficiency index of the underlying LIG and FT models as shown in Tables 7–9 and produces an HAHR classification model. The proposed algorithm is a generalized approach which balances the exploration through LIG and exploitation through FT to find a promising initial baseline and optimizes the results beyond this baseline. It leaves the choice of underlying LIG and FT members open to the user. A more advanced LIG or FT selection can further enhance the optimality of the overall model. Further study can be conducted to apply the proposed algorithm on datasets other than MAQC-II for wider comparisons.

For the LIG members, both majority-voting and soft-ensembles produced the same results. However, it is because the underlying classifiers return the predicted class labels instead of raw prediction values. It would be interesting to measure the impact of replacing the predicted class labels with the raw prediction values for soft ensembles. The advantage of soft ensembles was evident when used for FT members. Another future direction can be to cluster the erroneous instances separately and construct a focused model for those hard instances. Once a subset is trained on this cluster, it can be added to the beginning of the classification pipeline to bifurcate the instances accordingly. Use of GPUs/parallel computing for FSS generation and classification should be explored to reduce the overall execution time. Finally, the use of LIG as a filtering step for FT attack vectors should also be explored as potential areas of improvements for the ITO Algorithm.

Author Contributions: Conceptualization, J.Z. and K.Z.; methodology, J.Z.; software, J.Z.; validation, J.Z.; formal analysis, J.Z.; investigation, J.Z.; resources, J.Z. and K.Z.; data curation, J.Z.; writing—original draft preparation, J.Z.; writing—review and editing, J.Z. and K.Z.; visualization, J.Z.; supervision, K.Z. All authors have read and agreed to the published version of the manuscript.

Funding: This research received no external funding.

Acknowledgments: We would like to acknowledge and thank Usman Shahid for providing and maintaining the lab for experimentation. Sarim Zafar for assisting in Python setup and initial setup of experimentation. We would also like to acknowledge the following open-source contributions that were used as external libraries: Pairwise distance calculation. Vinnicyus Gracindo; PCA in Python http://stackoverflow.com/questions/13224362/principal-component-analysis-pca-in-python. Angle between two vectors (http://stackoverflow.com/questions/2827393/angles-between-two-n-dimensional-vectors-in-python) and (https://newtonexcelbach.wordpress.com/2014/03/01/the-angle-between-two-vectors-python-version/); parallelized MI/JMIM/MRMR Implementation (https://github.com/danielhomola/mifs); ACO based FSS (https://github.com/pjmattingly/ant-colony-optimization).

Conflicts of Interest: The authors declare no conflict of interest.

Abbreviations

The following abbreviations are used in this manuscript:

ITO	Infiltration Tactics Optimization algorithm.
MAQC-II	Microarray Quality Control study Phase II
mRMR	Minimum Redundancy Maximum Relevance.
MCC	Matthews Correlation Coefficient
HAHR	High Accuracy, High Reliability

References

1. Alanni, R.; Hou, J.; Azzawi, H.; Xiang, Y. Deep gene selection method to select genes from microarray datasets for cancer classification. *BMC Bioinform.* **2019**, *20*, 608.
2. Zhao, Z.; Morstatter, F.; Sharma, S.; Alelyani, S.; Anand, A.; Liu, H. Advancing feature selection research. *ASU Feature Sel. Repos.* **2010**, 1–28, doi 10.1.1.642.5862
3. Elloumi, M.; Zomaya, A.Y. *Algorithms in Computational Molecular Biology: Techniques, Approaches and Applications*; John Wiley & Sons: Hoboken, NJ, USA, 2011; Volume 21.
4. Bolón-Canedo, V.; Sánchez-Marono, N.; Alonso-Betanzos, A.; Benítez, J.M.; Herrera, F. A review of microarray datasets and applied feature selection methods. *Inf. Sci.* **2014**, *282*, 111–135.
5. Almugren, N.; Alshamlan, H. A survey on hybrid feature selection methods in microarray gene expression data for cancer classification. *IEEE Access* **2019**, *7*, 78533–78548.
6. Ding, C.; Peng, H. Minimum redundancy feature selection from microarray gene expression data. *J. Bioinform. Comput. Biol.* **2005**, *3*, 185–205.

7. Li, J.; Cheng, K.; Wang, S.; Morstatter, F.; Trevino, R.P.; Tang, J.; Liu, H. Feature selection: A data perspective. *ACM Comput. Surv. (CSUR)* **2017**, *50*, 94.
8. Peng, H.; Long, F.; Ding, C. Feature selection based on mutual information criteria of max-dependency, max-relevance, and min-redundancy. *IEEE Trans. Pattern Anal. Mach. Intell.* **2005**, *27*, 1226–1238.
9. Fakoor, R.; Ladhak, F.; Nazi, A.; Huber, M. Using deep learning to enhance cancer diagnosis and classification. In Proceedings of the International Conference on Machine Learning, Atlanta, GA, USA, 16–21 June 2013; ACM: New York, NY, USA, 2013; Volume 28.
10. Chen, Y.; Li, Y.; Narayan, R.; Subramanian, A.; Xie, X. Gene expression inference with deep learning. *Bioinformatics* **2016**, *32*, 1832–1839.
11. Sevakula, R.K.; Singh, V.; Verma, N.K.; Kumar, C.; Cui, Y. Transfer learning for molecular cancer classification using deep neural networks. *IEEE/ACM Trans. Comput. Biol. Bioinform.* **2018**, *16*, 2089–2100.
12. Shi, L.; Campbell, G.; Jones, W.D.; Campagne, F.; Wen, Z.; Walker, S.J.; Su, Z.; Chu, T.M.; Goodsaid, F.M.; Pusztai, L.; et al. The MicroArray Quality Control (MAQC)-II study of common practices for the development and validation of microarray-based predictive models. *Nat. Biotechnol.* **2010**, *28*, 827.
13. Djebbari, A.; Culhane, A.C.; Armstrong, A.J.; Quackenbush, J. *AI Methods for Analyzing Microarray Data*; Dana-Farber Cancer Institute: Boston, MA, USA, 2007.
14. Selvaraj, C.; Kumar, R.S.; Karnan, M. A survey on application of bio-inspired algorithms. *Int. J. Comput. Sci. Inf. Technol.* **2014**, *5*, 366–70.
15. Duncan, J.; Insana, M.; Ayache, N. Biomedical Imaging and Analysis In the Age of Sparsity, Big Data, and Deep Learning. *Proc. IEEE* **2020**, *108*, doi:10.1109/JPROC.2019.2956422.
16. Bojarski, M.; Del Testa, D.; Dworakowski, D.; Firner, B.; Flepp, B.; Goyal, P.; Jackel, L.D.; Monfort, M.; Muller, U.; Zhang, J.; et al. End to end learning for self-driving cars. *arXiv* **2016**, arXiv:1604.07316.
17. Huynh, B.Q.; Li, H.; Giger, M.L. Digital mammographic tumor classification using transfer learning from deep convolutional neural networks. *J. Med. Imaging* **2016**, *3*, 034501.
18. Spanhol, F.A.; Oliveira, L.S.; Petitjean, C.; Heutte, L. Breast cancer histopathological image classification using Convolutional Neural Networks. In Proceedings of the 2016 International Joint Conference on Neural Networks (IJCNN), Vancouver, BC, Canada, 24–29 July 2016; pp. 2560–2567. doi:10.1109/IJCNN.2016.7727519.
19. Han, Z.; Wei, B.; Zheng, Y.; Yin, Y.; Li, K.; Li, S. Breast cancer multi-classification from histopathological images with structured deep learning model. *Sci. Rep.* **2017**, *7*, 4172.
20. Lévy, D.; Jain, A. Breast mass classification from mammograms using deep convolutional neural networks. *arXiv* **2016**, arXiv:1612.00542.
21. Liao, Q.; Ding, Y.; Jiang, Z.L.; Wang, X.; Zhang, C.; Zhang, Q. Multi-task deep convolutional neural network for cancer diagnosis. *Neurocomputing* **2019**, *348*, 66–73.
22. Chapman, A. *Digital Games as History: How Videogames Represent the Past and Offer Access to Historical Practice*; Routledge Advances in Game Studies, Taylor & Francis: Abingdon, UK, 2016; pp. 185–185.
23. Ikeda, N.; Watanabe, S.; Fukushima, M.; Kunita, H. *Itô's Stochastic Calculus and Probability Theory*; Springer: Tokyo, Japan, 2012.
24. Sato, I.; Nakagawa, H. Approximation analysis of stochastic gradient Langevin dynamics by using Fokker–Planck equation and Ito process. In *International Conference on Machine Learning*; PMLR: Bejing, China, 2014; pp. 982–990.
25. Polley, E.C.; Van Der Laan, M.J. Super Learner in Prediction. U.C. Berkeley Division of Biostatistics Working Paper Series. Working Paper 266. May 2010. Available online: https://biostats.bepress.com/ucbbiostat/paper266/ (accessed on 15 March 2010).
26. Sollich, P.; Krogh, A. Learning with ensembles: How overfitting can be useful. In *Advances in Neural Information Processing Systems*; NIPS: Denver, CO, USA, 1995; pp. 190–196.
27. Shi, L.; Reid, L.H.; Jones, W.D.; Shippy, R.; Warrington, J.A.; Baker, S.C.; Collins, P.J.; De Longueville, F.; Kawasaki, E.S.; Lee, K.Y.; et al. The MicroArray Quality Control (MAQC) project shows inter-and intraplatform reproducibility of gene expression measurements. *Nat. Biotechnol.* **2006**, *24*, 1151.
28. Chen, J.J.; Hsueh, H.M.; Delongchamp, R.R.; Lin, C.J.; Tsai, C.A. Reproducibility of microarray data: A further analysis of microarray quality control (MAQC) data. *BMC Bioinform.* **2007**, *8*, 412.
29. Guilleaume, B. Microarray Quality Control. By Wei Zhang, Ilya Shmulevich and Jaakko Astola. *Proteomics* **2005**, *5*, 4638–4639.

30. Chicco, D.; Jurman, G. The advantages of the Matthews correlation coefficient (MCC) over F1 score and accuracy in binary classification evaluation. *BMC Genom.* **2020**, *21*, 6.
31. Su, Z.; Łabaj, P.P.; Li, S.; Thierry-Mieg, J.; Thierry-Mieg, D.; Shi, W.; Wang, C.; Schroth, G.P.; Setterquist, R.A.; Thompson, J.F.; et al. SEQC/MAQC-III Consortium: A comprehensive assessment of 521 RNA-seq accuracy, reproducibility and information content by the Sequencing Quality Control 522 Consortium. *Nat. Biotechnol.* **2014**, *32*, 903–914.
32. Nguyen, X.V.; Chan, J.; Romano, S.; Bailey, J. Effective global approaches for mutual information based feature selection. In Proceedings of the 20th ACM SIGKDD International Conference on Knowledge Discovery and Data Mining, New York, NY, USA, 24–27 August 2014; ACM: New York, NY, USA, 2014; pp. 512–521.
33. Potharaju, S.P.; Sreedevi, M. Distributed feature selection (DFS) strategy for microarray gene expression data to improve the classification performance. *Clin. Epidemiol. Glob. Health* **2019**, *7*, 171–176.
34. Wang, Z.; Palade, V.; Xu, Y. Neuro-fuzzy ensemble approach for microarray cancer gene expression data analysis. In Proceedings of the 2006 International Symposium on Evolving Fuzzy Systems, Ambleside, UK, 7–9 September 2006; pp. 241–246.
35. Chen, W.; Lu, H.; Wang, M.; Fang, C. Gene expression data classification using artificial neural network ensembles based on samples filtering. In Proceedings of the 2009 International Conference on Artificial Intelligence and Computational Intelligence, Shanghai, China, 7–8 November 2009; Volume 1, pp. 626–628.
36. Bosio, M.; Salembier, P.; Bellot, P.; Oliveras-Verges, A. Hierarchical clustering combining numerical and biological similarities for gene expression data classification. In Proceedings of the Engineering in Medicine and Biology Society (EMBC), 2013 35th Annual International Conference of the IEEE, Osaka, Japan, 3–7 July 2013; pp. 584–587.
37. Gashler, M.; Giraud-Carrier, C.; Martinez, T. Decision tree ensemble: Small heterogeneous is better than large homogeneous. In Proceedings of the 2008 Seventh International Conference on Machine Learning and Applications, San Diego, CA, USA, 11–13 December 2008; pp. 900–905.
38. Wu, Y. *Multi-Label Super Learner: Multi-Label Classification and Improving Its Performance Using Heterogenous Ensemble Methods*; Wellesley College: Wellesley, MA, USA, 2018.
39. Yu, Y.; Wang, Y.; Furst, J.; Raicu, D. Identifying Diagnostically Complex Cases Through Ensemble Learning. In *International Conference on Image Analysis and Recognition (ICIAR)*; Lecture Notes in Computer Science, Volume 11663; Springer: Cham Switzerland 2019; pp. 316–324.
40. Ayadi, W.; Elloumi, M. Biclustering of microarray data. In *Algorithms in Computational Molecular Biology: Techniques, Approaches and Applications*; John Wiley & Sons: Hoboken, NJ, USA, 2011; pp. 651–663.
41. Mohapatra, P.; Chakravarty, S.; Dash, P. Microarray medical data classification using kernel ridge regression and modified cat swarm optimization based gene selection system. *Swarm Evol. Comput.* **2016**, *28*, 144–160.
42. Ravishankar, H.; Sudhakar, P.; Venkataramani, R.; Thiruvenkadam, S.; Annangi, P.; Babu, N.; Vaidya, V. Understanding the mechanisms of deep transfer learning for medical images. *arXiv* **2017**, arXiv:1704.06040.
43. Polat, K.; Güneş, S. A novel hybrid intelligent method based on C4. 5 decision tree classifier and one-against-all approach for multi-class classification problems. *Expert Syst. Appl.* **2009**, *36*, 1587–1592.
44. Friedman, N.; Linial, M.; Nachman, I.; Pe'er, D. Using Bayesian networks to analyze expression data. *J. Comput. Biol.* **2000**, *7*, 601–620.
45. Hastie, T.; Rosset, S.; Zhu, J.; Zou, H. Multi-class adaboost. *Stat. Its Interface* **2009**, *2*, 349–360.
46. Kégl, B. The return of AdaBoost. MH: multi-class Hamming trees. *arXiv* **2013**, arXiv:1312.6086.
47. Geurts, P.; Ernst, D.; Wehenkel, L. Extremely randomized trees. *Mach. Learn.* **2006**, *63*, 3–42.
48. Breiman, L. Random forests. *Mach. Learn.* **2001**, *45*, 5–32.
49. LeCun, Y.; Bengio, Y.; Hinton, G. Deep learning. *Nature* **2015**, *521*, 436.
50. Jin, C.; Wang, L. Dimensionality dependent PAC-Bayes margin bound. In *Advances in Neural Information Processing Systems*; Curran Associates, Inc.: New York, NY, USA, , 2012; pp. 1034–1042.
51. Pedregosa, F.; Varoquaux, G.; Gramfort, A.; Michel, V.; Thirion, B.; Grisel, O.; Blondel, M.; Prettenhofer, P.; Weiss, R.; Dubourg, V.; et al. Scikit-learn: Machine Learning in Python. *J. Mach. Learn. Res.* **2011**, *12*, 2825–2830.
52. Brown, M.P.; Grundy, W.N.; Lin, D.; Cristianini, N.; Sugnet, C.W.; Furey, T.S.; Ares, M.; Haussler, D. Knowledge-based analysis of microarray gene expression data by using support vector machines. *Proc. Natl. Acad. Sci. USA* **2000**, *97*, 262–267.

53. Zhang, Y.; Gong, D.W.; Cheng, J. Multi-objective particle swarm optimization approach for cost-based feature selection in classification. *IEEE/ACM Trans. Comput. Biol. Bioinform.* **2015**, *14*, 64–75.
54. Annavarapu, C.S.R.; Dara, S.; Banka, H. Cancer microarray data feature selection using multi-objective binary particle swarm optimization algorithm. *EXCLI J.* **2016**, *15*, 460.
55. Plagianakos, V.; Tasoulis, D.; Vrahatis, M. Gene Expression Data Classification Using Computational Intelligence Techniques. 2005. Available online: https://thalis.math.upatras.gr/~dtas/papers/PlagianakosTV2005b.pdf (accessed on 15 March 2005).
56. Bosio, M.; Bellot, P.; Salembier, P.; Verge, A.O.; others. Ensemble learning and hierarchical data representation for microarray classification. In Proceedings of the 13th IEEE International Conference on BioInformatics and BioEngineering, Chania, Greece, 10–13 November 2013; pp. 1–4.
57. Luo, J.; Schumacher, M.; Scherer, A.; Sanoudou, D.; Megherbi, D.; Davison, T.; Shi, T.; Tong, W.; Shi, L.; Hong, H.; et al. A comparison of batch effect removal methods for enhancement of prediction performance using MAQC-II microarray gene expression data. *Pharmacogenomics J.* **2010**, *10*, 278–291.
58. Bosio, M.; Bellot, P.; Salembier, P.; Oliveras-Verges, A. Gene expression data classification combining hierarchical representation and efficient feature selection. *J. Biol. Syst.* **2012**, *20*, 349–375.

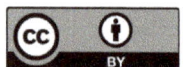

© 2020 by the authors. Licensee MDPI, Basel, Switzerland. This article is an open access article distributed under the terms and conditions of the Creative Commons Attribution (CC BY) license (http://creativecommons.org/licenses/by/4.0/).

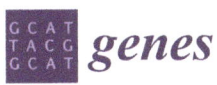

Article

DNA6mA-MINT: DNA-6mA Modification Identification Neural Tool

Mobeen Ur Rehman [1,2] and Kil To Chong [1,3,*]

1. Department of Electronics and Information Engineering, Jeonbuk National University, Jeonju 54896, Korea; cmobeenrahman@gmail.com or cmobeenrahman@jbnu.ac.kr
2. Department of Avionics Engineering, Air University, Islamabad 44000, Pakistan
3. Advanced Electronics and Information Research Center, Jeonbuk National University, Jeonju 54896, Korea
* Correspondence: kitchong@jbnu.ac.kr

Received: 3 July 2020; Accepted: 28 July 2020; Published: 5 August 2020

Abstract: DNA N^6-methyladenine (6mA) is part of numerous biological processes including DNA repair, DNA replication, and DNA transcription. The 6mA modification sites hold a great impact when their biological function is under consideration. Research in biochemical experiments for this purpose is carried out and they have demonstrated good results. However, they proved not to be a practical solution when accessed under cost and time parameters. This led researchers to develop computational models to fulfill the requirement of modification identification. In consensus, we have developed a computational model recommended by Chou's 5-steps rule. The Neural Network (NN) model uses convolution layers to extract the high-level features from the encoded binary sequence. These extracted features were given an optimal interpretation by using a Long Short-Term Memory (LSTM) layer. The proposed architecture showed higher performance compared to state-of-the-art techniques. The proposed model is evaluated on *Mus musculus*, Rice, and "Combined-species" genomes with 5- and 10-fold cross-validation. Further, with access to a user-friendly web server, publicly available can be accessed freely.

Keywords: DNA N6-methyladenine; Chou's 5-steps rule; Convolution Neural Network (CNN); Long Short-Term Memory (LSTM); computational biology

1. Introduction

In genomes of distinct species, DNA N^6-methyladenine (6mA) illustrates a crucial epigenetic transformation [1,2]. DNA 6mA is a non-canonical process that modifies the catalyzed adenine ring of DNA methyltransferases [3]. Alteration occurs at the sixth position of the adenine ring where a methyl group is additionally introduced. DNA 6mA holds a vital role in numerous biological processes, which includes DNA replication [4], DNA repair [5], DNA transcription [6], and others. Recent research established that uneven 6mA modification has a role in different diseases such as cancer [7], immune systems, and others. Therefore, this makes it necessary to identify a 6mA position in the genome sites. Mammalian 6mA largely originates from the genomic incorporation mediated by DNA polymerase, while the methylase-generated 6mA in mice remains elusive [8].

Silico prediction is considered to be a principal approach to encounter the aforementioned problem, while N^6-methyladenine prediction is its alternative. Intensive labor with extravagant experiments and expenses limits the use of silico prediction, making 6mA prediction an ideal solution for tracking modifications in the genome. For the identification of 6mA, diversified techniques can be found in the literature. Initially, ultraviolet absorption spectra, paper chromatographic movement, and electrophoretic mobility were combined to represent a complete mechanism. Although this method was not efficacious enough to be used for detecting 6mA transformations in animals [9], this led to an introduction of another technique for identifying 6mA modification using a restriction enzyme, but this approach was only capable of identifying transformed adenines that are present in the target motifs [10].

For the detection of 6mA sites in prokaryotes and eukaryotes, numerous techniques were proposed such as single molecule real-time (SMRT) sequencing [11], methylated DNA immunoprecipitation sequencing [12], ultra-high performance liquid chromatography with mass spectrometry [1], and metabolically generated stable isotope-labeled deoxynucleoside code [13]. Chlamydomonas genes carry 84% N^6-methyladenine modifications, which was identified after 6mA an immunoprecipitation sequencing experiment [14]. SMRT sequencing found out that adenines of methylated sites carry 2.8% of initial-diverged fungi [15]. Utilization of SMRT, 6mA immunoprecipitation, and mass spectrometry result in 0.2% of adenines being methylated [16].

The experimental techniques proved to be expensive and prolonged processes, therefore researchers tried to come up with computational techniques for prediction of DNA 6mA modifications. For this purpose, numerous prediction tools were proposed in the literature. iDNA6mA-PseKNC was the first ever N^6-methyladenine modification prediction tool for the *Mus musculus* genome [17]. iDNA6mA-PseKNC proposed sequence sample formulation for feature extraction and employed six different classifiers to identify the modification. csDMA is another reported tool that predicts the modification in N^6-adenine methylation, which used *K*-mer pattern, KSNPF frequency, nucleic shift density, binary code, and motif score matrix for extraction of the feature vector of the sequence [18]. Further, they deployed five different classifiers to evaluate the performance of the extracted feature set. Recently, 6mA-Finder was introduced as an online tool for predicting 6mA modification [19]. 6mA-Finder engaged seven sequence encoding schemes to get three types of physico-chemical features encoded. These encoded features were then embedded in seven different classifiers to evaluate the performance of encoded features. The i6mA-Pred is an identification tool for N^6-methyladenine modification in the rice genome [20].

FastFeatGen is another tool present in the literature that predicts DNA N^6 methyladenine sites [21]. FastFeatGen has used a parallel feature extraction technique followed by an exploratory feature selection algorithm to get the most relevant features. These features are then fed to Extra-Tree Classifier (ETC) for the prediction. Liang et al. proposed the i6mA-DNCP tool for the identification of 6mA sites [22]. i6mA-DNCP used optimized dinucleotide-based features with bagging classifier for the prediction model. Undoubtedly machine learning has illustrated high performance for many research problems, but the neural network has its benefits that need to be investigated for every research problem.

In recent years, Neural Network (NN)-based techniques, especially Convolution Neural Network (CNN), have shown tremendous improvement in many different research problems, e.g., in medical imaging [23,24] and bio-informatics [25–27], while the use of CNN for DNA-6mA modification identification is still in the infancy. Recently, a technique called iIM-CNN was reported by Wahab et al., which uses a CNN-based model for the N6-adenine methylation modification identification in genomes of different species [28]. The proposed CNN model in iIM-CNN carries two convolution layers with two max-pooling layers and a set of fully connected layers. iIM-CN showed high performance in prediction of N^6-methyladenine modification, somehow still, a research space is available where many aspects of CNN can be explored more.

This article aims to provide a CNN and Long Short-Term Memory (LSTM)-based efficient tool named DNA6mA-MINT, for DNA 6mA modification identification. The proposed model uses CNN for feature extraction while LSTM gives optimal interpretation to those features. The proposed architecture demonstrates higher performance than the existing state-of-the-art techniques on the "combined-species", *M. musculus* genome, and rice genome benchmark datasets. For better comparative analysis between DNA6mA-MINT and existing techniques, we have carried out performance analysis on 5- and 10-fold cross-validation. When compared with respective models available in the literature, Matthews Correlation Coefficient (MCC) for the "combined-species" benchmark dataset is noted with an increase of 20.83% for 5-fold cross-validation. The five steps are construction of dataset, encoding samples, constructing prediction model, evaluation of the proposed model, and establishing an online server. For the development of a useful and effective biological predictor, Chou's 5-steps rule needs to be followed [29,30]. These steps were followed by the previous researchers as well [17–20,28]. This research article follows Chou's 5-steps rule.

2. Benchmark Dataset

In this work, we used three datasets. The *M. musculus* genome database for DNA 6mA was proposed in 2018 by Feng et al. [17]. The dataset consists of 1934 samples for each positive and negative case. The 6mA sites available in the mouse genome were collected from MethSMRT database [31] with Gene Expression Omnibus (GEO) accession number GSE71866. Another dataset was on the rice genome, which was presented in 2019 by Chen et al. [20]. This dataset consists of 880 samples for each positive and negative case. The 6mA sites in rice genomes were provided by Zhou et al. [16] with GEO accession number GSE103145. Combining both aforementioned databases, a "combined-species" dataset is generated which contains 2768 samples for the positive cases and 2716 for negative cases. While the "combined-species" dataset did not contain sequence redundancy, which is eliminated by CD-HIT software [32], the rigorous sequence identity threshold was 0.80. Further, the dataset for training comprises 2214 positive samples and 2214 negative samples, while for the purpose of independent training 554 positive samples and 502 negative samples are taken into account. The length of all sequences in the datasets are 41 bp centered with the 6mA and non-6mA site.

3. Methodology

The proposed architecture was an efficient deep learning-based model comprised of several convolution layers, hidden layers, LSTM layers, and dense layers. Figure 1 is a visual representation of DNA6mA-MINT. This model holds the capability of extracting critical features from the input raw sequence, which are then used to carry prediction. The input sequence carries a combination of 4 nucleotides, A, T, C, and G, as can be seen in the dataset block of Figure 1. The NNs work on the numerical data only, therefore an encoding scheme is required here which can effectively convert the sequence-based data to a numerical representation. For the said purpose, binary encoding was taken into account. Where A, T, C, and G are represented as (1, 0, 0, 0), (0, 1, 0, 0), (0, 0, 1, 0), (0, 0, 0, 1), respectively.

Table 1 shows the architecture details of DNA6mA-MINT. The DNA6mA-MINT includes three convolution layers that use different parameters to extract the features from the input binary encoded sequence. The first convolution layer uses 32 filters with a filter size of five, followed by another convolution layer which uses 32 different filters with a filter size of four. The last convolution layer uses 16 filters of size four. Features extracted by the first two convolution layers undergo Batch normalization, Max-pooling layer, and a dropout layer discarding 40% of features, while the features extracted by the last convolution undergo Max-pooling and dropout of 20%. The number of filters for the convolution layer with their filter size, Stride length, pool-size, and the dropout ratio is decided after hyperparameter tuning. Therefore, the selected values of the parameters were capable of giving the best performance from the model.

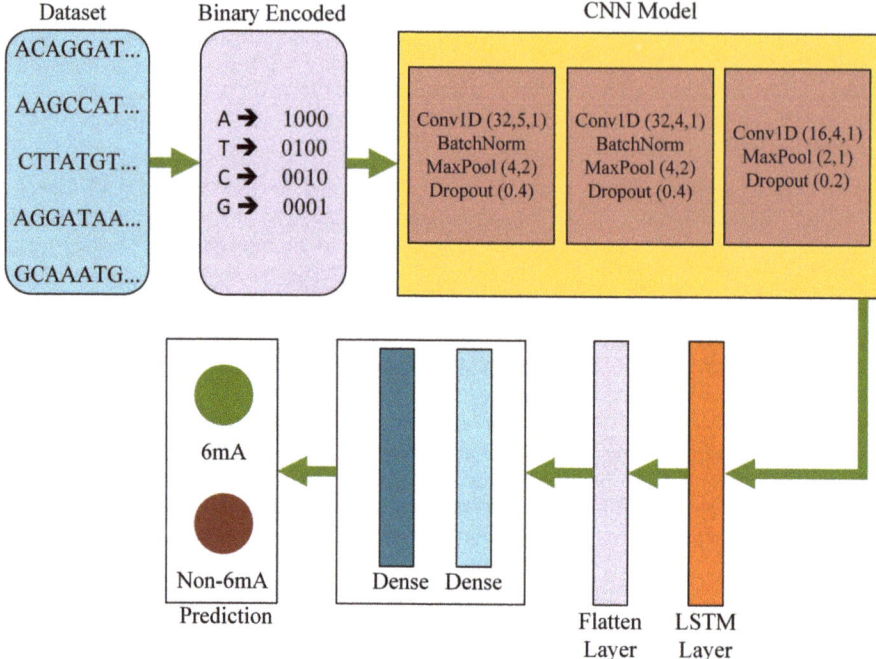

Figure 1. DNA6mA-MINT architecture for identification of DNA 6mA modification. Acronyms: Convolution 1 Dimension (Conv1D), BatchNormalization (BatchNorm), MaxPool (Max Pooling), Convolution Neural Network (CNN), Conv1d (number of filters, size of the filters, number of strides), MaxPool (pool size, number of strides), Dropout (ratio of features which needs to be discarded), and Long Short-Term Memory (LSTM).

Table 1. Architecture details of DNA6mA-MINT.

Layer	Output Shape	Number of Parameters
Input	(41,4)	-
Conv1D (32,5,1)	(37,32)	672
Batch Normalization	(37,32)	128
Max Pooling (4,2)	(17,32)	0
Dropout (0.4)	(17,32)	0
Conv1D (32,4,1)	(14,32)	4128
Batch Normalization	(14,32)	128
Max Pooling (4,2)	(6,32)	0
Dropout (0.4)	(6,32)	0
Conv1D (16,4,1)	(3,16)	2064
Max Pooling (2,1)	(1,16)	0
Dropout (0.2)	(1,16)	0
LSTM	(1,4)	336
Flatten	4	0
Dense	32	160
Dense	1	33

In CNN models a greater number of convolution layers represents the extraction of deeper features, but for the research problem under consideration, we cannot use more number of convolution layers, as by further increasing the convolution layers, the overfitting problem is observed. Using three convolution layers was an ideal solution to classify the input data we have, as this leads us to a high-performance architecture. All the convolution layers used ReLU as an activation function which eases the training process. At this stage, sigmoid or tanh are not used as an activation function, the reason being their vanishing gradient problem. The vanishing gradient problem makes the training process difficult, where ReLU solves this problem due to its unbounded nature.

The set of features extracted from the CNN model was fed into LSTM, which is a recurrent neural network (RNN). Here, the LSTM supports the sequence prediction. Therefore, the proposed model consists of two sub-models: the feature extractor which is the CNN model and the feature interpreter, which is the LSTM layer. In the proposed model, LSTM is used with a filter size of four, which is selected after hyperparameter tuning. The optimally interpreted feature set was converted to a single feature column by using a flattened layer. A single column feature set undergoes two dense layers with 32 and 1 neurons respectively to give the final classification output. The first dense layer uses the ReLU activation function while the second dense layer uses the sigmoid activation function. Sigmoid activation function makes the output range between 0 and 1 which is required for a binary classification problem. Below are the equations for ReLU and sigmoid functions.

$$ReLU(z) = max(0,z) \tag{1}$$

$$Sigmoid(z) = \frac{1}{1+exp(-z)} \tag{2}$$

DNA6mA-MINT is implemented on the Keras framework [33]. The output of the sigmoid activation function will be an input to the objective function. Binary cross-entropy is used as an objective function [34] and its equation is as follows,

$$BCE = -y_1 log(Sigmoid(z)) - (1-y_1)log(1-Sigmoid(z)) \tag{3}$$

where y_1 is the label for class sample. The loss can also be expressed as

$$BCE = \begin{cases} -log(Sigmoid(z)) & \text{if } y_1 = 1 \\ -log(1-Sigmoid(z)) & \text{if } y_1 = 0 \end{cases} \tag{4}$$

Stochastic gradient descent is used for optimizing the objective function. The equation below is used for calculating stochastic gradient descent,

$$\theta^{i+1} = \theta^i - \alpha \cdot \nabla_\theta Loss(\theta^i, y) \tag{5}$$

where θ^i is the current estimation of θ at iteration 'i', α is the learning rate, and $\nabla_\theta Loss(\theta^i, y)$ is computed gradient of the loss function.

Stochastic gradient descent reduces the computational complexity by achieving faster iterations [35]. In the optimization process, the learning rate and momentum were set to 0.004 and 0.9 respectively.

4. Figure of Merits

Evaluation of the DNA6mA-MINT is carried out using k-fold cross-validation where the value of k in our case is kept five and ten. In both cases, the whole dataset was divided into k subset. A single subset is chosen iteratively for the testing purpose where remaining subsets are used for training purposes. For the final performance estimation of the model, an average of k-trials is taken.

The figure of merits used in recent publications are listed with equations below,

$$Sensitivity = TPR = \frac{TP}{TP + FN} \tag{6}$$

$$Specificity = TNR = \frac{TN}{TN+FP} \tag{7}$$

$$Accuracy = \frac{TP+TN}{TP+TN+FP+FN} \tag{8}$$

$$MCC = \frac{TP \times TN - FP \times FN}{\sqrt{(TP+FP)(TP+FN)(TN+FP)(TN+FN)}} \tag{9}$$

where

TP = True Positive = 6mA correctly identified as 6mA
FP = False Positive = Non 6mA incorrectly identified as 6mA
TN = True Negative = Non 6mA correctly identified as Non 6mA
FN = False Negative = 6mA incorrectly identified as Non 6mA

Sensitivity, also known as True Positive Rate (TPR), is a statistical measure which calculates the ratio of positive samples identified as positive samples by the model. Specificity, also known as True Negative Rate (TNR), is also a statistical measure which calculates the ratio of negative samples identified as negative samples by the model. Accuracy measures the closeness of the model to the idle situation. While the Matthews correlation coefficient (MCC) depicts the quality of the model as a binary classifier, another figure of merit used in this study is the area under Receiver Operating Characteristics (auROC). It measures the performance of the model at various thresholds. The auROC indicates the capability of the model to distinguish two classes from each other.

5. Results and Discussion

The proposed model was evaluated on three datasets: *M. musculus* genome, rice genome, and "Combined-species". The state-of-the-art techniques in the literature carried out their results either using 5-fold cross-validation or 10-fold cross-validation. Therefore, we validated DNA6mA-MINT by using both numbers of folds so that a better comparative analysis can be derived. Therefore, it is important to compare 5-fold cross-validation results with the models that have reported their results on 5-fold cross-validation. Similarly, 10-fold results should be compared with the 10-fold cross-validated model in the literature. A greater number of folds depicts higher performance, the reason being that by increasing the number of folds, the training dataset gets a higher ratio of the data which increases the model performance.

Table 2 shows a comparison of the proposed model with existing techniques, while Figure 2 shows the graphical visualization of performance differences between existing techniques and the proposed technique in this study. In the case of *M. musculus* genomes, the DNA6mA-MINT achieved high results in all figures of merit when compared with models validated on 5-fold cross-validation. On the other hand, compared on 10-fold cross-validation, the 6mA-Finder exhibits higher auROC then the proposed model. However, in all other figures of merit the proposed model remains higher in performance.

For Rice genomes with 5-fold cross-validation, the DNA6mA-MINT depicts an increase in all figures of merit, while in 10-fold cross-validation, 6mA-Finder has not reported results for all figures of merit, but the reported auROC achieved by 6mA-Finder is lower than that achieved by the proposed model in 10-fold cross-validation.

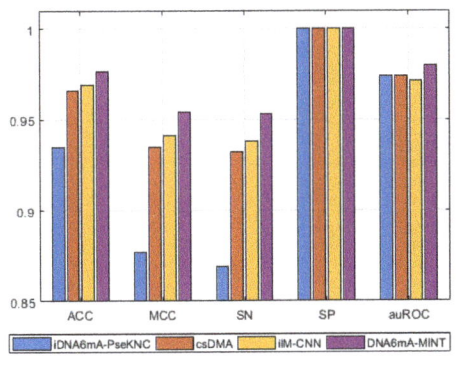

(a)

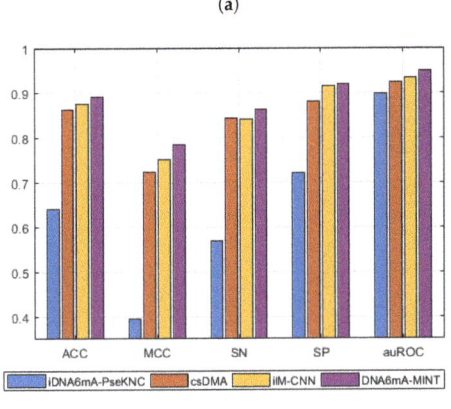

(b)

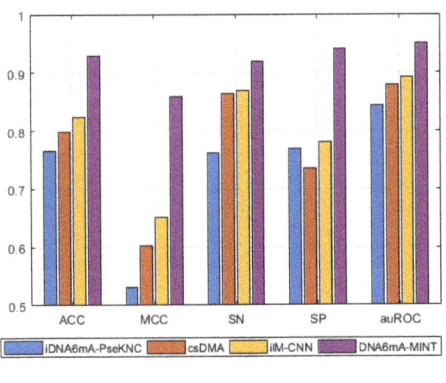

(c)

Figure 2. Graphical comparison of DNA6mA-MINT with state-of-the-art tools using five fold cross validation on different species. (**a**) *Mus musculus*, (**b**) Rice, (**c**) "Combined-species". Acronyms are Sensitivity (SN), Specificity (SP), Accuracy (ACC), Matthews Correlation Coefficient (MCC), and area under the Receiver Operating Characteristics (auROC).

Table 2. Performance comparison of DNA6mA-MINT with existing techniques on different species with 5- and 10-fold cross-validation.

Model	Species	Folds	SN	SP	ACC	MCC	auROC
iDNA6mA-PseKNC	M. musculus	5	0.869	1	0.935	0.877	0.974
	Rice	5	0.569	0.721	0.641	0.394	0.896
	Combined-species	5	0.762	0.769	0.765	0.531	0.844
csDMA	M. musculus	5	0.932	1	0.966	0.935	0.974
	Rice	5	0.842	0.880	0.861	0.723	0.923
	Combined-species	5	0.863	0.735	0.799	0.603	0.879
iIM-CNN	M. musculus	5	0.938	1	0.969	0.941	0.971
	Rice	5	0.841	0.914	0.875	0.752	0.934
	Combined-species	5	0.869	0.780	0.824	0.651	0.892
6mA-Finder	M. musculus	10	0.9349	1	0.9674	0.935	0.9954
	Rice	10	-	-	-	-	0.9394
	Combined-species	10	-	-	-	-	0.9207
DNA6mA-MINT	M. musculus	5	0.9531	1	0.9766	0.9543	0.980
	Rice	5	0.8621	0.9195	0.8908	0.7829	0.950
	Combined-species	5	0.9182	0.9409	0.9295	0.8593	0.950
DNA6mA-MINT	M. musculus	10	0.9427	1	0.9714	0.9444	0.98
	Rice	10	0.9425	0.908	0.9253	0.8511	0.950
	Combined-species	10	0.9318	0.9321	0.932	0.8639	0.960

"Combined-species" is another benchmark dataset for the evaluation of the proposed model. In "combined-species", the proposed model has shown a tremendous increase in performance when compared with existing techniques. In 5-fold cross-validated models, the DNA6mA-MINT increased the sensitivity, specificity, accuracy, MCC, and AuROC by 4.92%, 16.09%, 10.55%, 20.83%, and 5.8%, respectively. For 10-fold cross-validation, the proposed model illustrated an increase of 3.93% in auROC when compared with 6mA-Finder. The sharp increase in MCC depicts the higher quality of the DNA6mA-MINT in comparison to existing state-of-the-art tools.

Figure 3 shows the auROC curves for three species. As can be determined by the curves, the proposed model curves are approaching the ideal scenario. Especially in the case of *M. musculus*, which is almost near to ideal. Upon evaluation of DNA6mA-MINT on the "combined-species" independent dataset with 10-fold cross-validation, a massive increase of 8.99% is observed in auROC. The 6mA Finder has reported 87.01% auROC while the proposed model has achieved 96% auROC for "combined-species" independent dataset. The high performance shown by the DNA6mA-MINT depicts the reliability of the proposed tool.

For functional genomics, such an architecture should be used which can effectively model the DNA motifs with some insertion/deletion (indels). Keeping it in mind to unfold the quality of DNA6mA-MINT, the silico mutagenesis method is adopted. Nucleotides in the benchmark dataset are computationally mutated. The effect of this mutation in model prediction is studied. One by one the data at position "1-41" is mutated and the corresponding absolute difference is stored. Last, the averaged predicted score for all the mutations over all the sequences in the benchmark dataset is computed to construct the heat map. Figure 4 represents the constructed heat map illustrating the important position of the input sequence. As can be seen, the final prediction is more affected by the mutations occurring at the center of the sequence than the mutations happening on both sides of the sequence.

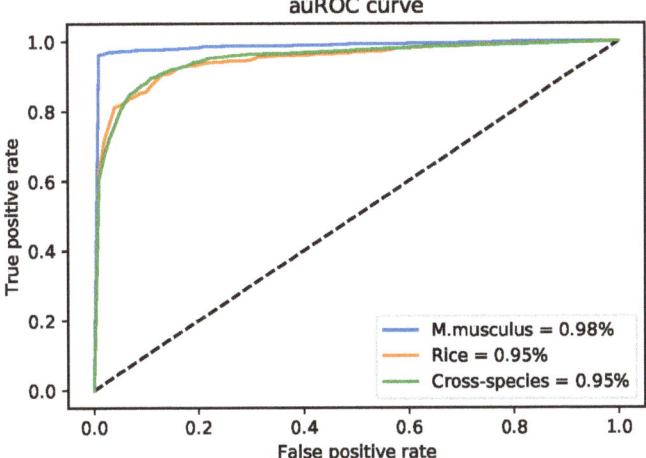

Figure 3. AuROC for *M. musculus*, Rice, and "Combined-species" genomes.

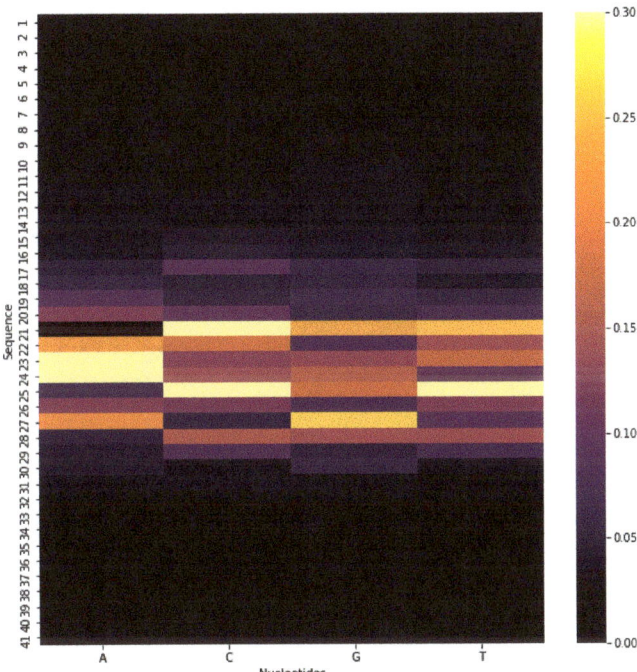

Figure 4. Heat Map to study the effect of mutation in model prediction.

In order to study the generalization of DNA6mA-MINT we have prepared additional dataset for Rice genome (which is a part of our future work) from the NCBI Gene Expression Omnibus (https://www.ncbi.nlm.nih.gov/geo/) under the accession number GSE103145. We have prepared from this repository 10,000 positive sequences and 10,000 negative sequences that are not 6mA.

Obtained values for sensitivity, specificity, and accuracy are 84.77, 82.78, and 83.76, respectively. The obtained results show that proposed model generalizes well to the new sequences.

6. Conclusions

DNA modification results in presiding form which is DNA N^6-methyladenine (6mA). DNA-6mA identification is necessary to explore different biological functions. This study proposed an effective computational tool for the identification of DNA-6mA using a Neural Network framework. The proposed model uses a CNN for feature extraction followed by the LSTM layer, which gives interpretation of the high-dimensional feature vector so that they can be optimally utilized for classification of methylated or non-methylated sites. For comparison purpose results are computed on five and ten folds for three datasets. The proposed model outperformed the results achieved by existing state-of-the-art models in the case of all the datasets. The aim to introduce this model is to utilize it for different research fields working in the development of medicine and bioinformatics. For the said reason, a web server is created which is publicly available at: http://home.jbnu.ac.kr/NSCL/DNA6mA-MINT.htm.

Author Contributions: Conceptualization, M.U.R. and K.T.C.; methodology, M.U.R.; software, M.U.R.; validation, M.U.R. and K.T.C.; investigation, M.U.R. and K.T.C.; writing—original draft preparation: M.U.R.; writing—review and editing, M.U.R. and K.T.C.; supervision, K.T.C. All authors have read and agreed to the published version of the manuscript.

Funding: This work was supported in part by the National Research Foundation of Korea (NRF) grant funded by the Korea government (MSIT) (No. 2020R1A2C2005612) and in part by the Brain Research Program of the National Research Foundation (NRF) funded by the Korean government (MSIT) (No. NRF-2017M3C7A1044816).

Conflicts of Interest: The authors declare no conflict of interest. The funders had no role in the design of the study; in the collection, analyses, or interpretation of data; in the writing of the manuscript; or in the decision to publish the results.

References

1. Greer, E.L.; Blanco, M.A.; Gu, L.; Sendinc, E.; Liu, J.; Aristizábal-Corrales, D.; Hsu, C.H.; Aravind, L.; He, C.; Shi, Y. DNA methylation on N^6-adenine in *C. elegans*. *Cell* **2015**, *161*, 868–878. [CrossRef] [PubMed]
2. Zhang, G.; Huang, H.; Liu, D.; Cheng, Y.; Liu, X.; Zhang, W.; Yin, R.; Zhang, D.; Zhang, P.; Liu, J.; et al. N^6-methyladenine DNA modification in *Drosophila*. *Cell* **2015**, *161*, 893–906. [CrossRef] [PubMed]
3. Luo, G.Z.; He, C. DNA N^6-methyladenine in metazoans: Functional epigenetic mark or bystander? *Nat. Struct. Mol. Biol.* **2017**, *24*, 503–506. [CrossRef]
4. Campbell, J.L.; Kleckner, N. *E. coli oriC* and the *dnaA* gene promoter are sequestered from *dam* methyltransferase following the passage of the chromosomal replication fork. *Cell* **1990**, *62*, 967–979. [CrossRef]
5. Pukkila, P.J.; Peterson, J.; Herman, G.; Modrich, P.; Meselson, M. Effects of high levels of DNA adenine methylation on methyl-directed mismatch repair in *Escherichia coli*. *Genetics* **1983**, *104*, 571–582. [PubMed]
6. Robbins-Manke, J.L.; Zdraveski, Z.Z.; Marinus, M.; Essigmann, J.M. Analysis of global gene expression and double-strand-break formation in DNA adenine methyltransferase-and mismatch repair-deficient *Escherichia coli*. *J. Bacteriol.* **2005**, *187*, 7027–7037. [CrossRef] [PubMed]
7. Xiao, C.L.; Zhu, S.; He, M.; Chen, D.; Zhang, Q.; Chen, Y.; Yu, G.; Liu, J.; Xie, S.Q.; Luo, F.; et al. N^6-methyladenine DNA modification in the human genome. *Mol. Cell* **2018**, *71*, 306–318. [CrossRef]
8. Liu, X.; Lai, W.; Li, Y.; Chen, S.; Liu, B.; Zhang, N.; Mo, J.; Lyu, C.; Zheng, J.; Du, Y.R.; et al. N^6-methyladenine is incorporated into mammalian genome by DNA polymerase. *Cell Res.* **2020**. [CrossRef]
9. Dunn, D.; Smith, J. Occurrence of a new base in the deoxyribonucleic acid of a strain of *Bacterium coli*. *Nature* **1955**, *175*, 336–337. [CrossRef]
10. Bird, A.P. Use of restriction enzymes to study eukaryotic DNA methylation: II. The symmetry of methylated sites supports semi-conservative copying of the methylation pattern. *J. Mol. Biol.* **1978**, *118*, 49–60. [CrossRef]
11. Flusberg, B.A.; Webster, D.R.; Lee, J.H.; Travers, K.J.; Olivares, E.C.; Clark, T.A.; Korlach, J.; Turner, S.W. Direct detection of DNA methylation during single-molecule, real-time sequencing. *Nat. Methods* **2010**, *7*, 461. [CrossRef] [PubMed]

12. Pomraning, K.R.; Smith, K.M.; Freitag, M. Genome-wide high throughput analysis of DNA methylation in eukaryotes. *Methods* **2009**, *47*, 142–150. [CrossRef]
13. Liu, B.; Liu, X.; Lai, W.; Wang, H. Metabolically generated stable isotope-labeled deoxynucleoside code for tracing DNA N^6-Methyladenine in human cells. *Anal. Chem.* **2017**, *89*, 6202–6209. [CrossRef] [PubMed]
14. Fu, Y.; Luo, G.Z.; Chen, K.; Deng, X.; Yu, M.; Han, D.; Hao, Z.; Liu, J.; Lu, X.; Doré, L.C.; et al. N^6-methyldeoxyadenosine marks active transcription start sites in *Chlamydomonas*. *Cell* **2015**, *161*, 879–892. [CrossRef]
15. Mondo, S.J.; Dannebaum, R.O.; Kuo, R.C.; Louie, K.B.; Bewick, A.J.; LaButti, K.; Haridas, S.; Kuo, A.; Salamov, A.; Ahrendt, S.R.; et al. Widespread adenine N6-methylation of active genes in fungi. *Nat. Genet.* **2017**, *49*, 964–968. [CrossRef] [PubMed]
16. Zhou, C.; Wang, C.; Liu, H.; Zhou, Q.; Liu, Q.; Guo, Y.; Peng, T.; Song, J.; Zhang, J.; Chen, L.; et al. Identification and analysis of adenine N6-methylation sites in the rice genome. *Nat. Plants* **2018**, *4*, 554–563. [CrossRef] [PubMed]
17. Feng, P.; Yang, H.; Ding, H.; Lin, H.; Chen, W.; Chou, K.C. iDNA6mA-PseKNC: Identifying DNA N^6-methyladenosine sites by incorporating nucleotide physicochemical properties into PseKNC. *Genomics* **2019**, *111*, 96–102. [CrossRef]
18. Liu, Z.; Dong, W.; Jiang, W.; He, Z. csDMA: An improved bioinformatics tool for identifying DNA 6mA modifications via Chou's 5-step rule. *Sci. Rep.* **2019**, *9*, 1–9.
19. Xu, H.; Hu, R.; Jia, P.; Zhao, Z. 6mA-Finder: A novel online tool for predicting DNA N6-methyladenine sites in genomes. *Bioinformatics* **2020**, *36*, 3257–3259. [CrossRef]
20. Chen, W.; Lv, H.; Nie, F.; Lin, H. i6mA-Pred: Identifying DNA N6-methyladenine sites in the rice genome. *Bioinformatics* **2019**, *35*, 2796–2800. [CrossRef]
21. Rahman, M.K. FastFeatGen: Faster Parallel Feature Extraction from Genome Sequences and Efficient Prediction of DNA N^6-Methyladenine Sites. In Proceedings of the International Conference on Computational Advances in Bio and Medical Sciences, Miami, FL, USA, 15–17 November 2019; pp. 52–64.
22. Kong, L.; Zhang, L. i6mA-DNCP: Computational identification of DNA N^6-methyladenine sites in the rice genome using optimized dinucleotide-based features. *Genes* **2019**, *10*, 828. [CrossRef] [PubMed]
23. Rehman, M.U.; Khan, S.H.; Abbas, Z.; Danish Rizvi, S.M. Classification of Diabetic Retinopathy Images Based on Customised CNN Architecture. In Proceedings of the 2019 Amity International Conference on Artificial Intelligence (AICAI), Dubai, UAE, 4–6 February 2019; pp. 244–248.
24. Rehman, M.U; Khan, S.H.; Rizvi, S.D.; Abbas, Z.; Zafar, A. Classification of skin lesion by interference of segmentation and convolotion neural network. In Proceedings of the 2018 2nd International Conference on Engineering Innovation (ICEI), Bangkok, Thailand, 5–6 July 2018; pp. 81–85.
25. Mahmoudi, O.; Wahab, A.; Chong, K.T. iMethyl-Deep: N6 methyladenosine identification of yeast genome with automatic feature extraction technique by using deep learning algorithm. *Genes* **2020**, *11*, 529. [CrossRef] [PubMed]
26. Wahab, A.; Mahmoudi, O.; Kim, J.; Chong, K.T. DNC4mC-Deep: Identification and analysis of DNA N4-methylcytosine sites based on different encoding schemes by using deep learning. *Cells* **2020**, *9*, 1756. [CrossRef] [PubMed]
27. Park, S.; Wahab, A.; Nazari, I.; Ryu, J.H.; Chong, K.T. i6mA-DNC: Prediction of DNA N6-Methyladenosine sites in rice genome based on dinucleotide representation using deep learning. *Chemom. Intell. Lab. Syst.* **2020**, *204*, 104102. [CrossRef]
28. Wahab, A.; Ali, S.D.; Tayara, H.; Chong, K.T. iIM-CNN: Intelligent identifier of 6mA sites on different species by using convolution neural network. *IEEE Access* **2019**, *7*, 178577–178583. [CrossRef]
29. Chou, K.C. Some remarks on protein attribute prediction and pseudo amino acid composition. *J. Theor. Biol.* **2011**, *273*, 236–247. [CrossRef]
30. Chou, K.C. Advances in predicting subcellular localization of multi-label proteins and its implication for developing multi-target drugs. *Curr. Med. Chem.* **2019**, *26*, 4918–4943. [CrossRef]
31. Ye, P.; Luan, Y.; Chen, K.; Liu, Y.; Xiao, C.; Xie, Z. MethSMRT: An integrative database for DNA N6-methyladenine and N4-methylcytosine generated by single-molecular real-time sequencing. *Nucleic Acids Res.* **2016**, gkw950. [CrossRef]
32. Fu, L.; Niu, B.; Zhu, Z.; Wu, S.; Li, W. CD-HIT: Accelerated for clustering the next-generation sequencing data. *Bioinformatics* **2012**, *28*, 3150–3152. [CrossRef]

33. Chollet, F.; Keras Special Interest Group. Keras: Deep Learning Library for Theano and Tensorflow. 2015, Volume 7, p. T1. Available online: https://keras.io/ (accessed on 1 August 2020).
34. De Boer, P.T.; Kroese, D.P.; Mannor, S.; Rubinstein, R.Y. A tutorial on the cross-entropy method. *Ann. Oper. Res.* **2005**, *134*, 19–67. [CrossRef]
35. Bottou, L.; Bousquet, O. The tradeoffs of large scale learning. In *Advances in Neural Information Processing Systems*; Neural Information Processing Systems Foundation (NIPS): Vancouver, BC, Canada, 2008; pp. 161–168.

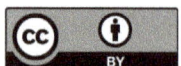

© 2020 by the authors. Licensee MDPI, Basel, Switzerland. This article is an open access article distributed under the terms and conditions of the Creative Commons Attribution (CC BY) license (http://creativecommons.org/licenses/by/4.0/).

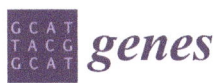

Article

Comparative Pathway Integrator: A Framework of Meta-Analytic Integration of Multiple Transcriptomic Studies for Consensual and Differential Pathway Analysis

Xiangrui Zeng [1,†], Wei Zong [2,†], Chien-Wei Lin [3], Zhou Fang [2], Tianzhou Ma [4], David A. Lewis [5], John F. Enwright [5] and George C. Tseng [2,*]

1. Computational Biology Department, Carnegie Mellon University, Pittsburgh, PA 15213, USA; xiangruz@andrew.cmu.edu
2. Department of Biostatistics, University of Pittsburgh, Pittsburgh, PA 15260, USA; WEZ97@pitt.edu (W.Z.); fangz.ark@gmail.com (Z.F.)
3. Division of Biostatistics, Medical College of Wisconsin, Wauwatosa, WI 53226, USA; chlin@mcw.edu
4. Department of Epidemiology and Biostatistics, University of Maryland, College Park, MD 20742, USA; tma0929@umd.edu
5. Department of Psychiatry, University of Pittsburgh, Pittsburgh, PA 15260, USA; lewisda@upmc.edu (D.A.L.); enwrightjf@upmc.edu (J.F.E.)
* Correspondence: ctseng@pitt.edu
† These authors contributed equally to this work.

Received: 16 May 2020; Accepted: 17 June 2020; Published: 24 June 2020

Abstract: Pathway enrichment analysis provides a knowledge-driven approach to interpret differentially expressed genes associated with disease status. Many tools have been developed to analyze a single study. However, when multiple studies of different conditions are jointly analyzed, novel integrative tools are needed. In addition, pathway redundancy introduced by combining multiple public pathway databases hinders interpretation and knowledge discovery. We present a meta-analytic integration tool, Comparative Pathway Integrator (CPI), to address these issues using adaptively weighted Fisher's method to discover consensual and differential enrichment patterns, a tight clustering algorithm to reduce pathway redundancy, and a text mining algorithm to assist interpretation of the pathway clusters. We applied CPI to jointly analyze six psychiatric disorder transcriptomic studies to demonstrate its effectiveness, and found functions confirmed by previous biological studies as well as novel enrichment patterns. CPI's R package is accessible online on Github metaOmics/MetaPath.

Keywords: pathway; meta-analysis; text mining

1. Introduction

In a typical transcriptomic study, a set of candidate genes associated with diseases or other outcomes are first identified through differential expression analysis. Then, to gain more insight into the underlying biological mechanism, pathway analysis (also known as gene set analysis) is usually applied to pursue functional annotation of the candidate biomarker list. The goal behind pathway analysis is to determine whether the detected biomarkers are enriched in pre-defined biological functional domains. These functional domains might come from one of the publicly available databases such as GO [1], Reactome [2] and KEGG [3], or one of the integrated pathway collection such as MSigDB [4] and Pathway Commons [5]. Three main categories of pathway analysis methods have been developed in the past decade. The first category of methods called "over-representation analysis" considers biomarkers under a certain cutoff of differential express (DE) evidence and statistically evaluates the fraction of DE genes in a particular pathway found among the background genes. Without a hard threshold, the second category "functional class scoring" takes the DE evidence scores of all genes in a pathway into account and aggregates them into a single pathway-specific statistics. The third category "pathway topology" further incorporates the information of gene-gene interaction and their cellular location in addition to the pathway database. Details of general pathway enrichment analysis review can be found in [6].

Many transcriptomic datasets have been generated with the rapid advances of high-throughput experimental technologies in the past decade. Meta-analysis, a set of statistical methods for combining multiple studies of a related hypothesis, has thus become popular [7]. Some methods have been developed for the pathway meta-analysis. Shen and Tseng [8] developed two approaches of meta-analysis for pathway enrichment by combining DE evidence at the gene level (MAPE_G) or at the pathway level (MAPE_P). Nguyen et al. [9] proposed a robust bi-level pathway meta-analysis by adding an intra-experiment level analysis and another data-driven meta-analysis approach, DANUBE [10], using unbiased empirical distribution. However, in many real applications, when multiple datasets for a common biological hypothesis are available but possibly performed under different conditions (e.g., different tissues, different cell composition or different experimental platforms), it becomes necessary to detect both pathways enriched consistently in all studies (consensually enriched pathways) and pathways enriched in partial studies (differentially enriched pathways). One naïve way is to identify the enriched pathways in each study individually and manually check whether a certain pathway is enriched in one or multiple studies (e.g., using Venn diagram for enriched pathways in each study under a certain FDR threshold). This approach is sensitive to the choice of FDR threshold and is ad hoc in drawing a final conclusion. To avoid an arbitrary significance threshold, Plaisieret et al. [11] and Cahill et al. [12] have proposed rank-rank hypergeometric overlap (RRHO) plot to visualize contrasting enrichment significance under all continuous significance level of two studies. This approach is, however, limited to comparing two studies. To the best of our knowledge, there is currently no available statistical tool that can achieve the goal of integrating pathway enrichment of multiple studies in an automated and systematic manner for characterizing consensually and differentially enriched pathways.

A second issue emerges with pathway enrichment analysis is the pathway redundancy across pathway databases. Researchers often have difficult time to infer and interpret the underlying biological mechanism without presumed bias due to the large number of pathways identified. This kind of redundancy frequently occurs in a regular pathway enrichment analysis since different pathway databases contain similar annotated pathways with highly overlapped genes. The DAVID Bioinformatics Resources [13] partially resolved this issue by clustering pathways based on a kappa statistic representing the pathway similarity. However, the users still had to manually inspect each pathway in a cluster. Due to the long and vague descriptions in many pathways, users can still struggle to reach a solid conclusion from the results.

In light of the aforementioned drawbacks in existing tools, we propose a meta-analytic integrative framework to combine multiple transcriptomic studies for identifying consensual and differential pathway enrichment, wrapped in a tool named Comparative Pathway Integrator (CPI). CPI incorporates 25 pathway databases, including GO [1], Reactome [2], KEGG [3] and MSigDB [4] or user-defined gene set lists, as reference of pathway analysis. In order to identify both consensual and differential enriched pathways across studies, we applied the adaptively weighted Fisher's method [14], which was originally developed to combine *p*-values from multiple omics studies for detecting homogeneous and heterogeneous differentially expressed genes. Next, cluster analysis based on pathway similarity (defined by gene overlap) is applied to remove the level of pathway redundancy. But unlike DAVID, we adopt a tight clustering algorithm similar to [15] to allow scattered pathways without being clustered and derive tight pathway clusters. Subsequently, we developed a text mining algorithm to automate the annotation of the tight pathway clusters by extracting keywords from pathway descriptions, which also offers more statistically valid summarization compared to leaving user to manually explore pathways in a cluster. Lastly, CPI provide users with both spreadsheets and graphical outputs for intuitive visualization, statistically solid presentation and insightful interpretation. CPI has a standalone R package as well as being disseminated into MetaOmics, an analysis pipeline and browser-based software suite for transcriptomic meta-analysis [16].

2. Materials and Methods

2.1. Workflow of Comparative Pathway Integrator (CPI)

CPI is a comprehensive tool incorporating several widely accepted mature methods as well as multiple novel algorithms/approaches. It is mainly composed of three steps (Figure 1). The first step (Section 2.2) performs meta-analytic pathway analysis, which integrates pathway enrichment analysis and meta-analysis. This step partially resembles the previous in-house work of R package MetaPath [8] but with advanced features. While MetaPath focuses on detecting consensually enriched pathways, CPI will detect both consensual and differentially enriched pathways, providing valuable information on how the patterns of pathway enrichment differ across studies. The second step (Section 2.3) implements pathway clustering. This step aims to reduce redundancy of the pathway information from commonly hundreds of enriched pathways to only handful (usually 5–10) pathway clusters. The results are more succinct and interpretable. The third step (Section 2.4) includes text mining based on pathway names and descriptions to find keywords characterizing the intrinsic biological functions of each pathway cluster. A permutation-based statistical test is performed to assess if a specific biological noun phrase appears significantly more than by chance. Without this step, it would be difficult to avoid subjective biases from users and to objectively identify the representative biological mechanisms for each pathway cluster since clustering of the pathways does not fundamentally reduce the total number of pathways under investigation. Finally, we generate graphical and spreadsheet outputs of pathway p-value matrices and pathway clustering details including gene composition and functional keywords.

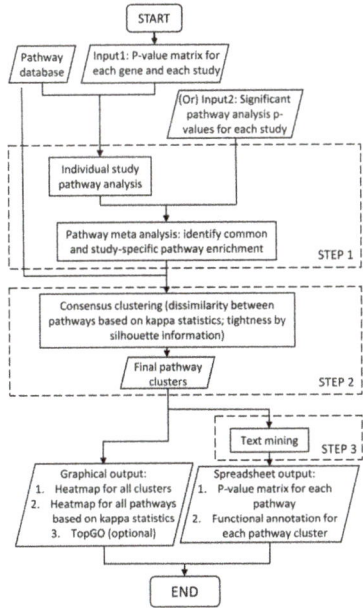

Figure 1. Workflow of Comparative Pathway Integrator (CPI).

2.2. Meta-Analytic Pathway Analysis

Compared to differential expression analysis, pathway enrichment analysis provides more biological insight in a more systematic and comprehensive manner. In CPI, we allow multiple methods of over representation analysis since recent comparative studies [17,18] have shown little additional advantages using sophisticated functional class scoring or pathway topology methods. But if such advanced pathway enrichment analysis is preferred, users can externally implement the pathway analysis and CPI can accept lists of significant pathways and the corresponding p-values as alternative input (Input 2 in Figure 1). Given pathway enrichment results, we perform adaptively-weighted Fisher's (AW-Fisher) method [14,19] for meta-analysis, to identify pathways significant in one or more studies/conditions. AW-Fisher not only increases statistical power, but also provides a 0/1 binary weight for each study, indicating whether a study contributes to the meta-analytic significance. Given a user-specified q-value cutoff, we obtain a list of significant pathways, with 0/1 binary weights indicating whether a pathway is significantly enriched across most or all studies/conditions (i.e., consensually enriched pathways) or only in partial studies (i.e., differentially enriched pathways). For example, in Section 3, the "GO:MF kinase activity" pathway has raw enrichment p-values $(0.26922, 0.17773, 0.06485, 2.04 \times 10^{-5}, 0.00449, 0.018922)$ for the six studies. AW-Fisher meta-analysis generates combined p-value $= 5.52 \times 10^{-6}$ (q-value = 0.00014) with adaptive weights = (0,0,1,1,1,1), showing enrichment in the last four bipolar studies or major depressive disorder studies but not in the first two schizophrenia studies.

2.3. Pathway Clustering for Reducing Redundancy and Enhancing Interpretation

Because of the nature of pathway definitions (e.g., hierarchy structure or overlapping functions), many genes are shared among different pathways. Similar pathways can also repeat in different pathway databases with slightly different gene composition, annotation or description. Such redundancies often stumble interpretation of pathway analysis results. In CPI, we perform pathway clustering to reduce the redundancy among detected pathways. The similarity between different pathways is calculated based on kappa statistics [20], which depends on how many genes are mutually identical or exclusive among those pathways. The kappa statistics represents the dissimilarity between two pathways based on the genes composing each pathway. Based on the dissimilarity matrix of all pathway pairs, consensus clustering [21] is used to estimate the number of clusters. Following the original consensus clustering method, an elbow plot and consensus CDF plot are generated to assist users to decide the number of clusters.

We next assign detected pathways into clusters. For most clustering algorithms including the aforementioned consensus clustering, all pathways are forced into clusters although it is well-known that leaving scattered subjects out of clusters often generate tighter clusters and improve the clustering performance in such high-dimensional data [15,22,23]. In CPI, we allow scattered pathways to form singletons, when its gene composition is largely different from representative pathway clusters, to avoid adding outliers to the pathway clusters. To improve the tightness of the clusters, we further calculated for each pathway the silhouette width [24], a measure of how tightly each pathway is grouped in its cluster, and removed the scattered pathways with low silhouette width iteratively until all pathways' silhouette widths are above a certain cutoff. The removing cutoff for silhouette width is estimated empirically based on its distribution as in our multi-disease application in Section 3 (we choose 0.1 in this paper). For the identified singleton pathways, we collected them to form a scattered pathway set instead of filtering them out. In general applications, we recommend users to investigate the identified tight pathway clusters first with the subsequent text mining tool introduced in the next subsection since these pathway clusters are better annotated in the pathway databases and are likely better studied in the current biological knowledge domain. We, however, do not discard pathways in the scattered set but recommend them in the secondary investigation.

2.4. Text Mining for Automated Annotation and Knowledge Retrieval of Pathway Clusters

2.4.1. Motivation and Problem Setting

Although the pathway cluster analysis in Section 2.3 can greatly reduce redundancy structure of the detected pathways, users still have to manually scan through all pathways in a cluster to grasp its major content and biologically driving mechanism, which can be labor-intensive and subject to the user's biased presumption. Therefore, we need a more rigorous and statistically meaningful summary of the pathway cluster to guide an unbiased interpretation. The above goal is expressed here as the text mining for key noun phrases of each pathway cluster: which noun phrase appears more frequently in a certain pathway cluster than by chance in statistical sense? We will therefore treat these noun phrases as the potentially representative entities (mechanism) for the pathway cluster. The entity is counted based on the number of pathways containing it, rather than the frequency of it appearing in all pathway descriptions in a cluster. For instance, in a certain cluster, if "T cell" occurs six times in 3 pathway descriptions: three times in pathway #1, twice in pathway #2 and once in pathway #3, T cell" is counted 3 occurrences even though it appears 6 times in total.

2.4.2. Pathway-Phrase Matrix

For each pathway description, we firstly extracted unique noun phrases from it. This step was done using the spacy_extract _nounphrases function from R package *spacyr* [25] which is an R wrapper around the Python *spaCy* package [26]. *spaCy* is an industrial strength text-mining package employing a large library database as well as some machine learning algorithms to detect information from texts. The stop words in English, such as "the", "a", "that", which are common and carry no important information, are removed from those noun phrases by using the English stop words database from R package *tm* [27]. After removing all stop words, the last word of each noun phrases, i.e., the central noun of a noun phrase, is lemmatized (converting plural form to singular form) by the lemmatize _words function in *textstem* [28]. The top 5000 common English words [29] were then filtered out from the result noun phrases of length one. A text mining process of an example sentence is shown in Figure 2.

In total, we provide 25 pathway databases (GO, KEGG, BioCarta, Reactome, Phenocarta, etc.) with 26,801 pathways in CPI for users to select in the analysis. The above preprocessing and filtering steps were repeated for each pathway to generate standard noun phrases for all pathways. Based on the results, we constructed a binary matrix where each row being a noun phrase and each column being a pathway with element $w_{ij} = 1$ indicating the pathway description j contains the noun phrase i and 0 otherwise.

Once the matrix was constructed, R package *wordnet* [30] was used to identify synonyms from row names of the matrix (noun phrases). When a pair of synonyms are identified, the phrase with lower occurrence in all pathways are combined with the phrase with higher occurrence. Then the row of less occurred phrase was deleted. Since in later text mining of pathway clusters, a phrase needs to at least occur in two pathways to be considered, all rows of phrases which occurred only once in the 26,801 pathways were deleted. As a result, a matrix of 36,037 rows and 26,801 columns was constructed.

For later penalized permutation test, the above text mining matrix construction procedure was also applied to pathway names of 26,801 pathways, producing a similar matrix of 36,037 rows and 26,801 columns with $v_{ij} = 1$ indicating the pathway name j contains the noun phrase i and 0 otherwise. For a given pathway (e.g., GO:0030964), the pathway name ("NADH dehydrogenase complex") is usually more concise while the pathway description ("An integral membrane complex that possesses NADH oxidoreductase activity. The complex is one of the components of the electron transport chain. It catalyzes the transfer of a pair of electrons from NADH to a quinone") gives a more detailed illustration of the pathway.

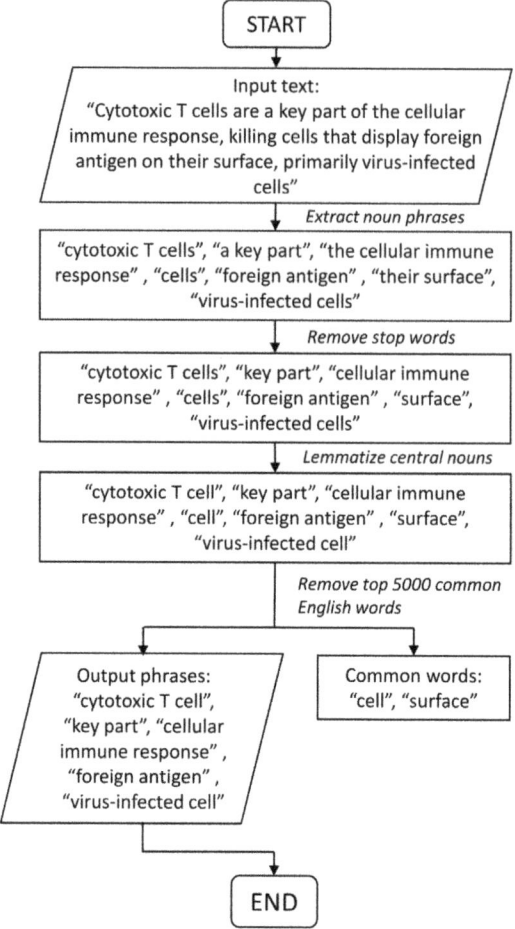

Figure 2. Workflow of noun phrase extraction.

2.4.3. Test Statistics for Noun Phrase Enrichment Analysis

A simple strategy to test for the significance of a phrase frequently appearing in a cluster is by simple counting and conducting Fisher exact test. Yet we found this method to be less powerful and less biologically justifiable from real data analysis, because the phrases in the term name or a shorter description of a pathway are deemed to be more representative than those in a full or longer description. In other words, phrases appearing in a pathway with shorter description should statistically contribute more weights than in a pathway with lengthy description because the latter is more likely to happen by chance. Therefore, we down-weighted the phrase count with long description by assigning a score between 0 and 1 to each pathway j to indicate whether it contains phrase i:

$$x_{ij} = \begin{cases} 1 & v_{ij} = 1 \text{ (phrase } i \text{ appeared in the } j\text{-th pathway name),} \\ exp(-\alpha \cdot |w_j|) & v_{ij} = 0 \text{ and } w_{ij} = 1 \text{ (phrase } i \text{ appeared only in the } j\text{-th pathway description),} \\ 0 & v_{ij} = w_{ij} = 0 \end{cases}$$

where $|w_j| = \sum_i w_{ij}$ is the number of unique noun phrases in the description of pathway j and α is a parameter controlling the degree of penalty. The greater α is, the greater the penalty is on longer description. When α equals to 0, there is no penalty and our test simplifies to Fisher's exact test with equal weight to pathway names and pathway descriptions. Based on evaluation in real data, $\alpha = 0.05$ is used in our package. Next, we define cluster score $T_i(C)$ to be the sum of scores of pathways in the cluster, i.e., for phrase i in a pathway cluster C, we define the test statistics:

$$T_i(C) = \sum_{j \in C} x_{ij}$$

2.4.4. Permutation Test

To test for the null hypothesis that a phrase is not enriched in a certain cluster, we adopt a permutation analysis. For each phrase i in the b-th permutation, pathways are randomly sampled to form subset S_b with the same cluster size as C. Test statistics $T_i(S_b)$ is recomputed at the end of each permutation. The operation is then repeated for a large number of times (say, $B = 10,000$ times). Finally, all $T_i(S_b)$'s form a null distribution and are compared to the observed statistics $T_i(C)$. And the p-value could be calculated by $p(T_i(C)) = \frac{\sum_{b=1}^{B} I(T_i(C) \geq T_i(S_b))}{B}$, indicating how extremely frequent phrase i is seen in cluster C. Multiple comparison is then corrected by Benjamini–Hochberg procedure [31] to control false discovery rate (FDR).

2.4.5. Graphical and Spreadsheet Output

In the final step, CPI outputs visualization tools, including (1) heatmap of kappa statistics matrix for pair-wise pathways (see Figure 3) (2) heatmap of pathway enrichment p-value matrix (pathways sorted by clusters on the rows and studies on the columns) (see Figure 4) (3) multi-dimensional scaling (MDS) plot of pathways and cluster assignment distributed by kappa statistics (see Supplementary Figure S3c) and (4) dendrograms of hierachical clustering (distance measured by pathway enrichment p-values) of studies in each cluster (see Figure 5). CPI also provides diagnostic tools such as CDF plot and scree plot to determine the number of clusters in consensus clustering.

2.4.6. Datasets and Databases

We provide 22 Homo sapiens pathway databases in CPI, including 14 pathway databases from MsigDB (containing GO, KEGG, Reactome, BioCarta, and others), 2 databases from Connectivity Map, transcription factor target database JASPAR, Protein-Protein interaction database and 3 microRNA target databases as options for enrichment analysis. In addition, GO and KEGG for Mus musculus and Saccharomyces cerevisiae, and JASPAR database for Mus musculus are also provided (see Supplementary Table S2). Users may choose to apply their own pathway databases with the extra computing cost of re-calculating the pathway-phrase matrix in Section 2.4.2.

3. Results

3.1. Application to Transcriptomic Data of Multiple Psychiatric Disorders

To demonstrate its utility, we applied CPI to an integrative analysis of a postmortem microarray dataset from three psychiatric disorders [32]. Briefly laser-microdissection was used to isolate pools of 100 pyramidal neurons from layers 3 (L3) and 5 (L5) from dorsolateral prefrontal cortex (DLPFC). Samples were collected from schizophrenia (SCZ), bipolar disorder (BP), and major depressive disorder (MDD) subjects and unaffected comparison subjects matched for age and sex. Samples consisted of both cell types from all subjects except for the L5 SCZ sample where two subjects were removed due to quality control issues. Following identification of differentially-expressed genes in each of the 6 diagnostic categories (cells from two layers and three different diagnoses) four default pathway databases in CPI (Gene Ontology, KEGG, Reactome and BioCarta) were used for this application.

Low expression and non-informative genes were first filtered out by quantile filtering and then differential expression (DE) analysis was conducted by limma embedded in the MAPE2.0 function from our package which allows both raw transcriptomic data input as well as DE p-value matrix provided by users. Pathway enrichment analysis was performed in each study using the top 400 DE genes and the results were meta analyzed by adaptively weighted Fisher's method in CPI to obtain the final integrative p-values and q-values in each pathway. We filtered out pathways containing less than 15 genes or more than 500 genes in the pathway databases. Of the 1901 pathways analyzed, 96 pathways had meta-analyzed q-values smaller than 0.0005 and were entered for pathway cluster analysis. The number of pathway clusters were selected to be 8 which was justified by the elbow plot and consensus CDF plot (see Supplementary Figure S2a,b) and 18 pathways were left out as scattered pathways.

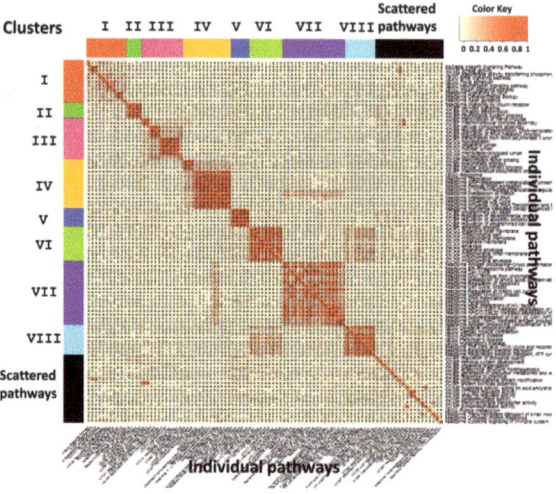

Figure 3. Heatmap of kappa statistics of pair-wise pathways in all clusters.

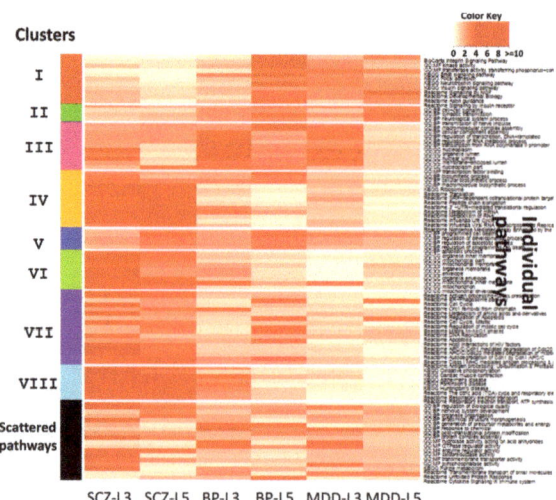

Figure 4. Heatmap of log10-scale pathway enrichment p-values of pathways annotated by eight pathway clusters (I-VIII) and a scattered pathway set (black).

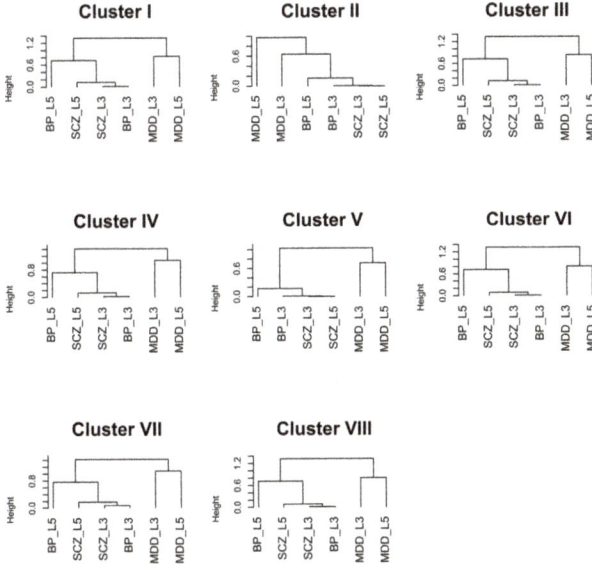

Figure 5. Hierarchical clustering of psychiatric studies in each cluster with distance defined by the log10-scale pathway enrichment *p*-values.

Figure 3 displays heatmap of kappa statistics of pair-wise pathways, sorted by the 8 identified pathway clusters and a scattered pathway set (black color). Figure 4 shows heatmap of log10-transformed pathway enrichment *p*-values with pathways on the rows and six studies on the columns. Dendrograms of hierachical clustering of studies in each cluster are shown in Figure 5. Table 1 contains 10 functionally annotated phrases identified from the penalized text mining algorithm for each pathway cluster. We note that, by our algorithm, heatmap pattern of pathways in the same cluster in Figure 4 may not visualize similarly since the pathway clusters are obtained by kappa statistics, representing similarity of gene content of any pair of pathways, rather than pathway enrichment *p*-values. But in general, we do observe clear pattern in almost all 8 clusters. For example, cluster VI, VII and VIII contain highly enriched pathways in SCZ-L3 and SCZ-L5, marginal enrichment in BP-L3 and BP-L5 but almost no significance in MDD-L3 and MDD-L5. Based on text mining results, clusters VI and VIII contain pathways related to *mitochondrion, ATP synthesis, NAD*, etc. Our results also suggest these alternations across DLPFC layer 3 and layer 5 are mainly related to ATP production rather than other aspects of mitochondrial function. Cluster VII with keywords *degradation, multiubiquitination, ubiquitin 26s proteasome system*, etc. is significantly altered in schizophrenia DLPFC layers and to a lesser extent in bipolar disorder. Similar results have been reported in a blood-based microarray investigation of both schizophrenia and bipolar disorder [33].

The result of cluster VI, VII and VIII is consistent to several biological findings in the literature. Firstly, our results are highly consistent with the original publication in [32]. Secondly, the paper [34] analyzed a mostly non-overlapping schizophrenia cohort and also showed that the differential expression genes at the layer 3 and/or layer 5 pyramidal cells in the DLPFC of schizophrenia subjects are mainly related to mitochondrial (MT) and ubiquitin-proteasome system (UPS) functions. The findings were followed up with qPCR validation in selected target genes. This is again consistent to our findings in cluster VI, VII and VIII. Finally, it has been shown that the synaptic area is particularly sensitive to MT and UPS deficits due to the high demand for ATP and for UPS activity at pre- and post-synaptic terminals [35], which is consistent with our results suggesting ATP production as the main aspect of the mitochondrial dysfunction in schizophrenia diseases.

Table 1. Ten significant keywords with q-value < 0.05 in each pathway cluster.

Cluster	Keywords
I	insulin, NGF, focal adhesion, BDNF, neurotrophins, Trk tyrosine kinase receptor, insulin receptor substrate, insulin receptor tyrosine kinase, Ras MAPK pathway, FAK
II	neuron
III	transcription, nucleoplasm, chromosome, nuclear content, nucleolus, RNA
IV	metabolism, mRNA, ribosome, replication, chemical reaction, cRNA, vRNA, viral protein, NUMB, nucleus
V	cell death, apoptotic process, activation, endogenous cellular process, programmed cell death, apoptosis
VI	mitochondrion, organelle, mitochondrial envelope, organelle envelope, lipid bilayer, inner e lumen facing lipid bilayer, semiautonomous self replicating organelle, tissue respiration, virtually eukaryotic cell, cytoplasm
VII	degradation, APC/C, apoptosis, CDC20, CDH1, mitotic protein, MHC, multiubiquitination, ubiquitin 26s proteasome system, exogenous antigen
VIII	respiratory electron transport, ATP synthesis, inner mitochondrial membrane, chemiosmotic gradient, brown fat, rotenone, FAD, mitochondrial matrix, body temperature, NAD

Abbreviation. NGF: *Nerve growth factor*, BDNF: *Brain-derived neurotrophic factor*, MAPK: *Mitogen-activated protein kinase*, FAK: *Focal adhesion kinase*, RNA: *Ribonucleic acid*, APC/C: *Anaphase-promoting complex*, MHC: *Major histocompatibility complex*, ATP: *Adenosine triphosphate*, FAD: *Flavin adenine dinucleotide*, NAD: *Nicotinamide adenine dinucleotide*, NUMB, CDC20, CDH1: *Gene names*.

Cluster I and cluster IV had a different pattern of pathway alterations. Cluster IV with keywords *metabolism, mRNA, ribosome, viral protein, NUMB,* etc. is significantly altered only in schizophrenia DLPFC layers, which indicates protein synthesis dysfunction. However, similar altered expression of gene sets related to protein synthesis has been found in postmortem hippocampus and orbitofrontal cortex of patients with major depression, bipolar disorder, and schizophrenia consensually [36]. This implies different degrees of protein synthesis pathway alterations in different brain tissues. Cluster I with keywords *insulin, NGF, BDNF, neurotrophins, Trk tyrosine kinase receptor,* etc. shows an enrichment pattern mainly in MDD and BP-L5 with little enrichment in SCZ of BP-L3. This suggests some similarity between the expression of these gene in layer 5 between BP and MDD subjects.

Pathways in cluster III are enriched in layer 3 of all three diseases (SCZ-L3, BP-L3 and MDD-L3) but to a lesser extent in layer 5 (SCZ-L5, BPL5 and MDD-L5). This cluster is annotated with keywords such as *transcription, nucleoplasm, chromosome, nuclear content, nucleolus, RNA,* indicating alterations in general aspects of nuclear function. Finally, cluster II and V with moderate enrichment in all six studies contain general neural disease related pathways with keywords such as *neuron, cell death and apoptotic process* and likely represent processes involved in neuronal survival.

Interestingly hierarchical clustering of the six categories of samples (cells from two layers and three different diagnoses) for each of the eight identified pathway clusters shows a similar pattern. Specifically, each of the 8 pathway clusters are most tightly clustered by diagnosis across layers suggesting similar alterations in layers 3 and 5 within a disease. Furthermore, across diagnoses BP and SCZ cluster more strongly with one another than with MDD. This is consistent with transcriptome [37–39] and genomic [40] findings suggesting similarities between SCZ and BP.

3.2. Justification to Penalize Pathway Description by Length in Text Mining

In pathway databases, some pathways come with only pathway names (usually less than 15 words) and some contains both pathway names and pathway descriptions (can be up to 1500 words). In Fisher's exact test by simple count, occurrences of a noun phrase are treated the same when appearing in these two extreme cases. In this case, signals of important mechanism terms in pathway names can be masked due to its frequent occurrence in pathway descriptions, while some non-informative terms can be falsely detected from long pathway descriptions. The penalization by pathway description length in Section 2.4.3 helps improve the sensitivity and reduce false positives. For example, in the real application in Section 3, the noun phrase *apoptosis* in cluster 7 was ranked low in the Fisher's exact test (r = 37, p = 0.051) while prioritized in permutation analysis of the penalized test statistics (r = 4, $p < 10^{-4}$) (see Supplementary Table S1). Some meaningless words such as et al in cluster 7 was ranked high in Fisher's exact test (r=11, $p = 5.08 \times 10^{-7}$), but ranked low by penalized statistics (r = 27 and p = 0.005). In our experience, $B = 10,000$ permutations are sufficient to obtain accurate p-value assessment while under a reasonable computing time. The entire permutation analysis for the example in Section 3 required only 1.5 min under parallel computing using ten cores.

4. Discussion

CPI has three advantages compared to existing methods. Firstly, CPI explores consensual and differential pathway enrichment pattern simultaneously when combining multiple related studies. To our knowledge, CPI is the first method for this purpose. Secondly, CPI clusters pathways by gene composition similarity (i.e., kappa statistics) to reduce pathway redundancy. Finally, CPI uses a statistically evaluated text mining method to annotate mechanisms of each pathway cluster automatically without subjective human interpretation. In addition, the proposed penalized text mining algorithm by permutation test was shown to outperform conventional Fisher's exact test in text mining. We applied the tool to six transcriptomic datasets spanning on three psychiatric disorders (SCZ, BP and MDD) and two layers in DLPFC (L3 and L5). The result identified multiple pathway clusters with enrichment patterns consistent with previous findings, such as mitochondrial ATP dysfunction in schizophrenia DLPFC layers, as well as other new findings.

The current CPI package has several limitations. Firstly, for single study pathway analysis, our tool currently only provides Fisher's exact test and Kolmogorov–Smirnov test. Users, however, can externally apply advanced methods such as GSEA [41] or others and take the result as alternative input. Secondly, our text mining algorithm relies on the descriptions provided by pathway databases. For pathway databases without detailed descriptions (e.g., in some KEGG pathways), text mining algorithm cannot annotate them well. Thirdly, computation time is not ignorable, especially in the text mining step. To incorporate more studies or more pathway databases, scalable computing algorithms will be needed.

5. Conclusions

In this article, we developed an integrative framework for combining and comparing pathway analyses from multiple transcriptomic studies, namely Comparative Pathway Integrator (CPI). CPI performs meta-analytic pathway analysis, reduces pathway redundancy to condense knowledge discovered from the results and conducts text mining to provide statistically solid inference on interpreting results. CPI has three major steps. In the first step, users can input either gene-based differential expression p-value matrix or pathway-based enrichment p-value matrix for each study to start with. If p-values of genes are entered, pathway enrichment analysis is applied first within each study. Enriched pathways are passed down to meta-analysis where AW-Fisher is applied to discover consensually and differentially enriched pathways. In the second step, significant pathways from AW-Fisher meta-analysis are clustered using consensus clustering, with consensus CDF plot and elbow plot to assist users to choose the number of clusters [21]. Silhouette information is used to achieve cluster tightness by removing scattered pathways without being clustered. In the third step, a penalized text mining algorithm is used to annotate each pathway cluster for an unbiased knowledge learning from the experimental data and pathway database. With the penalized matrix provided in package, CPI requires 2.8 min under parallel computing using ten cores to integrate six studies and 9888 genes in the psychiatric example with 1901 pathways in default pathway databases and B = 10,000 in permutation analysis. An R package is available at Github metaOmics/MetaPath.

In summary, CPI is a meta-analytic tool for integrating multiple related transcriptomic studies in pathway enrichment analysis. As more and more transcriptomic datasets accumulate in the public domain, the need of such integrative analysis will become more and more prevalent. CPI can fill the gap and provide biological insight in such comparative and integrative tasks. In addition to transcriptomic studies, the framework is readily extensible to integrate pathway analysis of multiple related proteomic studies or multiple metabolomics studies.

Supplementary Materials: The following are available online at http://www.mdpi.com/2073-4425/11/6/696/s1, Figure S1: p-values and q-values from individual pathway analysis and meta-analysis and AW-fisher weight for each pathway in each study, Figure S2: CDF plot of consensus clustering and delta plot of consensus clustering, Figure S3: Heatmap for Kappa statistic of pair-wise pathways and heatmap of log10-scale pathway enrichment p-values of pathways and MDS plot of pathways and cluster assignment distributed by kappa statistics and Hierarchical clustering of psychiatric studies in each cluster, Table S1: Fisher-exact test 2×2 table for "apoptosis" in cluster 7, Table S2: 22 Homo sapiens pathway database including 14 pathway database from MsigDB, 2 databases from Connectivity map, transcription factor target database JASPAR, Protein-Protein interaction database, 3 microRNA databases and 1 phenotype database as options for enrichment analysis.

Author Contributions: Conceptualization, C.-W.L., T.M. and G.C.T.; Methodology, X.Z., W.Z., C.-W.L., Z.F., T.M. and G.C.T.; Software, X.Z., W.Z. and C.-W.L.; Validation, W.Z., D.A.L., J.F.E. and G.C.T.; Data Curation, X.Z., D.A.L. and J.F.E.; Writing—Original Draft Preparation, X.Z., C.-W.L., Z.F., T.M. and G.C.T.; Writing—Review & Editing, W.Z., D.A.L., J.F.E. and G.C.T.; Supervision, G.C.T.; Funding Acquisition, D.A.L. and G.C.T. All authors have read and agreed to the published version of the manuscript.

Funding: This work was funded by the National Institute of Health R01CA190766 and R21LM012752 to X.Z., W.Z., C.-W.L., Z.F., T.M. and G.C.T.

Conflicts of Interest: The authors declare no conflict of interest.

References

1. Ashburner, M.; Ball, C.A.; Blake, J.A.; Botstein, D.; Butler, H.; Cherry, J.M.; Davis, A.P.; Dolinski, K.; Dwight, S.S.; Eppig, J.T.; et al. Gene Ontology: Tool for the unification of biology. *Nat. Genet.* **2000**, *25*, 25. [CrossRef] [PubMed]
2. Fabregat, A.; Sidiropoulos, K.; Garapati, P.; Gillespie, M.; Hausmann, K.; Haw, R.; Jassal, B.; Jupe, S.; Korninger, F.; McKay, S.; et al. The reactome pathway knowledgebase. *Nucleic Acids Res.* **2015**, *44*, D481–D487. [CrossRef]
3. Kanehisa, M.; Goto, S. KEGG: Kyoto encyclopedia of genes and genomes. *Nucleic Acids Res.* **2000**, *28*, 27–30. [CrossRef]
4. Liberzon, A.; Birger, C.; Thorvaldsdóttir, H.; Ghandi, M.; Mesirov, J.P.; Tamayo, P. The molecular signatures database hallmark gene set collection. *Cell Syst.* **2015**, *1*, 417–425. [CrossRef]
5. Rodchenkov, I.; Babur, O.; Luna, A.; Aksoy, B.A.; Wong, J.V.; Fong, D.; Franz, M.; Siper, M.C.; Cheung, M.; Wrana, M.; et al. Pathway Commons 2019 Update: Integration, analysis and exploration of pathway data. *Nucleic Acids Res.* **2020**, *48*, D489–D497. [CrossRef] [PubMed]
6. Khatri, P.; Sirota, M.; Butte, A.J. Ten years of pathway analysis: Current approaches and outstanding challenges. *PLoS Comput. Biol.* **2012**, *8*, e1002375. [CrossRef] [PubMed]
7. Tseng, G.C.; Ghosh, D.; Feingold, E. Comprehensive literature review and statistical considerations for microarray meta-analysis. *Nucleic Acids Res.* **2012**, *40*, 3785–3799. [CrossRef]
8. Shen, K.; Tseng, G.C. Meta-analysis for pathway enrichment analysis when combining multiple genomic studies. *Bioinformatics* **2010**, *26*, 1316–1323. [CrossRef]
9. Nguyen, T.; Tagett, R.; Donato, M.; Mitrea, C.; Draghici, S. A novel bi-level meta-analysis approach: Applied to biological pathway analysis. *Bioinformatics* **2016**, *32*, 409–416. [CrossRef]
10. Nguyen, T.; Mitrea, C.; Tagett, R.; Draghici, S. DANUBE: Data-driven meta-ANalysis using UnBiased empirical distributions—Applied to biological pathway analysis. *Proc. IEEE* **2016**, *105*, 496–515. [CrossRef]
11. Plaisier, S.B.; Taschereau, R.; Wong, J.A.; Graeber, T.G. Rank–rank hypergeometric overlap: Identification of statistically significant overlap between gene-expression signatures. *Nucleic Acids Res.* **2010**, *38*, e169. [CrossRef] [PubMed]
12. Cahill, K.M.; Huo, Z.; Tseng, G.C.; Logan, R.W.; Seney, M.L. Improved identification of concordant and discordant gene expression signatures using an updated rank-rank hypergeometric overlap approach. *Sci. Rep.* **2018**, *8*, 9588. [CrossRef] [PubMed]

13. Huang, D.W.; Sherman, B.T.; Tan, Q.; Kir, J.; Liu, D.; Bryant, D.; Guo, Y.; Stephens, R.; Baseler, M.W.; Lane, H.C.; et al. DAVID Bioinformatics Resources: Expanded annotation database and novel algorithms to better extract biology from large gene lists. *Nucleic Acids Res.* **2007**, *35*, W169–W175. [CrossRef] [PubMed]
14. Li, J.; Tseng, G.C. An adaptively weighted statistic for detecting differential gene expression when combining multiple transcriptomic studies. *Ann. Appl. Stat.* **2011**, *5*, 994–1019. [CrossRef]
15. Tseng, G.C.; Wong, W.H. Tight clustering: A resampling-based approach for identifying stable and tight patterns in data. *Biometrics* **2005**, *61*, 10–16. [CrossRef] [PubMed]
16. Ma, T.; Huo, Z.; Kuo, A.; Zhu, L.; Fang, Z.; Zeng, X.; Lin, C.W.; Liu, S.; Wang, L.; Liu, P.; et al. MetaOmics: Analysis pipeline and browser-based software suite for transcriptomic meta-analysis. *Bioinformatics* **2019**, *35*, 1597–1599. [CrossRef] [PubMed]
17. Tarca, A.L.; Bhatti, G.; Romero, R. A comparison of gene set analysis methods in terms of sensitivity, prioritization and specificity. *PLoS ONE* **2013**, *8*, e79217. [CrossRef]
18. Bayerlová, M.; Jung, K.; Kramer, F.; Klemm, F.; Bleckmann, A.; Beißbarth, T. Comparative study on gene set and pathway topology-based enrichment methods. *BMC Bioinform.* **2015**, *16*, 334. [CrossRef]
19. Huo, Z.; Tang, S.; Park, Y.; Tseng, G. p-value evaluation, variability index and biomarker categorization for adaptively weighted Fisher's meta-analysis method in omics applications. *Bioinformatics* **2019**, *36*, 524–532. [CrossRef]
20. Viera, A.J.; Garrett, J.M. Understanding interobserver agreement: The kappa statistic. *Fam. Med.* **2005**, *37*, 360–363.
21. Monti, S.; Tamayo, P.; Mesirov, J.; Golub, T. Consensus clustering: A resampling-based method for class discovery and visualization of gene expression microarray data. *Mach. Learn.* **2003**, *52*, 91–118. [CrossRef]
22. Maitra, R.; Ramler, I.P. Clustering in the Presence of Scatter. *Biometrics* **2009**, *65*, 341–352. [CrossRef] [PubMed]
23. Tseng, G.C. Penalized and weighted K-means for clustering with scattered objects and prior information in high-throughput biological data. *Bioinformatics* **2007**, *23*, 2247–2255. [CrossRef]
24. Rousseeuw, P.J. Silhouettes: A graphical aid to the interpretation and validation of cluster analysis. *J. Comput. Appl. Math.* **1987**, *20*, 53–65. [CrossRef]
25. Benoit, K.; Matsuo, A.; Benoit, M.K. R Package: 'spacyr'. 2018. Available online: https://cran.r-project.org/web/packages/spacyr/spacyr.pdf (accessed on 25 February 2020).
26. Honnibal, M.; Montani, I. spaCy 2: Natural language understanding with Bloom embeddings, convolutional neural networks and incremental parsing. *To Appear* **2017**, *7*.
27. Feinerer, I. Introduction to the tm Package Text Mining in R. 2013. Available online: https://cran.r-project.org/web/packages/tm/tm.pdf (accessed on 25 February 2020).
28. Rinker, T. R Package: 'textstem'. 2018. Available online: https://cran.r-project.org/web/packages/textstem/textstem.pdf (accessed on 25 February 2020).
29. Word Frequency Data. Top 5000 common English Words. 2017. Available online: http://www.wordfrequency.info (accessed on 25 February 2020).
30. Feinerer, I.; Hornik, K.; Wallace, M.; Hornik, M.K. Package 'wordnet'. 2017. Available online: https://cran.r-project.org/web/packages/wordnet/wordnet.pdf (accessed on 25 February 2020).
31. Benjamini, Y.; Hochberg, Y. Controlling the false discovery rate: A practical and powerful approach to multiple testing. *J. R. Stat. Soc. Ser. B (Methodol.)* **1995**, *57*, 289–300. [CrossRef]
32. Arion, D.; Huo, Z.; Enwright, J.F.; Corradi, J.P.; Tseng, G.; Lewis, D.A. Transcriptome alterations in prefrontal pyramidal cells distinguish schizophrenia from bipolar and major depressive disorders. *Biol. Psychiatry* **2017**, *82*, 594–600. [CrossRef]
33. Bousman, C.A.; Chana, G.; Glatt, S.J.; Chandler, S.D.; Lucero, G.R.; Tatro, E.; May, T.; Lohr, J.B.; Kremen, W.S.; Tsuang, M.T.; et al. Preliminary evidence of ubiquitin proteasome system dysregulation in schizophrenia and bipolar disorder: Convergent pathway analysis findings from two independent samples. *Am. J. Med. Genet. Part Neuropsychiatr. Genet.* **2010**, *153*, 494–502. [CrossRef]
34. Arion, D.; Corradi, J.P.; Tang, S.; Datta, D.; Boothe, F.; He, A.; Cacace, A.M.; Zaczek, R.; Albright, C.F.; Tseng, G.; et al. Distinctive transcriptome alterations of prefrontal pyramidal neurons in schizophrenia and schizoaffective disorder. *Mol. Psychiatry* **2015**, *20*, 1397–1405. [CrossRef]
35. Sheng, Z.H.; Cai, Q. Mitochondrial transport in neurons: Impact on synaptic homeostasis and neurodegeneration. *Nat. Rev. Neurosci.* **2012**, *13*, 77–93. [CrossRef]

36. Darby, M.; Yolken, R.H.; Sabunciyan, S. Consistently altered expression of gene sets in postmortem brains of individuals with major psychiatric disorders. *Transl. Psychiatry* **2016**, *6*, e890. [CrossRef] [PubMed]
37. Gandal, M.J.; Haney, J.R.; Parikshak, N.N.; Leppa, V.; Ramaswami, G.; Hartl, C.; Schork, A.J.; Appadurai, V.; Buil, A.; Werge, T.M.; et al. Shared molecular neuropathology across major psychiatric disorders parallels polygenic overlap. *Science* **2018**, *359*, 693–697. [CrossRef] [PubMed]
38. Lanz, T.A.; Reinhart, V.; Sheehan, M.J.; Rizzo, S.J.S.; Bove, S.E.; James, L.C.; Volfson, D.; Lewis, D.A.; Kleiman, R.J. Postmortem transcriptional profiling reveals widespread increase in inflammation in schizophrenia: A comparison of prefrontal cortex, striatum, and hippocampus among matched tetrads of controls with subjects diagnosed with schizophrenia, bipolar or major depressive disorder. *Transl. Psychiatry* **2019**, *9*, 1–13.
39. Ramaker, R.C.; Bowling, K.M.; Lasseigne, B.N.; Hagenauer, M.H.; Hardigan, A.A.; Davis, N.S.; Gertz, J.; Cartagena, P.M.; Walsh, D.M.; Vawter, M.P.; et al. Post-mortem molecular profiling of three psychiatric disorders. *Genome Med.* **2017**, *9*, 72. [CrossRef]
40. McGrath, L.M.; Cornelis, M.C.; Lee, P.H.; Robinson, E.B.; Duncan, L.E.; Barnett, J.H.; Huang, J.; Gerber, G.; Sklar, P.; Sullivan, P.; et al. Genetic predictors of risk and resilience in psychiatric disorders: A cross-disorder genome-wide association study of functional impairment in major depressive disorder, bipolar disorder, and schizophrenia. *Am. J. Med Genet. Part Neuropsychiatr. Genet.* **2013**, *162*, 779–788. [CrossRef]
41. Subramanian, A.; Tamayo, P.; Mootha, V.K.; Mukherjee, S.; Ebert, B.L.; Gillette, M.A.; Paulovich, A.; Pomeroy, S.L.; Golub, T.R.; Lander, E.S.; et al. Gene set enrichment analysis: A knowledge-based approach for interpreting genome-wide expression profiles. *Proc. Natl. Acad. Sci. USA* **2005**, *102*, 15545–15550. [CrossRef]

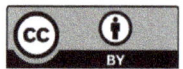

© 2020 by the authors. Licensee MDPI, Basel, Switzerland. This article is an open access article distributed under the terms and conditions of the Creative Commons Attribution (CC BY) license (http://creativecommons.org/licenses/by/4.0/).

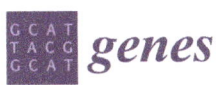

Review

Exercise and High-Fat Diet in Obesity: Functional Genomics Perspectives of Two Energy Homeostasis Pillars

Abdelaziz Ghanemi [1,2], Aicha Melouane [1,2], Mayumi Yoshioka [2] and Jonny St-Amand [1,2,*]

1. Department of Molecular Medicine, Faculty of Medicine, Laval University, Québec, QC G1V 0A6, Canada; abdelaziz.Ghanemi@crchudequebec.ulaval.ca (A.G.); rimca@live.fr (A.M.)
2. Functional Genomics Laboratory, Endocrinology and Nephrology Axis, CHU de Québec-Université Laval Research Center, Québec, QC G1V 4G2, Canada; mayumi.yoshioka@crchudequebec.ulaval.ca
* Correspondence: jonny.st-amand@crchudequebec.ulaval.ca; Tel.: +1-418-654-2296; Fax: +1-418-654-2761

Received: 17 June 2020; Accepted: 28 July 2020; Published: 31 July 2020

Abstract: The heavy impact of obesity on both the population general health and the economy makes clarifying the underlying mechanisms, identifying pharmacological targets, and developing efficient therapies for obesity of high importance. The main struggle facing obesity research is that the underlying mechanistic pathways are yet to be fully revealed. This limits both our understanding of pathogenesis and therapeutic progress toward treating the obesity epidemic. The current anti-obesity approaches are mainly a controlled diet and exercise which could have limitations. For instance, the "classical" anti-obesity approach of exercise might not be practical for patients suffering from disabilities that prevent them from routine exercise. Therefore, therapeutic alternatives are urgently required. Within this context, pharmacological agents could be relatively efficient in association to an adequate diet that remains the most efficient approach in such situation. Herein, we put a spotlight on potential therapeutic targets for obesity identified following differential genes expression-based studies aiming to find genes that are differentially expressed under diverse conditions depending on physical activity and diet (mainly high-fat), two key factors influencing obesity development and prognosis. Such functional genomics approaches contribute to elucidate the molecular mechanisms that both control obesity development and switch the genetic, biochemical, and metabolic pathways toward a specific energy balance phenotype. It is important to clarify that by "gene-related pathways", we refer to genes, the corresponding proteins and their potential receptors, the enzymes and molecules within both the cells in the intercellular space, that are related to the activation, the regulation, or the inactivation of the gene or its corresponding protein or pathways. We believe that this emerging area of functional genomics-related exploration will not only lead to novel mechanisms but also new applications and implications along with a new generation of treatments for obesity and the related metabolic disorders especially with the modern advances in pharmacological drug targeting and functional genomics techniques.

Keywords: obesity; differential genes expression; exercise; high-fat diet; pathways; potential therapeutic targets

---

1. Obesity as a Health Problem in Need of Novel Approaches

Obesity is defined as an abnormal or excessive fat accumulation [1] resulting from a broken energy homeostasis [2]. It has an epidemiological profile with a continuously increasing trend worldwide [3–5]. In the United States of America, at least 78.6 million people suffer from obesity [6]. Obesity is also linked to diabetes development (diabesity) [7]. In addition, not only many risk factors can increase obesity prevalence [8–10] but the obesity epidemic has also a major impact on health due to the complexity of its mechanisms, pathophysiology, and metabolic consequences [11]. Obesity has also been reported to increase risks and incidence of diseases and disorders such as advanced colorectal neoplasm [12], malnutrition [13], and mortality risk [14] in addition to decreasing life expectancy [15] among other diverse health impacts that could justify classifying obesity as a disease [16].

Diet control (caloric restriction), exercise, or the combination of both are the main anti-obesity approaches. For persons with morbid obesity, bariatric surgery can be an option [17] and medications are prescribed in some cases [18,19] as well. Although body weight management is a multibillion-dollar market, there are only few Food and Drug Administration-approved drugs available for long-term obesity treatment, but all have undesirable side effects [20,21].

In addition, some disabilities or heart diseases might limit the ability of individuals with obesity to exercise. In spite of the efforts of the diverse local, national, and international organizations in collaboration with health professionals and decision makers, obesity remains a major challenge with heavy consequences on life quality of the population and on healthcare budgets [22,23] especially that patients with obesity might require a specific or an adapted therapeutic care for some diseases compared to patients not suffering from obesity.

Therefore, there is an urgent need to further explore the obesity-related pathways in order to understand the underlying mechanisms and identify potential therapeutic targets. Herein, we focus on exercise and high-fat (HF) diet as they represent key factors for obesity prevention, development, and treatment area. We highlight how functional genomics allows exploring these factors via illustrative examples along with the research, pharmacological and clinical possible outcomes, and implications.

2. Exercise-Related Genes and Pathways: Towards an Exercise Pill

2.1. Exercise and Health

Along with resting energy expenditure, exercise-induced energy expenditure represents a key component of the total energy expenditure [24]. In addition to its place within the energy balance as the most variable part [24], exercise has benefits at different levels even for the older population [25]. Regular exercise contributes to reduced body weight, blood pressure, low-density lipoprotein, and total cholesterol and increases high-density lipoprotein cholesterol, muscular function, and strength as well as insulin sensitivity [26,27]. This makes exercise an important therapy both to prevent and manage obesity [28]. Although the purpose remains to create an accumulative negative caloric balance leading to weight loss [29], intensity, regularity, and duration of an exercise defines its type and the related outcomes and benefits.

The choice of exercise types depends on what we want to achieve in terms of muscle strength, fat mass loss, mitochondrial function enhancement, etc., as well as the ability of the individual depending on factors like age, cardiovascular health, and disability. For instance, an elderly person with cardiovascular disease would go for a walk to burn calories because of their limited exercise capacity [30]. The key metabolic tissue used during exercise is the skeletal muscle and its health represents a key factor for both an improved metabolic performance as well as a healthy ageing [31] which are two risk factors of obesity.

Exercise has a crucial role in maintaining skeletal muscle homeostasis [32] especially for the older population [33]. Biochemical profile of muscles is highly determined by protein synthesis (muscle contraction) and energy metabolism (energy expenditure) that govern the ability of energy usage via locomotion, which is a principle component of anti-obesity therapy involving exercise. Importantly, both body size and body composition, which are shaped by exercise, are determinants of resting energy expenditure. This shows that the benefits of exercise in terms of caloric use goes beyond the exercise-related energy expenditure. In addition, the benefits of exercise are not limited to energy metabolism, lipoprotein profile, or obesity treatment. Indeed, studies have shown how exercise could help to improve the prognosis, therapy, or prevent (reduce the risk) the onset of diverse diseases and conditions such as cancers [34,35], cancer-induced cardiac cachexia [36], multiple sclerosis [37], stroke [38], breast cancer-related lymphedema [39], as well as to counteract some treatments side effects [40] and can even be prescribed as a complimentary therapy (e.g., exercise oncology) [41].

2.2. Exercise Impacts Gene Expression

Identifying genes that are regulated by exercise (exercise-induced genes, especially in the skeletal muscle) has been among the focus of different research groups that have already identified a number of key exercise-related transcriptomes. For instance, numerous studies have obtained data that defined the effects of exercise on genes that are related to exercise benefits at the biochemical and metabolic levels. Indeed, they have shown that exercise induces the expression of genes that regulate or are related to mitochondrial biogenesis [42], oxidative phosphorylation (OXPHOS) [43], antioxidant defense mechanism [44], cell proliferation [45], and the amelioration of insulin resistance [46] which indicates links between exercise outcomes and transcriptome modifications.

Furthermore, other gene expression-based studies, mainly comparative [47] and under different conditions including exercise [48] and resting [49] have allowed the collation of data and increase our understanding of the skeletal muscle transcriptome and functions in diverse contexts and depending on the population category. This contributes to a more precise mechanistic understanding of the genetic and biochemical changes at the molecular level. Thus, could guide to a muscle-targeting therapy development for obesity by defining the pathway associations with genes to optimize other therapies and even improve the pharmacovigilance based on genetic profiling. Beyond that, identifying exercise-induced genes would support further progress in understanding and treating different diseases other than those only depending on energy homeostasis which would expend the benefits of "exercise pills".

2.3. Gene Expression Patterns Underlie Muscular Adaptation to Exercise

Exploring such exercise-induced genes and pathways contributes to understand the molecular profiles that govern the adaptive responses of muscles to exercise. In addition, advances in epigenetics of muscle [50] in relation to exercise [51,52], diet [52], and aging [53] would further strengthen this field beyond genomics and put each of these pillars within a complementary network of data via which we can investigate potential therapies. For instance, exercise during pregnancy induces offspring changes [54,55], indicating that mother physical activity (intensity and frequency) impacts the health of the unborn child which opens an area in molecular pediatrics research.

Our team has also focused on gene expression in the skeletal muscle of endurance athletes compared to sedentary men and identified 33 genes that are differentially expressed [56]. This study, which supports the data reported above, highlight the global muscle gene expression including genes mostly related to muscle contraction and energy metabolism (two parameters improved by exercise). Moreover, these data further support our previous characterization of the global gene expression profile of sprinter's muscle, that shows transcripts mainly involved in contraction and energy metabolism as the most expressed in muscles of sprinters [57]. Such genetic expression pattern reflects a functional and metabolic adaptation of athletes toward an increased muscle contractile function along with an enhanced energy expenditure in the context of exercise training-induced muscle adaptations [58]. Furthermore, another study, involving healthy men, shows that moderate-intensity exercise at the lactate threshold induces the expression of transcriptomes involved in the tricarboxylic acid cycle, β-oxidation, antioxidant enzymes, contractile apparatus, and electron transport in the skeletal muscle [59].

Following the same line of thought, it was demonstrated that after 6 weeks of endurance training at lactate threshold intensity, the regulation of skeletal muscle transcriptome in elderly men includes increased expression of genes related to oxidative OXPHOS [60]. All these changes reflect an increase in the energy expenditure ability via an enhanced mitochondrial activity with an increased usage of biofuels which would be combined to reduced energy storage and lead to protection from obesity. This study [60] has also highlighted the importance of mitochondrial OXPHOS and extracellular matrix (ECM) remodeling in the skeletal muscle adaptation which correlates with a previously reported work in which genes of both ECM and calcium binding are upregulated and those related to diabetes are modulated in human skeletal muscle following a 6 wks aerobic training [61]. We note that the exercise-induced genes are associated with a profile that counteracts the ageing process. Indeed, whereas ageing (risk factor for obesity) decreases metabolic performance (e.g., mitochondrial dysfunction [62]) and the strength of the muscle [63] and increases oxidative stress [64], exercise improves those biological patterns in the muscle.

One of the mild endurance training induced genes that draws particular attention is the secreted protein acidic and rich in cysteine (SPARC). This gene was characterized as an exercise-induced gene [60] as well as electrical pulse stimulation (considered as the in vitro form of exercise)-induced gene in C2C12 myoblasts [65]. In addition, studies have shown that SPARC increased in the skeletal muscle during training [66–68]. This same protein plays diverse roles in energy metabolism especially in the muscle [69,70], ECM remodeling and myoblast differentiation [71–74], inflammation [75], and cancer development [76], which would indicate that SPARC plays a role in exercise-induced benefit related processes involving inflammation, cancer, and tissue remodeling.

All these gene expression changes help to understand, at least in part, exercise-induced pathways of mitochondrial biogenesis [77] and mitochondrial biochemistry [78] as well as muscle adaptation [79] and how exercise can reverse ageing impacts on skeletal muscle [80]. Such genomics studies are supported and complemented by proteomics studies that have explored the variations in protein expression in muscle depending on the physical activity [66,81–83] and reflects an adaptation of the proteinic profile, comparable to the transcriptomic changes, as well. This includes the increase in the expression of a peroxisome proliferator-activated receptor γ coactivator 1 α isoform PGC-1α4 that is involved in the regulation of skeletal muscle hypertrophy [84] which reflects an aspect from the correlation and complementarity between the functional genomics and functional proteomics.

Moreover, studies of exercise-related genes can be categorized depending on exercise type, e.g., endurance-based exercise and resistance-based exercise [85]. The transcriptomic signature of exercised muscle is also variable depending on muscle fibers and age [86]. This indicates a need of a classification strategy depending of the variables (age, muscle fibers, exercise type, etc.) that modify gene expression response to exercise. Such classification could also be extrapolated to the therapeutic target identification depending on the suitable pharmacological effects (enhance the metabolism, increase muscle strength, etc.).

2.4. Implications

Such exercise-related gene expression patterns explain some of the exercise benefits, including those seen even after detraining [87], including increased muscle contraction and energy metabolism improvement, thereby providing molecular and mechanistic links between the exercise benefits and the genes (over) expressed with or following exercise which could potentially be used for drug development towards an "exercise pill" (Figure 1).

Importantly, the exercise benefits and their clinical outcomes are precisely what clinicians hope to observe in their patients (with obesity, diabetes, etc.) such as an improved blood lipoprotein profile [88,89], increased usage of lipids and glucose, ameliorated insulin resistance, as well as an enhanced energy expenditure. Obtaining these effects is exactly what functional genomics-based therapies aim to achieve via pharmacological agents. Indeed, identifying exercise-specific genes and exploring the pathways they control would allow the development of exercise pills. Such pills could therapeutically mimic the effects of exercise via targeting these "exercise-genes" pathways through pharmacological agents and thus, obtain the benefits of exercise without intensive training. This is of a particular importance for old (and suffering from heart diseases) or disabled individuals who have limited ability to exercise but who therapeutically require the benefits of exercise. Therefore, such "exercise pill" would allow to overcome this limitation of applying exercise as a therapy for obesity.

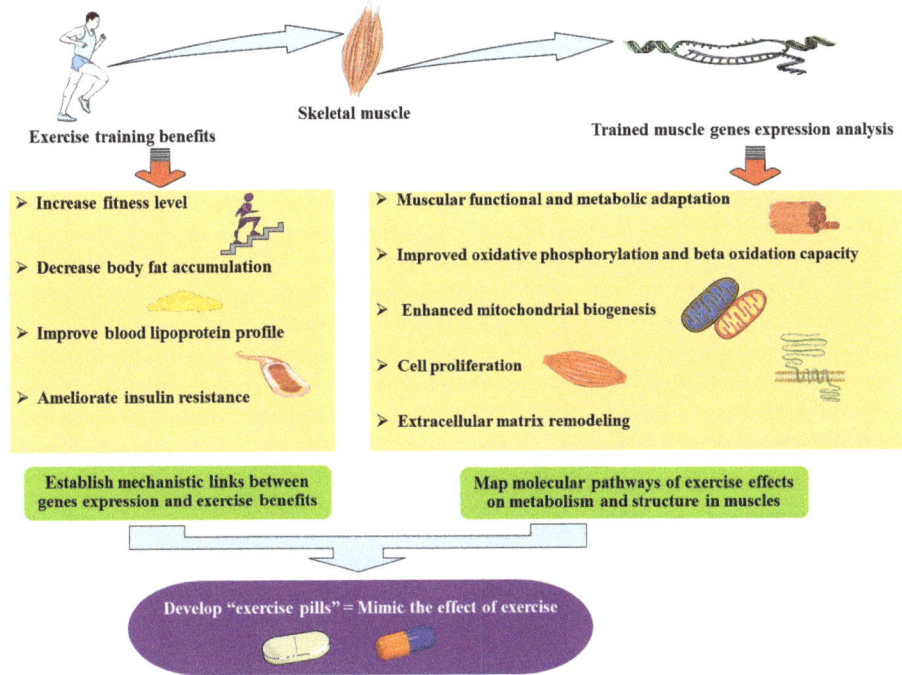

Figure 1. The implications of identifying genes differentially expressed during exercise training: exercise-induced genes.

3. Diet-Related Genes: A Focus on High-Fat Diet to Identify a Lipid-Specific Signal

3.1. High-Fat Diet Particularities in Obesity Context

As diet is the other pillar in obesity research and represents the energy intake and a key part of anti-obesity therapy, it is also an important factor for gene expression studies in the context of obesity. The diverse properties and impacts the diet has on metabolism pattern and biochemical adaptations made the identification and the exploration of associated specific gene expression patterns an important element in obesity molecular research. The effect of diet on obesity development is well known especially for HF diet [90–92]. The reason behind the focus on fat, beyond the concept of excess caloric intake, is that this nutrient, compared to both carbohydrates and proteins, has limited effect on satiety, is associated with high palatability, and has a high caloric density [93]. In addition, the lipid content in the modern Western diet increases fat consumption and is part of the unhealthy lifestyle. Indeed, following a HF meal ingestion, both caloric intake and energy expenditure favor weight gain because of the palatability, high caloric density, and low satiety effect of HF nutrients, as well as the weak potency for fat oxidation and energy expenditure associated with elevated fat intake [94–96]. The other pattern associated with HF diet is that the offspring have obesity risk and gene expression alterations [97] as a consequence of the maternal HF diet. This highlights the need to focus on HF diet especially as it impacts gene expression and epigenetics profile [98] as exemplified by studies showing that epigenetic changes can be consequences of the maternal HF diet [99–101]

The control of food intake represents a major determinant in the etiology of obesity especially with HF meals which acutely disrupt energy balance [102,103]. Feeding behavior is controlled by short-term circulating nutrients and hormones as well as signals derived from peripheral tissues in response to a meal and changes in energy stores. Within this context, the hypothalamus is a key brain center upon which all these peripheral signals converge to regulate feeding behavior and energy intake, thus it controls short-term as well as long-term energy balance and steady-state body weight [104,105]. Therefore, screening the changes in gene level following acute HF meal ingestions would reveal new elements within the gut–brain axis leading to the development of novel approaches for the understanding and the control of energy homeostasis. In particular, the identification of transcriptomic changes induced by HF diet both in digestive and peripheral tissues as well as within the central energy metabolism control centers in the brain.

3.2. Digestive System (First Food "Receptors")

Differentially expressed genes in the stomach and intestine are key elements since these two tissues represent the sites of most of the digestive processes and where the nutrients are first available in the simplest forms (that interact with endocrine system and different receptors). Thus, stomach and intestine represent the starting point of signals controlling energy balance (including food intake). Importantly, variations (gene expression) within the digestive system may reflect changes at the digestive process that could impact the availability, the absorbance ratio, as well as the biochemical and endocrine effects of the diet nutrients. Since HF diet-induced transcriptomes would require more attention than the low-fat (LF) induced genes, it is of a great importance to identify and more precisely distinguish between HF and LF specific genes. Therefore, the particularity of selected studies we report first herein is that fasting status was the reference (control) to study both HF and LF-specific genes. In fact, numerous previous studies that investigated HF-specific changes used LF conditions as a reference, therefore, were not able to characterize LF-specific genes nor to distinguish HF-specific from LF-specific transcriptomes. We first report a transcriptomic study that identified the peripheral signals of appetite and satiety from mice duodenum by investigating the transcriptomic changes in the duodenum mucosa 30 min, 1 h, and 3 h (to explore acute impact rather than chronic gene expression modifications) following HF and LF meal ingestion [106]. This study reveals that energy, protein, and fat intake transcriptome expression changes were higher in the HF groups compared to LF groups [106,107]. These data correlate with an intestinal mucosal mRNA analysis that demonstrates changes in the expression of genes related to anabolic and catabolic lipid metabolism pathways [108] and a recent paper shows that the expression of genes related to the uptake and transport of lipid and cholesterol as well as glucose storage are upregulated in the duodenum [109]. This changes specific patterns of HF-diet compared to LF-diet. Digestive mucosa is the first tissue that interacts with nutrients during the first digestive processes and has the ability to produce signal molecules that can act as hormones within the gut–brain axis [110]. Therefore, the key concept beyond identifying digestive mucosal diet-induced genes is to eventually identify new signals and responses to nutrient ingestion controlling food intake and energy expenditure. As an example of a potential signal molecule, the trefoil factor 2 (*Tff2*) has been identified as a newly found HF-specific gene [106] for which its deficiency in mice leads to a protection from HF diet-induced obesity [111,112]. Among the hundreds of genes that are modulated after HF or LF meal ingestion [106,113–116], we put a spotlight on the *Tff2* and its pathway as a potential targetable pathway for obesity molecular therapies. Indeed, this gene is upregulated by HF (and not LF) diet [106] which suggests it is a specific acute HF-induced signals that may impact food intake regulation. At the peripheral level, HF-diet decreases the expression of genes involved in metabolizing glucose in porcine perirenal and subcutaneous adipose tissues [116] which would indicate the switch (as an adaptation) of the metabolism toward less glucose usage in the presence of lipid intake, probably to increase lipid metabolism following a LF diet intake. In addition, it has been shown that in mesenteric adipose tissue, only LF meal upregulated transcripts implicated in lipid biosynthesis, whereas transcripts involved in lipid utilization and glucose production were downregulated in both HF and LF meals following 3 h of meal ingestion [114], also pointing a metabolic adaptation of lipid metabolism depending of lipid ratio within the diet.

3.3. Adipose Tissue (Energy-Stocking Tissue) and Skeletal Muscle (Energy-Usage Tissue)

HF diet induces an increase in the expression of genes related to inflammation, whereas it downregulates genes related to lipid metabolism, adipocyte differentiation markers, and detoxification processes, and cytoskeletal structural components in mouse adipose tissue [117]. These observations highlight how the metabolic function reacts to HF diet in terms of adaptation and at the same time emphasizes health problems associated with obesity such as inflammation. These results, further indicate that the metabolism is shifted toward the usage of lipids rather than glucose, are in agreement with other studies showing that HF diet enhances the expression of genes related to lipid catabolism in the skeletal muscle [118]. Such data illustrate how the metabolic cellular system can adapt to the type and the quantity of nutrients received through different diets and the activated metabolic processes are chosen depending on such factors. Exploring such "diet-oriented" metabolic pathways might allow the development of pharmacological approaches that could mimic such pathways in order to increase lipid store usage by tissues as a part of anti-obesity therapies. Importantly, knowing the metabolism-related genes regulated by diet could optimize pharmacotherapies and diet-based therapies by selecting the type and the quantity of specific nutrients that could act towards a suitable metabolic phenotype for a specific patient. Herein, it is worth emphasizing that in order to correctly design a study, selecting the control group remains critical. Indeed, to study HF or LF diet, it is important to define the reference whether it is fasting status or fed control. In case of fed control, not only the caloric content but also the fat type and its chemical nature are also to be taken into account when reaching conclusions.

3.4. Brain (Energy Balance-Control Centers)

Besides identifying diet-related peripheral signals, changes induced by the diet at the central level have also been studied. For instance, the study of HF and LF meal ingestion-induced changes in the hypothalamic transcriptome reveals that 3 h after the beginning of meal ingestion, 12 transcripts were regulated by food intake including two involved in mitochondrial functions [115]. This work also reveals the increased expression of the major urinary protein 1 (*Mup1*) gene in the hypothalamus of LF fed mice compared to fasting mice. MUP1 is a protein involved in metabolic profile improvement including energy balance toward skeletal muscle with increased mitochondrial function and energy expenditure in diabetic mice [119]. These MUP1 effects on metabolism regulation [120] including glucose and lipid metabolism [121], might explain the benefits of the LF diet. Such benefits are not only explained by the limited caloric intake in LF diet compared to HF diet but results from the switch of the metabolic profile toward more fuel usage and energy expenditure. In addition, we might also suggest that *Mup1*, with biochemical effects protecting from obesity, is involved in the pathways that are blunted during obesity which would further increase energy storage and decrease energy expenditure. Indeed, in another study, a 8–12 d dietary restriction in LF-diet groups of mice led to a downregulation of *Mup1* in adipose tissue [122] which could be an adaptation to the dietary restriction in order to conserve energy stores and limit energy usage since the organism is under caloric privation. This further highlights the importance of *Mup1* in energy balance, both in energy expenditure and energy conservation, and presents its function as a potential molecular target for obesity as well.

Furthermore, regarding the hypothalamic (center of energy homeostasis control) transcriptome, high-fructose diet fed to Wistar rats throughout development lead to the remodeling of 966 genes and enhanced both depressive-like and anxiety-like behaviors [123] which could lead individuals to manifest either increase or loss of their appetite. In addition, the hypothalamic transcriptome pattern under HF diet condition (over 2 wks) exploring the neuropeptides involved in energy balance explains how ingesting a HF meal contributes to remodeling the expression of neuropeptide Y, agouti-related protein, and proopiomelanocortin over time [124]. This last element is extremely important to understand the establishment and the development of obesity by studying key molecular signals at different steps and reveal the underlying paths. Importantly, the data generated on preferentially expressed genes in the hypothalamus and pituitary gland [125,126] improve the understanding of the central control of energy metabolism and diet impact on gene expression.

3.5. Potential Applications

The characterization of novel fat-specific genes may contribute to the development of new therapeutic targets for appetite and satiety controls. Herein, it is worth mentioning that the existence of two levels of diet-dependent energy metabolism control (peripheral and central) provides wider therapeutic options and further choices depending on the patient's physiological or pathophysiological status. For instance, a patient with obesity suffering from a functional gastrointestinal disease might not respond well for an obesity therapy targeting the peripheral signals and would require targeting the central pathways. Mapping how the metabolic profiles (governed by selected genes) change according to the type of diet and the time between meal ingestion and gene expression analysis (and eventually at which time the meal is ingested) would allow the identification of selected signals that are specific and/or time dependent (Figure 2). Such data could allow to improve precise personal therapies for individuals.

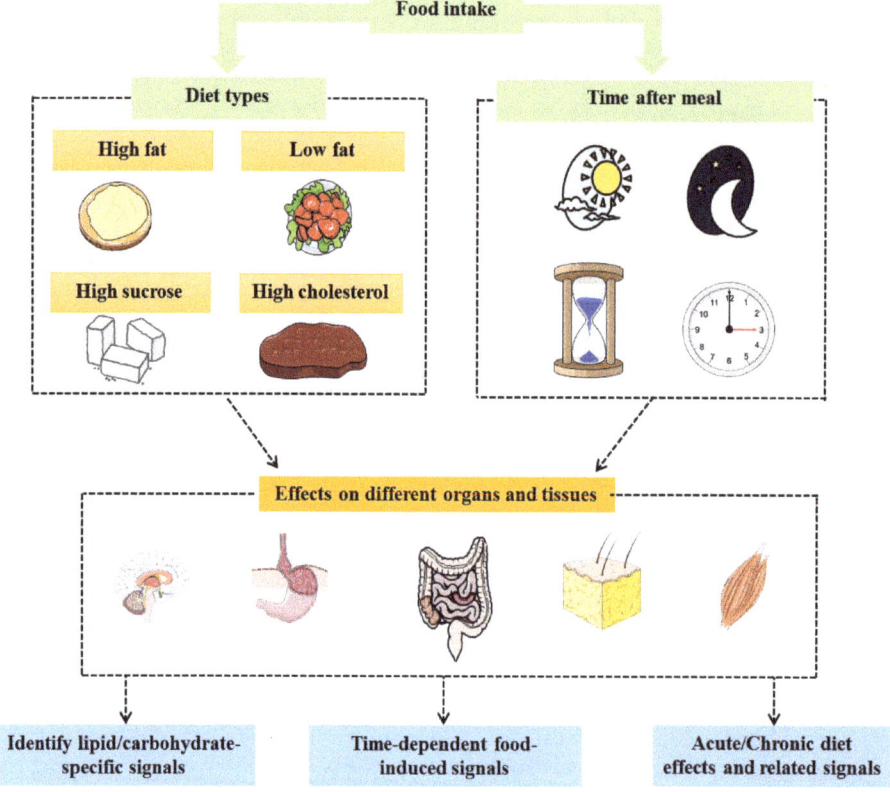

Figure 2. Studying the effects (expressed genes and the associated pathways) of different types of diets on the different organs/tissues involved in energy balance at different times allow to identify time-dependent specific signals (such as lipid-specific signals) regulating metabolism homeostasis.

Additional studies have examined the interaction between diet and gene expression regulation. HF and high-cholesterol (HFHC) diet, and HFHC plus high-sucrose diet [127] have been explored within the context of differentially expressed genes. Unlike the previous examples, blood RNA analysis was performed and revealed differential hyperlipidemia gene expression profiles even though levels of fasting plasma lipids and glucose corresponding to these two diets was similar [127]. This indicates that gene expression might not reflect phenotypic changes and that corresponding in vivo metabolic and biochemical exploration is required to understand gene expression modifications. In addition to studying the effects of diet itself, it is highly relevant to explore the impacts of drugs that modify the effects and distribution of nutrients in vivo. For example, Salomäki et al. (2014), showed that administering metformin (prescribed to regulate glucose blood levels [128]) to pregnant female mice that were on a HF diet resulted in transcriptome related to mitochondrial ATP production and adipocytes differentiation of the offspring [129] resulting in an improved metabolic phenotype. From a therapeutic viewpoint (pharmacology and nutrition), understanding the pathways stimulated or deactivated depending of the type of diets would allow nutritionists and clinicians to adapt the diet for their patients based on the therapy they are following or based on their lifestyle to avoid possible adverse interactions between the diets, therapies, and activated pathways (genes, enzymes, etc.). This would help mitigate therapeutic failure, or pharmacotoxicity by reducing the drug clearance (metabolism) that could lead to a toxic accumulation. The goal herein remains to reach and adapt to the clinical and therapeutic needs.

Finally, the main potential application beyond focusing on HF-diet-induced genes remains the fact that lipid metabolism-related feedback hormones (mainly leptin) do not have an acute effect. In fact, their effects develop after a relatively long period of time compared to carbohydrate-induced hormones (for instance insulin) that are stimulated immediately following a carbohydrate intake. This highlights the importance of elucidating changes that are both acute and specific to HF diet intake in order to identify acute signals of lipid intake; based on which therapies (hormonal or pharmacological) can be developed. In addition, HF diet changed the expression of genes related to neurogenesis, calcium signaling, and synapse, in the brain cortex [130]. Such ability of the diet to impact neuronal-specific gene patterns could explain how diet and obesity establishment affect the ability of the brain to control energy balance and would require comparable studies in the hypothalamic region, the center of metabolic homeostasis control. Combining the study of changes in the intestinal mucosa (first tissue that comes in contact with the food) with those in the brain (centers that receive peripheral signals and control food intake) would provide the best combination to identify acute HF-specific signals of food intake regulation and, therefore, optimize the therapies based on these axes.

4. Conclusions, Discussion, and Perspectives

Overall, identifying such differentially expressed genes related to exercise and high-fat diet and their related pathways could suggest potential novel therapeutic targets for obesity treatments after elucidating the mechanisms linking those genes to the diverse energy metabolism phenotypes. Functional genomics would, therefore, lead to a new generation of therapeutic approaches that would, through targeting selected energy balance pathways, mimic the benefits and outcomes of physical activity, suitable diets, or even hormones.

For the diet, due to the properties of lipids (high caloric density, low satiety effect, etc.), we believe that one of the best strategies to develop pharmacotherapies for obesity would be to target HF intake at the appetizer time. Therefore, one of the primary strategies is to identify and study the HF diet-induced satiety hormone; usually transcriptionally regulated 30 min to 3 h after HF meal and to deliver it at the time of appetizer in order to control HF intake, obesity, and the related complex diseases and conditions. Herein, it is important to emphasize that adequate diet control is the key solution for obesity (especially if combined with exercise [131,132]) and that pharmacological options remain complementary in selected cases. Regarding identifying pathways of the exercise-induced genes is important for development of exercise pills (long-term objective) that could therapeutically mimic the effects of exercise via targeting these "exercise-genes" pathways through pharmacological agents and, thus, obtain the benefits of exercise without intensive training. This is of a great importance for individuals who are not able to perform exercise because of physical handicap or diseases like heart failure.

Importantly, data generated by functional genomics, especially if combined with functional proteomics and the dynamic-dependent studies of the diverse related pathways will not only provide new insight into therapeutic options and research applications but also into clinical implications. Such implications will cover exercise, HF diet, but also other obesity-related factors such as hormones which are worth exploring within the functional genomics context.

Author Contributions: A.G. designed the review structure and wrote the review. A.G., A.M., M.Y., and J.S.-A. discussed the content and exchanged ideas and suggestions (concepts to add, figures, references selection, etc.) throughout the writing process and edited (and critically revised) the review. J.S.-A. gave the final approval of the version to be published. All authors have read and agreed to the published version of the manuscript.

Funding: This research received no external funding.

Acknowledgments: The graphical abstract and Figure 1; Figure 2 of this manuscript were created using images from: http://smart.servier.com. Servier Medical Art by Servier is licensed under a Creative Commons Attribution 3.0 Unported License.

Conflicts of Interest: The authors declare no conflict of interest.

Abbreviations

ECM: extracellular matrix; HF, high-fat; HFHC, HF and high-cholesterol; LF, low-fat; MUP1/Mup1, major urinary protein 1; OXPHOS, oxidative phosphorylation; PGC1α (also known as PPARGC1A), peroxisome proliferator-activated receptor γ coactivator 1 α; *SPARC*/SPARC, secreted protein acidic and rich in cysteine; *Tff2*, trefoil factor 2.

References

1. Obesity: Preventing and managing the global epidemic. Report of a WHO consultation. In *WHO Technical Report Series 894*; World Health Organization: Geneva, Switzerland, 2000; pp. i-xii, 1-253.
2. Ghanemi, A.; Yoshioka, M.; St-Amand, J. Broken Energy Homeostasis and Obesity Pathogenesis: The Surrounding Concepts. *J. Clin. Med.* **2018**, *7*, 453. [CrossRef] [PubMed]
3. Inoue, Y.; Qin, B.; Poti, J.; Sokol, R.; Gordon-Larsen, P. Epidemiology of Obesity in Adults: Latest Trends. *Curr. Obes. Rep.* **2018**, *7*, 276–288. [CrossRef] [PubMed]
4. Ng, M.; Fleming, T.; Robinson, M.; Thomson, B.; Graetz, N.; Margono, C.; Mullany, E.C.; Biryukov, S.; Abbafati, C.; Abera, S.F.; et al. Global, regional, and national prevalence of overweight and obesity in children and adults during 1980–2013: A systematic analysis for the Global Burden of Disease Study 2013. *Lancet* **2014**, *384*, 766–781. [CrossRef]
5. Ghanemi, A.; Yoshioka, M.; St-Amand, J. Will an obesity pandemic replace the coronavirus disease-2019 (COVID-19) pandemic? *Med. Hypotheses* **2020**, *144*, 110042. [CrossRef]
6. Andolfi, C.; Fisichella, P.M. Epidemiology of Obesity and Associated Comorbidities. *J. Laparoendosc. Adv. Surg. Tech. A* **2018**, *28*, 919–924. [CrossRef]
7. Bhupathiraju, S.N.; Hu, F.B. Epidemiology of Obesity and Diabetes and Their Cardiovascular Complications. *Circ. Res.* **2016**, *118*, 1723–1735. [CrossRef]
8. Wang, J.; Wu, Y.; Xiong, G.; Chao, T.; Jin, Q.; Liu, R.; Hao, L.; Wei, S.; Yang, N.; Yang, X. Introduction of complementary feeding before 4 months of age increases the risk of childhood overweight or obesity: A meta-analysis of prospective cohort studies. *Nutr. Res.* **2016**, *36*, 759–770. [CrossRef]
9. Segal, M.; Eliasziw, M.; Phillips, S.; Bandini, L.; Curtin, C.; Kral, T.V.E.; Sherwood, N.E.; Sikich, L.; Stanish, H.; Must, A. Intellectual disability is associated with increased risk for obesity in a nationally representative sample of U.S. children. *Disabil. Health J.* **2016**, *9*, 392–398. [CrossRef]
10. Michopoulos, V. Stress-Induced alterations in estradiol sensitivity increase risk for obesity in women. *Physiol. Behav.* **2016**. [CrossRef]
11. Heymsfield, S.B.; Wadden, T.A. Mechanisms, Pathophysiology, and Management of Obesity. *N. Engl. J. Med.* **2017**, *376*, 254–266. [CrossRef]
12. Kim, J.Y.; Park, D.I.; Yu, J.; Jung, Y.S.; Park, J.H.; Kim, H.J.; Cho, Y.K.; Sohn, C.I.; Jeon, W.K.; Kim, B.I.; et al. Increased Risk of Advanced Colorectal Neoplasia Among Korean Men With Metabolic Abnormality and Obesity. *Clin. Gastroenterol. Hepatol.* **2016**, *14*. [CrossRef] [PubMed]
13. Fu, M.C.; D'Ambrosia, C.; McLawhorn, A.S.; Schairer, W.W.; Padgett, D.E.; Cross, M.B. Malnutrition Increases With Obesity and Is a Stronger Independent Risk Factor for Postoperative Complications: A Propensity-Adjusted Analysis of Total Hip Arthroplasty Patients. *J. Arthroplast.* **2016**. [CrossRef] [PubMed]

14. Ricketts, T.A.; Sui, X.; Lavie, C.J.; Blair, S.N.; Ross, R. Addition of Cardiorespiratory Fitness Within an Obesity Risk Classification Model Identifies Men at Increased Risk of All-Cause Mortality. *Am. J. Med.* **2016**, *129*, 536.e13–536.e20. [CrossRef] [PubMed]
15. Fontaine, K.R.; Redden, D.T.; Wang, C.; Westfall, A.O.; Allison, D.B. Years of life lost due to obesity. *JAMA* **2003**, *289*, 187–193. [CrossRef] [PubMed]
16. Ghanemi, A.; St-Amand, J. Redefining obesity toward classifying as a disease. *Eur. J. Intern. Med.* **2018**, *55*, 20–22. [CrossRef] [PubMed]
17. le Roux, C.W.; Heneghan, H.M. Bariatric Surgery for Obesity. *Med. Clin. N. Am.* **2018**, *102*, 165–182. [CrossRef]
18. Nuffer, W. Chapter 5-Pharmacologic Agents Chapter for Abdominal Obesity. In *Nutrition in the Prevention and Treatment of Abdominal Obesity*, 2nd ed.; Watson, R.R., Ed.; Academic Press: Cambridge, MA, USA, 2019; pp. 51–66. [CrossRef]
19. Kim, G.W.; Lin, J.E.; Blomain, E.S.; Waldman, S.A. Antiobesity pharmacotherapy: New drugs and emerging targets. *Clin. Pharmacol. Ther.* **2014**, *95*, 53–66. [CrossRef]
20. Gadde, K.M.; Pritham Raj, Y. Pharmacotherapy of Obesity: Clinical Trials to Clinical Practice. *Curr. Diab. Rep.* **2017**, *17*, 34. [CrossRef]
21. Gadde, K.M.; Apolzan, J.W.; Berthoud, H.R. Pharmacotherapy for Patients with Obesity. *Clin. Chem.* **2017**. [CrossRef]
22. Canella, D.S.; Novaes, H.M.; Levy, R.B. Medicine expenses and obesity in Brazil: An analysis based on the household budget survey. *BMC Public Health* **2016**, *16*, 54. [CrossRef]
23. Verhaeghe, N.; De Greve, O.; Annemans, L. The potential health and economic effect of a Body Mass Index decrease in the overweight and obese population in Belgium. *Public Health* **2016**. [CrossRef] [PubMed]
24. Westerterp, K.R. Control of Energy Expenditure in Humans. In *Endotext*; Feingold, K.R., Anawalt, B., Boyce, A., Chrousos, G., Dungan, K., Grossman, A., Hershman, J.M., Kaltsas, G., Koch, C., et al., Eds.; MDText.com, Inc.: South Dartmouth, MA, USA, 2000.
25. Galloza, J.; Castillo, B.; Micheo, W. Benefits of Exercise in the Older Population. *Phys. Med. Rehabil. Clin. N Am.* **2017**, *28*, 659–669. [CrossRef] [PubMed]
26. Myers, J. Cardiology patient pages. Exercise and cardiovascular health. *Circulation* **2003**, *107*, e2–e5. [CrossRef]
27. Tran, Z.V.; Weltman, A. Differential effects of exercise on serum lipid and lipoprotein levels seen with changes in body weight. A meta-Analysis. *Jama* **1985**, *254*, 919–924. [CrossRef] [PubMed]
28. Blundell, J.E.; Gibbons, C.; Caudwell, P.; Finlayson, G.; Hopkins, M. Appetite control and energy balance: Impact of exercise. *Obes. Rev.* **2015**, *16* (Suppl. 1), 67–76. [CrossRef]
29. Chin, S.H.; Kahathuduwa, C.N.; Binks, M. Physical activity and obesity: What we know and what we need to know. *Obes. Rev.* **2016**, *17*, 1226–1244. [CrossRef] [PubMed]
30. Marcin, T.; Eser, P.; Prescott, E.; Mikkelsen, N.; Prins, L.F.; Kolkman, E.K.; Lado-Baleato, Ó.; Cardaso-Suaréz, C.; Bruins, W.; van der Velde, A.E.; et al. Predictors of pre-Rehabilitation exercise capacity in elderly European cardiac patients-The EU-CaRE study. *Eur. J. Prev. Cardiol.* **2019**. [CrossRef]
31. McLeod, M.; Breen, L.; Hamilton, D.L.; Philp, A. Live strong and prosper: The importance of skeletal muscle strength for healthy ageing. *Biogerontology* **2016**, *17*, 497–510. [CrossRef]
32. Brook, M.S.; Wilkinson, D.J.; Phillips, B.E.; Perez-Schindler, J.; Philp, A.; Smith, K.; Atherton, P.J. Skeletal muscle homeostasis and plasticity in youth and ageing: Impact of nutrition and exercise. *Acta Physiol. (Oxf.)* **2016**, *216*, 15–41. [CrossRef]
33. Shad, B.J.; Wallis, G.; van Loon, L.J.; Thompson, J.L. Exercise prescription for the older population: The interactions between physical activity, sedentary time, and adequate nutrition in maintaining musculoskeletal health. *Maturitas* **2016**, *93*, 78–82. [CrossRef]
34. Figueira, A.C.C.; Figueira, M.C.; Silva, C.; Padrao, A.; Oliveira, P.A.; Ferreira, R.P.; Duarte, J.A. Exercise Training-Induced Modulation in Microenvironment of Rat Mammary Neoplasms. *Int. J. Sports Med.* **2018**. [CrossRef] [PubMed]
35. Pedersen, L.; Idorn, M.; Olofsson, G.H.; Lauenborg, B.; Nookaew, I.; Hansen, R.H.; Johannesen, H.H.; Becker, J.C.; Pedersen, K.S.; Dethlefsen, C.; et al. Voluntary Running Suppresses Tumor Growth through Epinephrine- and IL-6-Dependent NK Cell Mobilization and Redistribution. *Cell Metab.* **2016**, *23*, 554–562. [CrossRef] [PubMed]

36. Antunes, J.M.M.; Ferreira, R.M.P.; Moreira-Goncalves, D. Exercise Training as Therapy for Cancer-Induced Cardiac Cachexia. *Trends Mol. Med.* **2018**, *24*, 709–727. [CrossRef] [PubMed]
37. Wesnes, K.; Myhr, K.M.; Riise, T.; Cortese, M.; Pugliatti, M.; Bostrom, I.; Landtblom, A.M.; Wolfson, C.; Bjornevik, K. Physical activity is associated with a decreased multiple sclerosis risk: The EnvIMS study. *Mult. Scler.* **2018**, *24*, 150–157. [CrossRef]
38. Han, P.; Zhang, W.; Kang, L.; Ma, Y.; Fu, L.; Jia, L.; Yu, H.; Chen, X.; Hou, L.; Wang, L.; et al. Clinical Evidence of Exercise Benefits for Stroke. *Adv. Exp. Med. Biol.* **2017**, *1000*, 131–151. [CrossRef]
39. Panchik, D.; Masco, S.; Zinnikas, P.; Hillriegel, B.; Lauder, T.; Suttmann, E.; Chinchilli, V.; McBeth, M.; Hermann, W. The Effect of Exercise on Breast Cancer-Related Lymphedema: What the Lymphatic Surgeon Needs to Know. *J. Reconstr. Microsurg.* **2018**. [CrossRef]
40. Keilani, M.; Hasenoehrl, T.; Baumann, L.; Ristl, R.; Schwarz, M.; Marhold, M.; Sedghi Komandj, T.; Crevenna, R. Effects of resistance exercise in prostate cancer patients: A meta-analysis. *Support Care Cancer* **2017**, *25*, 2953–2968. [CrossRef]
41. Hart, N.H.; Galvao, D.A.; Newton, R.U. Exercise medicine for advanced prostate cancer. *Curr. Opin. Support Palliat. Care* **2017**, *11*, 247–257. [CrossRef]
42. Erlich, A.T.; Brownlee, D.M.; Beyfuss, K.; Hood, D.A. Exercise induces TFEB expression and activity in skeletal muscle in a PGC-1alpha-Dependent manner. *Am. J. Physiol. Cell Physiol.* **2017**. [CrossRef]
43. Vainshtein, A.; Tryon, L.D.; Pauly, M.; Hood, D.A. Role of PGC-1alpha during acute exercise-Induced autophagy and mitophagy in skeletal muscle. *Am. J. Physiol. Cell Physiol.* **2015**, *308*, C710–C719. [CrossRef]
44. Wang, P.; Li, C.G.; Qi, Z.; Cui, D.; Ding, S. Acute exercise stress promotes Ref1/Nrf2 signalling and increases mitochondrial antioxidant activity in skeletal muscle. *Exp. Physiol.* **2016**, *101*, 410–420. [CrossRef] [PubMed]
45. Choi, S.; Liu, X.; Li, P.; Akimoto, T.; Lee, S.Y.; Zhang, M.; Yan, Z. Transcriptional profiling in mouse skeletal muscle following a single bout of voluntary running: Evidence of increased cell proliferation. *J. Appl. Physiol. (Bethesda, Md. 1985)* **2005**, *99*, 2406–2415. [CrossRef] [PubMed]
46. Hu, Z.; Zhou, L.; He, T. Potential effect of exercise in ameliorating insulin resistance at transcriptome level. *J. Sports Med. Phys. Fit.* **2017**. [CrossRef] [PubMed]
47. Larose, M.; St-Amand, J.; Yoshioka, M.; Belleau, P.; Morissette, J.; Labrie, C.; Raymond, V.; Labrie, F. Transcriptome of mouse uterus by serial analysis of gene expression (SAGE): Comparison with skeletal muscle. *Mol. Reprod. Dev.* **2004**, *68*, 142–148. [CrossRef] [PubMed]
48. Vissing, K.; Schjerling, P. Simplified data access on human skeletal muscle transcriptome responses to differentiated exercise. *Sci. Data* **2014**, *1*, 140041. [CrossRef] [PubMed]
49. Lindholm, M.E.; Huss, M.; Solnestam, B.W.; Kjellqvist, S.; Lundeberg, J.; Sundberg, C.J. The human skeletal muscle transcriptome: Sex differences, alternative splicing, and tissue homogeneity assessed with RNA sequencing. *FASEB J.* **2014**, *28*, 4571–4581. [CrossRef]
50. Seaborne, R.A.; Strauss, J.; Cocks, M.; Shepherd, S.; O'Brien, T.D.; van Someren, K.A.; Bell, P.G.; Murgatroyd, C.; Morton, J.P.; Stewart, C.E.; et al. Human Skeletal Muscle Possesses an Epigenetic Memory of Hypertrophy. *Sci. Rep.* **2018**, *8*, 1898. [CrossRef]
51. Lindholm, M.E.; Marabita, F.; Gomez-Cabrero, D.; Rundqvist, H.; Ekstrom, T.J.; Tegner, J.; Sundberg, C.J. An integrative analysis reveals coordinated reprogramming of the epigenome and the transcriptome in human skeletal muscle after training. *Epigenetics* **2014**, *9*, 1557–1569. [CrossRef]
52. Sharples, A.P.; Stewart, C.E.; Seaborne, R.A. Does skeletal muscle have an 'epi'-memory? The role of epigenetics in nutritional programming, metabolic disease, aging and exercise. *Aging Cell* **2016**, *15*, 603–616. [CrossRef]
53. Gensous, N.; Bacalini, M.G.; Pirazzini, C.; Marasco, E.; Giuliani, C.; Ravaioli, F.; Mengozzi, G.; Bertarelli, C.; Palmas, M.G.; Franceschi, C.; et al. The epigenetic landscape of age-related diseases: The geroscience perspective. *Biogerontology* **2017**, *18*, 549–559. [CrossRef]
54. Li, S.; Chen, Y.; Zhang, Y.; Zhang, H.; Wu, Y.; He, H.; Gong, L.; Zeng, F.; Shi, L. Exercise during pregnancy enhances vascular function via epigenetic repression of Ca(V)1.2 channel in offspring of hypertensive rats. *Life Sci.* **2019**, *231*, 116576. [CrossRef] [PubMed]
55. Hopkins, S.A.; Baldi, J.C.; Cutfield, W.S.; McCowan, L.; Hofman, P.L. Exercise training in pregnancy reduces offspring size without changes in maternal insulin sensitivity. *J. Clin. Endocrinol. Metab.* **2010**, *95*, 2080–2088. [CrossRef]

56. Yoshioka, M.; Tanaka, H.; Shono, N.; Snyder, E.E.; Shindo, M.; St-Amand, J. Serial analysis of gene expression in the skeletal muscle of endurance athletes compared to sedentary men. *FASEB J.* **2003**, *17*, 1812–1819. [CrossRef] [PubMed]
57. Yoshioka, M.; Tanaka, H.; Shono, N.; Shindo, M.; St-Amand, J. Gene expression profile of sprinter's muscle. *Int. J. Sports Med.* **2007**, *28*, 1053–1058. [CrossRef] [PubMed]
58. Cochran, A.J.; Percival, M.E.; Tricarico, S.; Little, J.P.; Cermak, N.; Gillen, J.B.; Tarnopolsky, M.A.; Gibala, M.J. Intermittent and continuous high-intensity exercise training induce similar acute but different chronic muscle adaptations. *Exp. Physiol.* **2014**, *99*, 782–791. [CrossRef]
59. Nishida, Y.; Tanaka, H.; Tobina, T.; Murakami, K.; Shono, N.; Shindo, M.; Ogawa, W.; Yoshioka, M.; St-Amand, J. Regulation of muscle genes by moderate exercise. *Int. J. Sports Med.* **2010**, *31*, 656–670. [CrossRef]
60. Riedl, I.; Yoshioka, M.; Nishida, Y.; Tobina, T.; Paradis, R.; Shono, N.; Tanaka, H.; St-Amand, J. Regulation of skeletal muscle transcriptome in elderly men after 6 weeks of endurance training at lactate threshold intensity. *Exp. Gerontol.* **2010**, *45*, 896–903. [CrossRef]
61. Timmons, J.A.; Larsson, O.; Jansson, E.; Fischer, H.; Gustafsson, T.; Greenhaff, P.L.; Ridden, J.; Rachman, J.; Peyrard-Janvid, M.; Wahlestedt, C.; et al. Human muscle gene expression responses to endurance training provide a novel perspective on Duchenne muscular dystrophy. *Faseb J.* **2005**, *19*, 750–760. [CrossRef]
62. Huang, J.H.; Hood, D.A. Age-Associated mitochondrial dysfunction in skeletal muscle: Contributing factors and suggestions for long-Term interventions. *IUBMB Life* **2009**, *61*, 201–214. [CrossRef]
63. Marzetti, E.; Lawler, J.M.; Hiona, A.; Manini, T.; Seo, A.Y.; Leeuwenburgh, C. Modulation of age-induced apoptotic signaling and cellular remodeling by exercise and calorie restriction in skeletal muscle. *Free Radic Biol. Med.* **2008**, *44*, 160–168. [CrossRef]
64. Lourenço Dos Santos, S.; Baraibar, M.A.; Lundberg, S.; Eeg-Olofsson, O.; Larsson, L.; Friguet, B. Oxidative proteome alterations during skeletal muscle ageing. *Redox Biol.* **2015**, *5*, 267–274. [CrossRef] [PubMed]
65. Melouane, A.; Yoshioka, M.; Kanzaki, M.; St-Amand, J. Sparc, an EPS-induced gene, modulates the extracellular matrix and mitochondrial function via ILK/AMPK pathways in C2C12 cells. *Life Sci.* **2019**, *229*, 277–287. [CrossRef] [PubMed]
66. Norheim, F.; Raastad, T.; Thiede, B.; Rustan, A.C.; Drevon, C.A.; Haugen, F. Proteomic identification of secreted proteins from human skeletal muscle cells and expression in response to strength training. *Am. J. Physiol. Endocrinol. Metab.* **2011**, *301*, E1013–E1021. [CrossRef] [PubMed]
67. Melouane, A.; Carbonell, A.; Yoshioka, M.; Puymirat, J.; St-Amand, J. Implication of SPARC in the modulation of the extracellular matrix and mitochondrial function in muscle cells. *PLoS ONE* **2018**, *13*, e0192714. [CrossRef]
68. Aoi, W.; Naito, Y.; Takagi, T.; Tanimura, Y.; Takanami, Y.; Kawai, Y.; Sakuma, K.; Hang, L.; Mizushima, K.; Hirai, Y.; et al. A novel myokine, secreted protein acidic and rich in cysteine (SPARC), suppresses colon tumorigenesis via regular exercise. *Gut* **2013**, *62*, 882–889. [CrossRef]
69. Ghanemi, A.; Melouane, A.; Yoshioka, M.; St-Amand, J. Secreted protein acidic and rich in cysteine and bioenergetics: Extracellular matrix, adipocytes remodeling and skeletal muscle metabolism. *Int. J. Biochem. Cell Biol.* **2019**, *117*, 105627. [CrossRef]
70. Ghanemi, A.; Yoshioka, M.; St-Amand, J. Secreted Protein Acidic and Rich in Cysteine: Metabolic and Homeostatic Properties beyond the Extracellular Matrix Structure. *Appl. Sci.* **2020**, *10*, 2388. [CrossRef]
71. Sage, H.; Vernon, R.B.; Funk, S.E.; Everitt, E.A.; Angello, J. SPARC, a secreted protein associated with cellular proliferation, inhibits cell spreading in vitro and exhibits Ca+2-dependent binding to the extracellular matrix. *J. Cell Biol.* **1989**, *109*, 341–356. [CrossRef]
72. Francki, A.; Motamed, K.; McClure, T.D.; Kaya, M.; Murri, C.; Blake, D.J.; Carbon, J.G.; Sage, E.H. SPARC regulates cell cycle progression in mesangial cells via its inhibition of IGF-Dependent signaling. *J. Cell Biochem.* **2003**, *88*, 802–811. [CrossRef]
73. Mason, I.J.; Taylor, A.; Williams, J.G.; Sage, H.; Hogan, B.L. Evidence from molecular cloning that SPARC, a major product of mouse embryo parietal endoderm, is related to an endothelial cell 'culture shock' glycoprotein of Mr 43,000. *Embo J.* **1986**, *5*, 1465–1472. [CrossRef]
74. Cho, W.J.; Kim, E.J.; Lee, S.J.; Kim, H.D.; Shin, H.J.; Lim, W.K. Involvement of SPARC in in vitro differentiation of skeletal myoblasts. *Biochem. Biophys. Res. Commun.* **2000**, *271*, 630–634. [CrossRef] [PubMed]

75. Ghanemi, A.; Yoshioka, M.; St-Amand, J. Secreted protein acidic and rich in cysteine and inflammation: Another homeostatic property? *Cytokine* **2020**, *133*, 155179. [CrossRef] [PubMed]
76. Ghanemi, A.; Yoshioka, M.; St-Amand, J. Secreted protein acidic and rich in cysteine and cancer: A homeostatic hormone? *Cytokine* **2020**, *127*, 154996. [CrossRef]
77. Hood, D.A. Mechanisms of exercise-induced mitochondrial biogenesis in skeletal muscle. *Appl. Physiol. Nutr. Metab.* **2009**, *34*, 465–472. [CrossRef] [PubMed]
78. Hoffman, N.J.; Parker, B.L.; Chaudhuri, R.; Fisher-Wellman, K.H.; Kleinert, M.; Humphrey, S.J.; Yang, P.; Holliday, M.; Trefely, S.; Fazakerley, D.J.; et al. Global Phosphoproteomic Analysis of Human Skeletal Muscle Reveals a Network of Exercise-Regulated Kinases and AMPK Substrates. *Cell Metab.* **2015**, *22*, 922–935. [CrossRef]
79. Hamilton, M.T.; Booth, F.W. Skeletal muscle adaptation to exercise: A century of progress. *J. Appl. Physiol. (1985)* **2000**, *88*, 327–331. [CrossRef]
80. Melov, S.; Tarnopolsky, M.A.; Beckman, K.; Felkey, K.; Hubbard, A. Resistance exercise reverses aging in human skeletal muscle. *PLoS ONE* **2007**, *2*, e465. [CrossRef]
81. Petriz, B.A.; Gomes, C.P.; Almeida, J.A.; de Oliveira, G.P., Jr.; Ribeiro, F.M.; Pereira, R.W.; Franco, O.L. The Effects of Acute and Chronic Exercise on Skeletal Muscle Proteome. *J. Cell Physiol.* **2017**, *232*, 257–269. [CrossRef]
82. Holloway, K.V.; O'Gorman, M.; Woods, P.; Morton, J.P.; Evans, L.; Cable, N.T.; Goldspink, D.F.; Burniston, J.G. Proteomic investigation of changes in human vastus lateralis muscle in response to interval-Exercise training. *Proteomics* **2009**, *9*, 5155–5174. [CrossRef]
83. Burniston, J.G. Changes in the rat skeletal muscle proteome induced by moderate-intensity endurance exercise. *Biochim. Biophys. Acta* **2008**, *1784*, 1077–1086. [CrossRef]
84. Ruas, J.L.; White, J.P.; Rao, R.R.; Kleiner, S.; Brannan, K.T.; Harrison, B.C.; Greene, N.P.; Wu, J.; Estall, J.L.; Irving, B.A.; et al. A PGC-1alpha isoform induced by resistance training regulates skeletal muscle hypertrophy. *Cell* **2012**, *151*, 1319–1331. [CrossRef] [PubMed]
85. Coffey, V.G.; Hawley, J.A. Concurrent exercise training: Do opposites distract? *J. Physiol.* **2017**, *595*, 2883–2896. [CrossRef] [PubMed]
86. Raue, U.; Trappe, T.A.; Estrem, S.T.; Qian, H.R.; Helvering, L.M.; Smith, R.C.; Trappe, S. Transcriptome signature of resistance exercise adaptations: Mixed muscle and fiber type specific profiles in young and old adults. *J. Appl. Physiol. (1985)* **2012**, *112*, 1625–1636. [CrossRef] [PubMed]
87. St-Amand, J.; Yoshioka, M.; Nishida, Y.; Tobina, T.; Shono, N.; Tanaka, H. Effects of mild-exercise training cessation in human skeletal muscle. *Eur. J. Appl. Physiol.* **2012**, *112*, 853–869. [CrossRef] [PubMed]
88. Jacobs, K.A.; Krauss, R.M.; Fattor, J.A.; Horning, M.A.; Friedlander, A.L.; Bauer, T.A.; Hagobian, T.A.; Wolfel, E.E.; Brooks, G.A. Endurance training has little effect on active muscle free fatty acid, lipoprotein cholesterol, or triglyceride net balances. *Am. J. Physiol. Endocrinol. Metab.* **2006**, *291*, E656–E665. [CrossRef] [PubMed]
89. Shono, N.; Urata, H.; Saltin, B.; Mizuno, M.; Harada, T.; Shindo, M.; Tanaka, H. Effects of low intensity aerobic training on skeletal muscle capillary and blood lipoprotein profiles. *J. Atheroscler. Thromb.* **2002**, *9*, 78–85. [CrossRef]
90. Laguna-Camacho, A. Influence on Adiposity and Atherogenic Lipaemia of Fatty Meals and Snacks in Daily Life. *J. Lipids* **2017**, *2017*, 1375342. [CrossRef]
91. Ribaroff, G.A.; Wastnedge, E.; Drake, A.J.; Sharpe, R.M.; Chambers, T.J.G. Animal models of maternal high fat diet exposure and effects on metabolism in offspring: A meta-regression analysis. *Obes. Rev.* **2017**, *18*, 673–686. [CrossRef]
92. Flatt, J.P. The difference in the storage capacities for carbohydrate and for fat, and its implications in the regulation of body weight. *Ann. N. Y. Acad. Sci.* **1987**, *499*, 104–123. [CrossRef]
93. Maher, T.; Clegg, M.E. Dietary lipids with potential to affect satiety: Mechanisms and evidence. *Crit. Rev. Food Sci. Nutr.* **2018**, 1–26. [CrossRef]
94. Lissner, L.; Levitsky, D.A.; Strupp, B.J.; Kalkwarf, H.J.; Roe, D.A. Dietary fat and the regulation of energy intake in human subjects. *Am. J. Clin. Nutr.* **1987**, *46*, 886–892. [CrossRef] [PubMed]
95. Flatt, J.P.; Ravussin, E.; Acheson, K.J.; Jequier, E. Effects of dietary fat on postprandial substrate oxidation and on carbohydrate and fat balances. *J. Clin. Investig.* **1985**, *76*, 1019–1024. [CrossRef] [PubMed]

96. Schutz, Y.; Flatt, J.P.; Jequier, E. Failure of dietary fat intake to promote fat oxidation: A factor favoring the development of obesity. *Am. J. Clin. Nutr.* **1989**, *50*, 307–314. [CrossRef] [PubMed]
97. Keleher, M.R.; Zaidi, R.; Shah, S.; Oakley, M.E.; Pavlatos, C.; El Idrissi, S.; Xing, X.; Li, D.; Wang, T.; Cheverud, J.M. Maternal high-fat diet associated with altered gene expression, DNA methylation, and obesity risk in mouse offspring. *PLoS ONE* **2018**, *13*, e0192606. [CrossRef]
98. Keleher, M.R.; Zaidi, R.; Hicks, L.; Shah, S.; Xing, X.; Li, D.; Wang, T.; Cheverud, J.M. A high-Fat diet alters genome-Wide DNA methylation and gene expression in SM/J mice. *BMC Genom.* **2018**, *19*, 888. [CrossRef]
99. Suter, M.A.; Ma, J.; Vuguin, P.M.; Hartil, K.; Fiallo, A.; Harris, R.A.; Charron, M.J.; Aagaard, K.M. In utero exposure to a maternal high-Fat diet alters the epigenetic histone code in a murine model. *Am. J. Obstet. Gynecol.* **2014**, *210*, 463.E1–463.E11. [CrossRef]
100. Wankhade, U.D.; Zhong, Y.; Kang, P.; Alfaro, M.; Chintapalli, S.V.; Thakali, K.M.; Shankar, K. Enhanced offspring predisposition to steatohepatitis with maternal high-Fat diet is associated with epigenetic and microbiome alterations. *PLoS ONE* **2017**, *12*, e0175675. [CrossRef]
101. Glendining, K.A.; Fisher, L.C.; Jasoni, C.L. Maternal high fat diet alters offspring epigenetic regulators, amygdala glutamatergic profile and anxiety. *Psychoneuroendocrinology* **2018**, *96*, 132–141. [CrossRef]
102. Smilowitz, J.T.; German, J.B.; Zivkovic, A.M. Food Intake and Obesity: The Case of Fat. In *Fat Detection: Taste, Texture, and Post Ingestive Effects*; Montmayeur, J.P., le Coutre, J., Eds.; CRC Press/Taylor & Francis: Boca Raton, FL, USA, 2010.
103. Astrup, A. The role of dietary fat in the prevention and treatment of obesity. Efficacy and safety of low-Fat diets. *Int. J. Obes. Relat. Metab. Disord. J. Int. Assoc. Study Obes.* **2001**, *25* (Suppl. 1), S46–S50. [CrossRef]
104. Liu, L.; Wang, Q.; Liu, A.; Lan, X.; Huang, Y.; Zhao, Z.; Jie, H.; Chen, J.; Zhao, Y. Physiological Implications of Orexins/Hypocretins on Energy Metabolism and Adipose Tissue Development. *ACS Omega* **2020**, *5*, 547–555. [CrossRef]
105. Milbank, E.; López, M. Orexins/Hypocretins: Key Regulators of Energy Homeostasis. *Front. Endocrinol.* **2019**, *10*, 830. [CrossRef] [PubMed]
106. Yoshioka, M.; Bolduc, C.; Raymond, V.; St-Amand, J. High-Fat meal-Induced changes in the duodenum mucosa transcriptome. *Obes. (Silver Spring Md.)* **2008**, *16*, 2302–2307. [CrossRef] [PubMed]
107. Mucunguzi, O.; Melouane, A.; Ghanemi, A.; Yoshioka, M.; Boivin, A.; Calvo, E.L.; St-Amand, J. Identification of the principal transcriptional regulators for low-fat and high-fat meal responsive genes in small intestine. *Nutr. Metab.* **2017**, *14*, 66. [CrossRef] [PubMed]
108. Douglass, J.D.; Malik, N.; Chon, S.H.; Wells, K.; Zhou, Y.X.; Choi, A.S.; Joseph, L.B.; Storch, J. Intestinal mucosal triacylglycerol accumulation secondary to decreased lipid secretion in obese and high fat fed mice. *Front. Physiol.* **2012**, *3*, 25. [CrossRef] [PubMed]
109. Smolders, L.; Mensink, R.P.; Boekschoten, M.V.; de Ridder, R.J.J.; Plat, J. The acute effects on duodenal gene expression in healthy men following consumption of a low-Fat meal enriched with theobromine or fat. *Sci. Rep.* **2018**, *8*, 1700. [CrossRef] [PubMed]
110. Martin, C.R.; Osadchiy, V.; Kalani, A.; Mayer, E.A. The Brain-Gut-Microbiome Axis. *Cell Mol. Gastroenterol. Hepatol.* **2018**, *6*, 133–148. [CrossRef]
111. De Giorgio, M.R.; Yoshioka, M.; Riedl, I.; Moreault, O.; Cherizol, R.G.; Shah, A.A.; Blin, N.; Richard, D.; St-Amand, J. Trefoil factor family member 2 (Tff2) KO mice are protected from high-Fat diet-Induced obesity. *Obes. (Silver Spring)* **2013**, *21*, 1389–1395. [CrossRef]
112. Ghanemi, A.; Melouane, A.; Mucunguzi, O.; Yoshioka, M.; St-Amand, J. Energy and metabolic pathways in trefoil factor family member 2 (Tff2) KO mice beyond the protection from high-Fat diet-Induced obesity. *Life Sci.* **2018**, *215*, 190–197. [CrossRef]
113. De Giorgio, M.R.; Yoshioka, M.; St-Amand, J. Feeding regulates the expression of pancreatic genes in gastric mucosa. *J. Obes.* **2010**, *2010*, 371950. [CrossRef]
114. Bolduc, C.; Yoshioka, M.; St-Amand, J. Acute molecular mechanisms responsive to feeding and meal constitution in mesenteric adipose tissue. *Obes. (Silver Spring)* **2010**, *18*, 410–413. [CrossRef]
115. De Giorgio, M.R.; Yoshioka, M.; St-Amand, J. Feeding induced changes in the hypothalamic transcriptome. *Clin. Chim. Acta* **2009**, *406*, 103–107. [CrossRef] [PubMed]
116. Gondret, F.; Vincent, A.; Houee-Bigot, M.; Siegel, A.; Lagarrigue, S.; Louveau, I.; Causeur, D. Molecular alterations induced by a high-Fat high-Fiber diet in porcine adipose tissues: Variations according to the anatomical fat location. *BMC Genom.* **2016**, *17*, 120. [CrossRef]

117. Moraes, R.C.; Blondet, A.; Birkenkamp-Demtroeder, K.; Tirard, J.; Orntoft, T.F.; Gertler, A.; Durand, P.; Naville, D.; Bégeot, M. Study of the Alteration of Gene Expression in Adipose Tissue of Diet-Induced Obese Mice by Microarray and Reverse Transcription-Polymerase Chain Reaction Analyses. *Endocrinology* **2003**, *144*, 4773–4782. [CrossRef] [PubMed]
118. Perez-Schindler, J.; Kanhere, A.; Edwards, L.; Allwood, J.W.; Dunn, W.B.; Schenk, S.; Philp, A. Exercise and high-fat feeding remodel transcript-metabolite interactive networks in mouse skeletal muscle. *Sci. Rep.* **2017**, *7*, 13485. [CrossRef] [PubMed]
119. Hui, X.; Zhu, W.; Wang, Y.; Lam, K.S.; Zhang, J.; Wu, D.; Kraegen, E.W.; Li, Y.; Xu, A. Major urinary protein-1 increases energy expenditure and improves glucose intolerance through enhancing mitochondrial function in skeletal muscle of diabetic mice. *J. Biol. Chem.* **2009**, *284*, 14050–14057. [CrossRef]
120. Zhou, Y.; Rui, L. Major urinary protein regulation of chemical communication and nutrient metabolism. *Vitam. Horm.* **2010**, *83*, 151–163. [CrossRef]
121. Zhou, Y.; Jiang, L.; Rui, L. Identification of MUP1 as a regulator for glucose and lipid metabolism in mice. *J. Biol. Chem.* **2009**, *284*, 11152–11159. [CrossRef]
122. van Schothorst, E.M.; Keijer, J.; Pennings, J.L.; Opperhuizen, A.; van den Brom, C.E.; Kohl, T.; Franssen-van Hal, N.L.; Hoebee, B. Adipose gene expression response of lean and obese mice to short-Term dietary restriction. *Obes. (Silver Spring)* **2006**, *14*, 974–979. [CrossRef]
123. Harrell, C.S.; Burgado, J.; Kelly, S.D.; Johnson, Z.P.; Neigh, G.N. High-Fructose diet during periadolescent development increases depressive-Like behavior and remodels the hypothalamic transcriptome in male rats. *Psychoneuroendocrinology* **2015**, *62*, 252–264. [CrossRef]
124. Ziotopoulou, M.; Mantzoros, C.S.; Hileman, S.M.; Flier, J.S. Differential expression of hypothalamic neuropeptides in the early phase of diet-Induced obesity in mice. *Am. J. Physiol. Endocrinol. Metab.* **2000**, *279*, E838–E845. [CrossRef]
125. St-Amand, J.; Yoshioka, M.; Tanaka, K.; Nishida, Y. Transcriptome-Wide identification of preferentially expressed genes in the hypothalamus and pituitary gland. *Front. Endocrinol.* **2011**, *2*, 111. [CrossRef] [PubMed]
126. Bedard, K.; Bedard, J.; Rocheleau, G.; Ferland, G.; Gaudreau, P. Aging and diets regulate the rat anterior pituitary and hypothalamic transcriptome. *Neuroendocrinology* **2013**, *97*, 146–159. [CrossRef] [PubMed]
127. Takahashi, J.; Waki, S.; Matsumoto, R.; Odake, J.; Miyaji, T.; Tottori, J.; Iwanaga, T.; Iwahashi, H. Oligonucleotide microarray analysis of dietary-induced hyperlipidemia gene expression profiles in miniature pigs. *PLoS ONE* **2012**, *7*, e37581. [CrossRef] [PubMed]
128. Maruthur, N.M.; Tseng, E.; Hutfless, S.; Wilson, L.M.; Suarez-Cuervo, C.; Berger, Z.; Chu, Y.; Iyoha, E.; Segal, J.B.; Bolen, S. Diabetes Medications as Monotherapy or Metformin-Based Combination Therapy for Type 2 Diabetes: A Systematic Review and Meta-analysis. *Ann. Intern. Med.* **2016**, *164*, 740–751. [CrossRef]
129. Salomaki, H.; Heinaniemi, M.; Vahatalo, L.H.; Ailanen, L.; Eerola, K.; Ruohonen, S.T.; Pesonen, U.; Koulu, M. Prenatal metformin exposure in a maternal high fat diet mouse model alters the transcriptome and modifies the metabolic responses of the offspring. *PLoS ONE* **2014**, *9*, e115778. [CrossRef]
130. Yoon, G.; Cho, K.A.; Song, J.; Kim, Y.-K. Transcriptomic Analysis of High Fat Diet Fed Mouse Brain Cortex. *Front. Genet.* **2019**, *10*. [CrossRef]
131. Hansen, D.; Dendale, P.; Berger, J.; van Loon, L.J.; Meeusen, R. The effects of exercise training on fat-mass loss in obese patients during energy intake restriction. *Sports Med.* **2007**, *37*, 31–46. [CrossRef]
132. Miller, C.T.; Fraser, S.F.; Levinger, I.; Straznicky, N.E.; Dixon, J.B.; Reynolds, J.; Selig, S.E. The effects of exercise training in addition to energy restriction on functional capacities and body composition in obese adults during weight losss: A systematic review. *PLoS ONE* **2013**, *8*, e81692. [CrossRef]

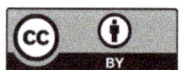

© 2020 by the authors. Licensee MDPI, Basel, Switzerland. This article is an open access article distributed under the terms and conditions of the Creative Commons Attribution (CC BY) license (http://creativecommons.org/licenses/by/4.0/).

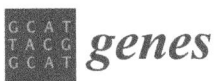 *genes*

Article

A Comparative Study of Supervised Machine Learning Algorithms for the Prediction of Long-Range Chromatin Interactions

Thomas Vanhaeren [1], Federico Divina [1], Miguel García-Torres [1], Francisco Gómez-Vela [1], Wim Vanhoof [2] and Pedro Manuel Martínez-García [3,4,*]

- [1] Division of Computer Science, Universidad Pablo de Olavide, 41013 Sevilla, Spain; vtho@alu.upo.es (T.V.); fdivina@upo.es (F.D.); mgarciat@upo.es (M.G.-T.); fgomez@upo.es (F.G.-V.)
- [2] Faculty of Computer Science, University of Namur, 5000 Namur, Belgium; wim.vanhoof@unamur.be
- [3] Centro Andaluz de Biología Molecular y Medicina Regenerativa (CABIMER), CSIC-Universidad de Sevilla-Universidad Pablo de Olavide, 41092 Sevilla, Spain
- [4] Facultad de Ciencias y Tecnología, Universidad Isabel I, 09003 Burgos, Spain
- [*] Correspondence: pedromanuel.martinez@ui1.es

Received: 8 June 2020; Accepted: 20 August 2020; Published: 24 August 2020

Abstract: The role of three-dimensional genome organization as a critical regulator of gene expression has become increasingly clear over the last decade. Most of our understanding of this association comes from the study of long range chromatin interaction maps provided by Chromatin Conformation Capture-based techniques, which have greatly improved in recent years. Since these procedures are experimentally laborious and expensive, in silico prediction has emerged as an alternative strategy to generate virtual maps in cell types and conditions for which experimental data of chromatin interactions is not available. Several methods have been based on predictive models trained on one-dimensional (1D) sequencing features, yielding promising results. However, different approaches vary both in the way they model chromatin interactions and in the machine learning-based strategy they rely on, making it challenging to carry out performance comparison of existing methods. In this study, we use publicly available 1D sequencing signals to model cohesin-mediated chromatin interactions in two human cell lines and evaluate the prediction performance of six popular machine learning algorithms: decision trees, random forests, gradient boosting, support vector machines, multi-layer perceptron and deep learning. Our approach accurately predicts long-range interactions and reveals that gradient boosting significantly outperforms the other five methods, yielding accuracies of about 95%. We show that chromatin features in close genomic proximity to the anchors cover most of the predictive information, as has been previously reported. Moreover, we demonstrate that gradient boosting models trained with different subsets of chromatin features, unlike the other methods tested, are able to produce accurate predictions. In this regard, and besides architectural proteins, transcription factors are shown to be highly informative. Our study provides a framework for the systematic prediction of long-range chromatin interactions, identifies gradient boosting as the best suited algorithm for this task and highlights cell-type specific binding of transcription factors at the anchors as important determinants of chromatin wiring mediated by cohesin.

Keywords: machine-learning; chromatin interactions; prediction; genomics; genome architecture

1. Introduction

Mammalian genomes stretch for more than two meters and are formed by around three billion base pairs that are tightly packed within the nucleus, which has a width on the order of micrometers. Strikingly, this level of compaction is compatible with a proper accessibility to the cellular machinery required for essential metabolic processes such as replication or transcription. Over recent years, it has become clear that such seemingly counterintuitive events can be explained by the architectural organization of the genome, which forms 3D structures with several levels of complexity [1,2]. Beyond nucleosome-nucleosome interactions, chromatin loops represent the smallest scale of genome organization. Loops bring distal genomic loci into close physical proximity and typically range from one to several hundreds of kilobases [3,4]. On a larger scale, chromosomes are spatially segregated into structures called topologically associating domains (TADs). TADs are blocks of chromatin where all pairs of loci interact with each other more frequently than with neighboring regions [5,6]. At a higher level, the interactions of TADs with one another make up megabase-scale structures that extend to whole chromosomes and are known as nuclear compartment [7]. Since there is not yet a well characterized biological delineation between such orders of genome organization, in this study we will use the term 'loop' to refer indistinctly to chromatin interactions at any level of this hierarchy. Accordingly, we will refer to the pair of distal loci that are brought together as 'loop anchors'.

Recent findings have revealed that 3D genome organization is more complex than anticipated [3]. Indeed, genome architecture can vary between cell types and is dynamic during cell differentiation and development [8]. Evidence also points to an essential role of the 3D genome in the control of gene expression by allowing communications between promoters and distal enhancers [9–12]. In addition, the insulator protein CCCTC-binding factor (CTCF) and the ring-shaped cohesin complex have been shown to highly co-localize both at the borders of TADs and at the anchors of intra-TADs chromatin interactions in mammalian cells, which likely indicates that these factors work together to shape chromatin architecture [3,5–7]. A plausible hypothesis of how TADs and loops are formed postulates that cohesin extrudes DNA loops until it encounters an obstacle such as convergently oriented loop anchor DNA sequences actively bound by CTCF [13,14]. This hypothesis places cohesin as the main player in the so-called loop extrusion model [13–16]. Interestingly, recent evidence has revealed that cohesin is moved to CTCF sites by transcription [17], suggesting that RNA polymerase II (Pol II) might be a driving force for this mechanism.

Most of the advances in our understanding of how high order genome organization links to essential cellular metabolic processes comes from the development of Chromatin Conformation Capture (3C)-based technologies [18], which has provided the scientific community with high resolution genome-wide chromatin interaction maps for several mammalian cell types. Despite technical improvements, experimental profiling of such maps not only remains difficult and expensive, but also requires a remarkably high sequencing depth for the achievement of high resolution [3,19]. Therefore, in silico predictions that take advantage of the wealth of publicly available sequencing data emerges as a rational strategy to generate virtual chromatin interaction maps in new cell types for which experimental maps are still lacking. To date, several studies have been devoted to predict chromatin loops based on one-dimensional (1D) genomic information with accurate results [20–25]. In such works, authors have modeled loops using different designs and machine learning approaches. Accordingly, they reached different conclusions regarding which chromatin features are most predictive and whether information within the loops (away from the anchors) contributes to the predictive power.

Here, we model cohesin-mediated chromatin loops using an integrative approach based on ENCODE 1D sequencing datasets to test the performance of six different machine learning algorithms: decision trees (DT), random forests (RF), gradient boosting (XGBoost), Support Vector Machines (SVMs), multi-layer perceptron (MLP) and deep learning Artificial Neural Network (DL-ANN). We find that XGBoost achieves the best performance, with precision scores of around 0.95. We also show that, although architectural features at the anchors display the greatest predictive power, transcription-associated features accurately predict chromatin loops. Among these features, transcription factors are the most informative and their contribution resides mainly at the anchors and varies across human cell lines.

2. Materials and Methods

2.1. Processing Publicly Available Data

The experimental data used in this study is summarized in Table S1. With the exception of Hi-C, which was used for visualization purposes, the rest of the datasets were batch-downloaded from ENCODE [26]. BAM files were used for ChIP-seq, RNA-seq and DNase-seq, while tsv tables labeled as 'long range chromatin interactions' were used for ChIA-PET experiments targeting RAD21. Figures 1 and S1 show genome browser views displaying a selection of these datasets. All the analyses were performed in K562 and GM12878 cell lines using human assembly hg19.

2.2. Identification of RAD21-Associated Loops

RAD21 loops in K562 were extracted from ENCODE dataset ENCFF002ENO. For the identification of RAD21 loops in GM12878, two replicates were considered (datasets ENCFF002EMO and ENCFF002EMQ) and only overlapping loops were retained. We defined overlapping loops as those that share both anchors, allowing a maximum gap of 2 kb. Following this approach, we identified 3290 and 5486 loops in K562 and GM12878, respectively. For machine learning classification, we generated the same number of negative loops for each cell line. In order to build robust models that were able to accurately separate loops from random genomic regions, we generated an initial set of negative loops by randomly combining pairs of RAD21 ChIP-seq peaks (see Figure 2a). Then, loops that overlapped experimental ones were filtered out. Since genomic distance highly influences chromatin interactions, the resulting set of negative loops were passed through a regression model trained to capture the distribution of genomic distances between anchors of experimental loops. Finally, 3290 and 5486 loops were randomly selected from the K562 and GM12878 negative sets, respectively. In this way, the number of positive and negative loops in the final datasets were equal and with similar genomic distance distributions. Since we used pairs of RAD21 peaks to generate the initial set of background loops, we examined RAD21 (and CTCF) ChIP-seq reads at the anchors of our positive and negative loops. We observed a clear read enrichment of both signals (Figure S1), indicating that final loop sets are adequate for subsequent training.

2.3. Machine Learning Data Matrix

To model loops using chromatin features, we quantified 23 sequencing datasets within and adjacent to each loop using a modified version of the approach described by Handoko et al. [27]. Given a loop with length L, we extended L base pairs to its left and right and the extended region (with length 3L) was splitted into 1500 bins (Figure 2b, top). Then, we scored the sequencing experiments (Table S1) within each bin (Figure 2b, bottom). The scoring was performed by counting reads that aligned to each bin and normalizing by bin genomic length and sequencing library size. For each cell line, we obtained a final data matrix with rows representing loops and columns representing quantification of chromatin features at each bin.

The 23 chromatin feature datasets (Table S1) included marks associated with chromatin accessibility (DNAse-seq), expression (RNA-seq), RNA Pol2 binding (POLR2A, POLR2AphosphoS5), active promoters (H3k4me2, H3k4me3, H3k9ac), enhancers (H3k4me1), active gene bodies and elongation (H3k36me3, H4k20me1), transcriptional repression (H3k27me3, H3k9me3), architectural components (CTCF, RAD21) and transcription factors (ATF3, CEBPB, JUND, MAX, REST, SIN3A, SP1, SRF, YY1). The motivation of selecting these datasets was to keep a wide set of chromatin features representing different molecular events. Only datasets from ENCODE common to both cell lines were selected.

2.4. Supervised Learning

In this work, we used six Machine Learning strategies in order to induce a classification model for the data. Each of the model is applied to a training set and then the prediction models are evaluated on a test set. We briefly describe each method in the following subsections.

2.4.1. Decision Trees (DT)

We have used the algorithm implementation provided by [28,29]. A decision tree (DT) algorithm iteratively builds a classification tree by adding a node to the tree. Features are used within internal nodes in order to classify examples.

A DT algorithm induces a tree by splitting the original dataset into smaller sets based on a test applied to the features. This process is repeated recursively on each smaller set and is complete when the small set present in one node presents the same value as the target label or when no more gain in predictive power is obtained by splitting further. Such a process is known as recursive partitioning.

The features selected depend on a measure used in order to assess the importance of a feature. The Gini Impurity measure was used, which is defined as:

$$1 - \sum_{i=1}^{n} p^2(c_i) \qquad (1)$$

where $p(c_i)$ s the probability of class c_i in a node. We have also run several experiments on the datasets used in the paper with the Entropy, and the results were basically the same with the two measures.

In this paper, we used the implementation provided by the library Scikit Learn (Sklearn) library [28]. The maximum depth parameter has been set to 10. The criterion was set to Entropy, while Gini is in theory intended for continuous attributes, Entropy is intended for attributes occurring in classes but since Entropy uses logarithmic functions slower to compute. For the training of the K562 DT, both criteria were tested and compared.

2.4.2. Random Forests (RF)

This strategy [30] belongs to the family of ensemble learning algorithms, based on a divide and conquer approach that improves performance. The principle behind ensemble methods is that a group of weak models are put together to form a stronger model. This is due to the fact that ensemble strategies reduce variance, improving the prediction power. RF algorithms induce a set of trees, which are then used in order to produce the final output, using a voting scheme. The trees are built one at a time. Each tree is obtained using a randomly selected training subset and a randomly selected subset of features. It follows that the trees depend on the values of an independently sampled input data set, using the same distribution for all trees.

In this case we also used the implementation provided in [29]. We have set the number of estimators to 250, even if we noticed that the results show little variation with estimators between 50 and 250. The maximum depth of the trees was set to 8, and the criteria used was the Entropy.

2.4.3. XGBoost

This algorithm, as well as other gradient boosting algorithms such as the well known Gradient Boosting Method (GBM), sequentially assembles weak models to produce a predictive model [31]. During this sequential procedure, a gradient descend procedure is applied. This procedure is repeated until a given number of trees has been induced, or when no improvement is registered. An important aspect of XGBoost is how the algorithm controls over-fitting, which is a a known issue in gradient boosting algorithms. XGBoost adopts a more regularized model formalization, which allows the algorithm to obtain better results than GBM. XGBoost is a method that has recently received much attention in the data science community, as it has been successfully applied in different domains. This popularity is mostly due to the scalability of the method. In fact, XGBoost can run up to ten times faster than other popular approaches on a single machine. Again, we used the Scikit-learn library for this algorithm. In this case the number of estimators was set to 100, the learning rate to 0.1 and the maximum depth to 3.

2.4.4. Deep Learning

Deep learning [32] is a subset of machine learning that incorporates computational models and algorithms that mimic the architecture of biological neural networks in the brain, such as Artificial Neural Networks (ANNs). In a rough analogy with biological learning system, ANNs consist of densely interconnected units, called neurons [33]. Each neuron receives several real valued input, e.g., from other neurons of the network, and produces a single real valued output. The output depends on an activation function used in each unit, which introduces non-linearity to the output. The activation function is used only if the input received by a unit is higher than a given activation threshold. If this is not the case, then no output is produced. Normally, an ANN consists of different layers of neurons. The term "Deep" refers to the number of such layers and complexity of an ANN. There are three types of layers: the input layer, the output layer, and the hidden layer (which extracts the patterns within the data). Therefore, as the data moves from one hidden layer to another, the features are recombined and recomposed into complex features. Because of this, deep learning works especially well with unstructured data, but requires a huge volume of training data. Deep learning has proven to be successful in different applications fields such as acoustics, imaging or natural language processing.

In this paper, we used the Multi-layer Perceptron (MLP) classifier provided by Sklearn library [28]. In particular, for the experiments performed on the K562 cellular line, we used an Alpha (regularization term) of 0.001, with an adaptive learning rate and a network consisting of 40 layers with 10 neurons on the first layer. Alpha forces the parameters to have small values for robustness. The optimal hyper-parameters used to train the MLP classifier for the GM12878 cell dataset were the same as for the K562 cell, except for the Hidden Layer Sizes which was set to 100 layers, with 20 neurons on the first layer. These parameters were experimentally determined.

We have also used the implementation offered by Keras library [34]. For K562 loops, we first tested a neural network made of two hidden layers: Layer 1, 120 neurons, relu activation; Layer 2, 10 neurons, relu activation; Layer 3 (output), 1 neuron, sigmoid activation. The resulting accuracy was 0.99 for training and 0.77 for testing, hinting at a possible overfit. We have also tested the same network architecture with a reduced dataset (removing features associated with RAD21 and CTCF), and obtained 0.99 for testing and 0.69 for testing. Since it is probable that the model has overfitted, we have decided to try out a separate architecture on the K562 cell line, that also included Dropout layers; specifically, the architecture looked like this: Layer 1, 120 neurons, relu activation; Layer D1, Dropout 0.2; Layer 2, 30 neurons, relu activation; Layer D2, Dropout 0.2; Layer 3, 10 neurons, relu activation; Layer 4 (output), 1 neuron, sigmoid activation. The results slightly improved, obtaining for the full dataset on training 0.99 and testing 0.79 (0.02 improvement). The results for the reduced dataset stayed the same.

For GM12878 loops, we obtained an accuracy of 0.99 on the full dataset for training and 0.81 for testing. When we tried the reduced dataset, the models yielded an accuracy of 0.99 for training and 0.66 for testing. Given the low difference between the accuracies of an architecture that includes Dropout layers, we decided not to train GM12878 on a dropout-enabled neural network. Then again, the proposed architecture probably overfits, but the accuracies obtained stay in line with the those obtained using other algorithms presented in this paper.

2.4.5. Support Vector Machines (SVM)

This supervised technique tries to find an hyperplane in a n-dimensional space (being n the number of features), capable of separating the training examples [35]. Several such hyperplanes may exist, and SVM aims at finding the one that maximazes the distance between data points of the classes. The hyperplane is basically the classification model, with data falling on one side of the hyperplane being assigned a class, while data falling on the other side are assigned the other class. Data are not always linearly separable, and in these cases, a kernel function is used in order to transform the original data points with the aim of mapping the original data points into a higher dimensional space where we can find a hyperplane that can separate the samples.

In this study we used the Radial Basis Function (RBF) kernel. The RBF kernel is an often used kernel for classification tasks [36]. In particular, the C-value for the RBF function was set to 100, after having performed several preliminary experiments.

To evaluate the methods, we used four popular measures [37]:

$$Accuracy = \frac{TP + TN}{TP + TN + FP + FN} \tag{2}$$

$$Precision = \frac{TP}{TP + FP} \tag{3}$$

$$Recall = \frac{TP}{TP + FN} \tag{4}$$

$$F1\text{-}Score = \frac{2 \times Precision \times Recall}{Precision + Recall} \tag{5}$$

In the above equation we used the following terminology:

- True Positive (TP): a true positive represents the case when the actual class matches the predicted class;
- True Negative (TN): a true negative is similar to a true positive, the only difference being that the actual and predicted classes are part of the negative examples;
- False Positive (FP): a false positive is the case when the actual class negative, but the example is classified as positive;
- False Negative (FN): similar to false positive, but it this case this refers to the case where a positive example is classified as negative.

3. Results and Discussion

3.1. Association of Genomic and Epigenomic Features with Chromatin Loops

We started by assessing the genomic and epigenomic landscape of chromatin loops. We used published ChIA-PET datasets targeting the cohesin complex component RAD21 [38] from two human cancer cell lines (Table S1), K562 and GM12878, identifying 3,290 and 5,486 chromatin loops, respectively. 1D sequencing datasets from ENCODE (ENCODE Project Consortium, 2012) were also collected in order to represent the chromatin features associated with loops and their genomic neighbourhoods (Figures 1 and S2). As expected, we observed a large colocalization of CTCF and RAD21 architectural proteins with loop anchors, in agreement with previously reported data [5,39]. On the other hand, whereas the repressive mark H3K27me3 and the gene body mark H3K36me3 were found to be dispersed along loops and across loop anchors, other regulatory marks were enriched both at loop anchors and inside the loops. Such is the case of Pol2, open chromatin measured by DNase-seq and several transcription factors. The same stands for H3K4me1 and H3K4me3, two well known markers for enhancers and promoters. These observations suggest that regulatory features measured by high-throughput sequencing provide a valuable source of information for the prediction of chromatin loops.

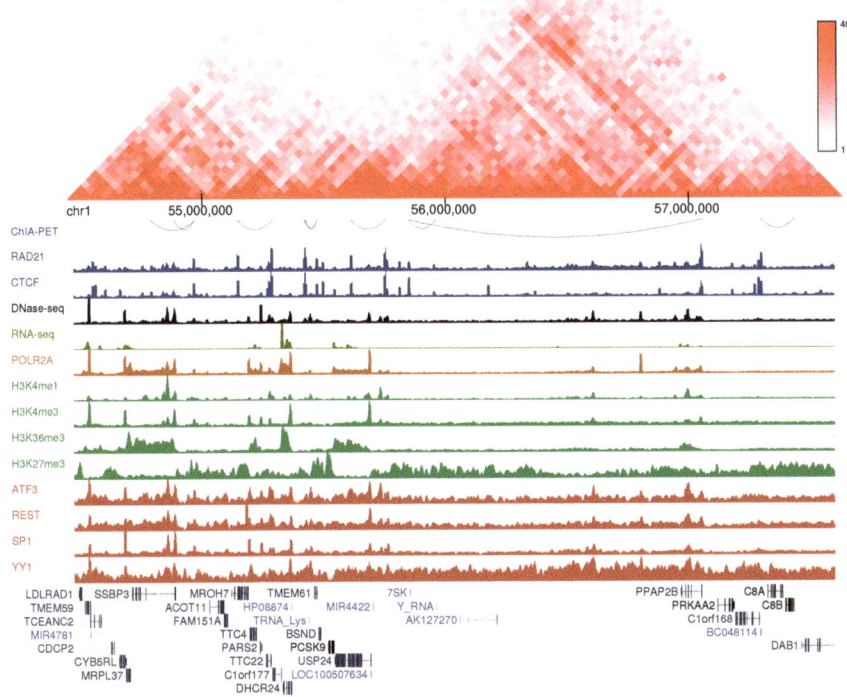

Figure 1. Chromatin features associated with RAD21 loops in GM12878 cell line. Hi-C interaction frequencies are shown in the top panel and ChIA-PET interactions are represented as blue arcs in the second panel. Then, a genome browser view for relevant chromatin features is displayed, including architectural factors (blue), DNase-seq (black), RNA-seq (yellow), RNA Pol2 (orange), histone marks (green) and transcription factors (red).

3.2. An Integrative Approach to Predict Chromatin Loops

To integrate sequencing features data into a predictive model of chromatin loops, we applied the computational framework of Figure 2. We first generated positive and negative sets of RAD21-associated chromatin loops. We used the experimental loops from the previous section as the positive set and the negative set was generated by combining pairs of RAD21 ChIP-seq peaks from ENCODE that do not overlap experimental loop anchors (see Material and Methods). Given the relative distribution of regulatory marks with respect to chromatin loops (Figure 1), we argued that these marks may affect loops not only at the anchors but also at the region between them. Therefore, to comprehensively measure the occupancy of chromatin features within and adjacent to each loop, we based our strategy on the approach of [27]. Given a loop with length L, we extended L base pairs to its left and right and the extended region (with length 3L) was partitioned into 1500 bins. For each bin, 23 high-throughput sequencing experiments (Table S1) were scored, resulting in a data matrix with rows representing loops and columns representing the scored experiments at each bin. Finally, we trained and tested classifiers in both cell lines using six machine learning algorithms. This design based on multi bins allowed us to measure the position-specific ability of sequencing data to predict chromatin loops with an unprecedented resolution. As a result, we ended up with model matrices of 34,500 columns and either 3290 (K562) or 5486 (GM12878) rows (Figure 2).

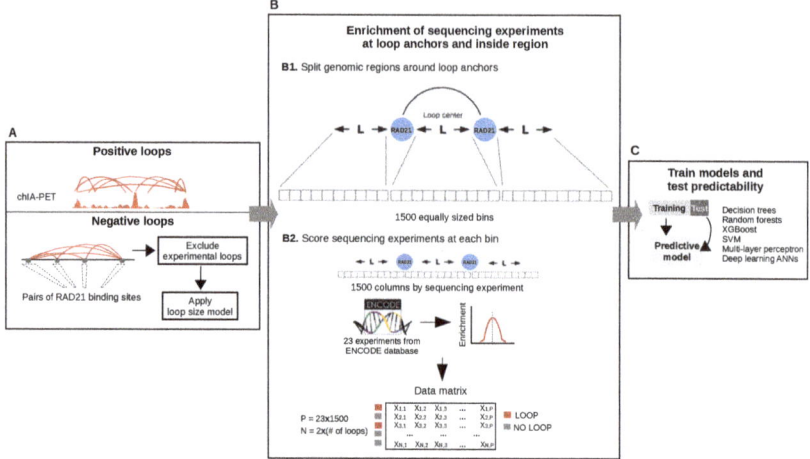

Figure 2. Illustration of the integrative machine learning schema for the prediction of chromatin loops. (**A**) Positive and negative RAD21-associated loops were first identified (see Methods). (**B**) Then, given a loop with length L, we extended L base pairs to its left and right and the extended region (with length 3L) was partitioned into 1500 bins. For each bin, 23 high-throughput sequencing experiments were scored, resulting in a data matrix with rows representing loops and columns representing the scored features. (**C**) Finally, we trained and tested classifiers using six machine learning algorithms. XGBoost: Gradient boosting; SVM: Support Vector Machines; ANN: Artificial Neural Networks.

3.3. Model Performance

The final feature matrices were divided into training (80%) and test (20%) and six classification algorithms were applied: decision trees, random forests, XGBoost, SVM, MLP and DL-ANN. To evaluate the performance of classification, trained models were applied to the test sets and several metrics were calculated including accuracy (Acc), precision, recall and F1-score. Accurate predictions were obtained by the six algorithms, with almost no differences on the performance metrics and with similar values in both cell lines (Tables 1 and 2). The smallest accuracies were obtained by DL-ANN, with values of 0.81 and 0.79 for GM12878 and K562, respectively. On the other hand, XGBoost significantly outperformed the rest of the methods, achieving accuracies of 0.95 and 0.96 for GM12878 and K562, respectively. As a matter of fact, the other four classification algorithms achieved very similar performance for GM12878 cell line, with Acc ranging from 0.81 to 0.83, while for K562 they ranged from 0.82 to 0.87. These results demonstrate that chromatin loops can be accurately predicted using our integrative approach and indicate that gradient boosting by XGBoost provides the best performance for this task.

Table 1. Machine learning performance of the proposed models in K562 cell line.

Algorithm	Accuracy	Precision	Recall	F1-Score
Decision Trees	0.8698	0.8707	0.8699	0.8698
Random Forests	0.8424	0.8469	0.8425	0.8419
XGBoost	0.9634	0.9638	0.9635	0.9635
SVM	0.8219	0.8224	0.8219	0.8218
MLP	0.8226	0.8231	0.8227	0.8226
Deep learning ANN	0.7930	0.7944	0.7930	0.7928

Table 2. Machine learning performance of the proposed models in GM12878 cell line.

Algorithm	Accuracy	Precision	Recall	F1-Score
Decision Trees	0.8313	0.8314	0.8313	0.8313
Random Forests	0.8262	0.8284	0.8263	0.8261
XGBoost	0.9474	0.9485	0.9475	0.9474
SVM	0.8087	0.8088	0.8088	0.8087
MLP	0.8322	0.8328	0.8323	0.8322
Deep learning ANN	0.8064	0.8065	0.8065	0.8065

3.4. Loop Anchors Are the Most Informative Regions

Next, we explored the most informative features for predicting chromatin loops. The design of our approach based on Handoko et al. [27] represents each chromatin feature as a 1500-bin array (Figure 2), which allowed us to comprehensively evaluate the contribution of a given feature according to its relative position within and at both sides of loops. Among the six methods we compared, DT, RF and XGBoost assign an importance measure during the training process, providing information on which repertoire of features are the most relevant in the classification. For this reason, and given that these algorithms showed better overall performance than SVM and MLP (Tables 1 and 2), the latter were excluded from this analysis. As expected, binding of architectural components (CTCF, RAD21) showed the highest predictive power in both cell lines and regardless the learning algorithm (Figures 3 and S3). We observed that the relative positions of the most informative features are highly biased towards genomic bins close to loop anchors. This is true for the top 10 important bins of both cell lines and for the three tested algorithms, suggesting that chromatin information between anchors in only modestly predictive.

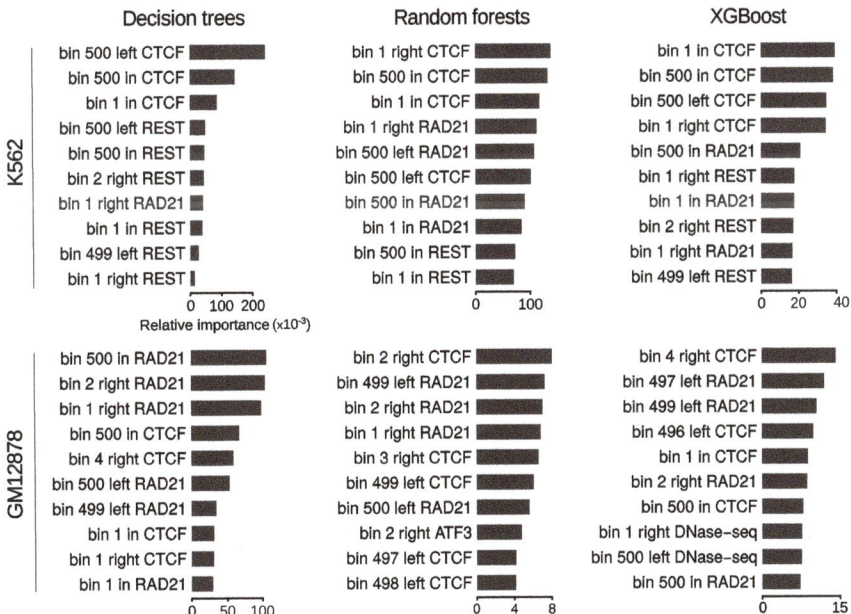

Figure 3. Ranking of top 10 important features for the prediction of RAD21 chromatin loops. Horizontal bars represent relative importances of featured bins. The terms 'left', 'in' and 'right' are used for bins from 1 to 500, 501 to 1000 and 1001 to 1500, respectively. The relative position of the bins within one of these 3 windows is also included in the feature names.

Although the three methods overall agreed on the top important features, while for DT the predictive power is concentrated in ~10 bins, this is not the case of RF and XGBoost, where it seemed to be more widely distributed (Figure S3). Among the top 10 important features of each algorithm in GM12878, bins associated with CTCF and RAD21 binding around loop anchors were largely predominant (Figure 3, bottom panel). The only exception was a bin associated with the transcription factor ATF3 at the right anchors, which was identified as the 8th most important feature by RF. On the other hand, in K562 REST was found together with CTCF and RAD21 among the top 10 important features by the three methods (Figure 3, top panel). Bins associated with this transcriptional repressor at loop anchors, although less informative, are as frequent as those associated with CTCF and RAD21.

The contribution of features that do not belong to the top 10 important ones greatly varies from one method to another. For example, DT and XGBoost reported several bins associated with histone marks among the top 30 important features in both cell lines, while this was never the case for RF (Figure S3). On the other hand, RF seemed to assign some predictive importance to DNase-seq and, in a lesser extent, to YY1, whereas these features were rarely found among the top 30 important features when using DT and XGBoost. These observations are likely to indicate that the contribution of such features is negligable compared to the top important ones.

Our design also allowed us to represent the contribution of each chromatin feature according to its relative position within and at both sides of loops (Figures 4, 5 and S4A–F). In agreement with the importance analysis, most of the predictive information for the majority of the evaluated chromatin datasets resides at the anchors and their close genomic vicinity. Besides the architectural components CTCF and RAD21, this is particularly prominent for DNase I hypersensitivity and transcription factors (Figures 4 and 5). Altogether, these results suggest that, in addition to architectural components, transcriptional features at the anchors contribute to chromatin wiring in RAD21-mediated loops.

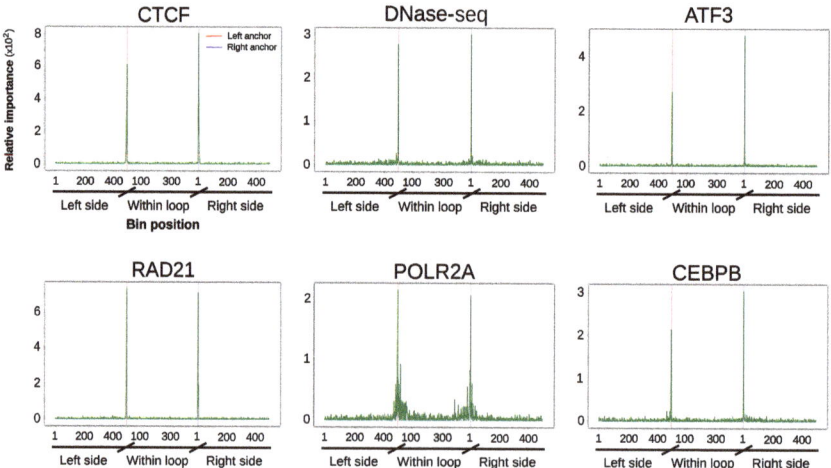

Figure 4. Position specific importance of selected high-throughput sequencing datasets in GM12878 cell line. Random forests importance score is shown for the 1500 bins corresponding to the most informative experiments. Coordinates of the x-axis are similar to those of Figure 5. Figure S4D–F display similar plots for all the tested datasets as well as for Decision Trees and XGBoost algorithms. CTCF: CCCTC-binding factor

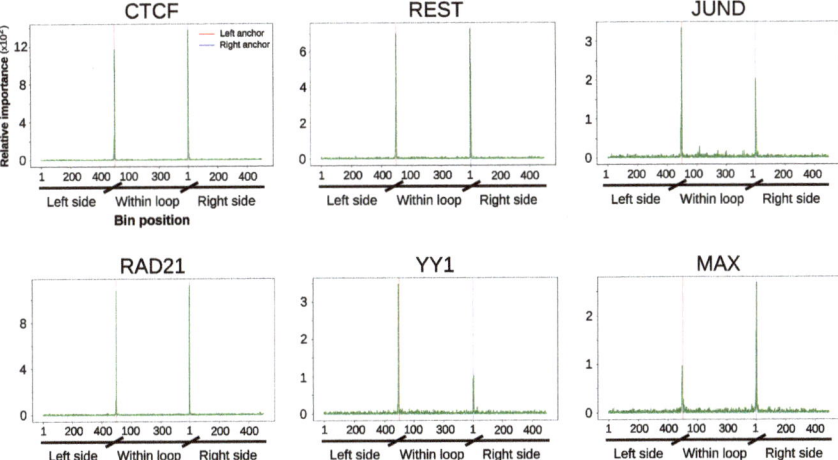

Figure 5. Position specific importance of selected high-throughput sequencing datasets in K562 cell line. Random forests importance score is shown for the 1500 bins corresponding to the most informative experiments. Coordinates of the x-axis are similar to those described in Figure 3, with left and right anchor position represented as red and blue vertical lines, respectively. Figure S4A–C display similar plots for all the tested datasets as well as for Decision Trees and XGBoost algorithms.

3.5. Removing Architectural Features Has a Modest Effect on XGboost Performance for K562

Given the importance of transcription associated factors in the final predictions, we next investigated whether these features alone can be used in order to predict chromatin loops. To this aim, we removed CTCF and RAD21 from the matrices and evaluated models trained with the rest of the datasets. We observed that the six algorithms decreased their performance, with significant differences in the acquired predictions and GM12878 showing more pronounced drops (Tables 3 and 4). The highest decrease was reported by DT in GM12878 cell line, which yielded an accuracy of 0.68, while when the whole set of features was used, the accuracy achieved was of 0.83 (Table 2). SVM, MLP and DL-ANN performance in both cell lines also seemed to be drastically affected by the removal of architectural factors. While these methods exhibited accuracies of 0.79–0.83 in the previous analysis, these values decreased to 0.66–0.73 after removing CTCF and RAD21 ChIP-seq data. Although its performance sensibly decreased in GM12878, XGboost was found again to achieve the best predictions. Strikingly, the performance of this algorithm was almost not affected by the removal of architectural components in K562 cell line, yielding an accuracy of 0.95 (Table 3). This result agrees with our previous analysis of relative importance, in which the binding of REST transcription factor at loop anchors was found to be among the most predictive features. We can then conclude that, at least in K562, transcription information alone is enough for the prediction of RAD21-mediated chromatin interactions.

Exploration of the most informative features in the new DT, RF and XGBoost models reveals that most of the predictive power resides in transcription factor binding and, to a lesser extend, DNase I hypersensitivity and Pol II binding (Figures 6 and S5). Again, we observed that the relative positions of these features were biased towards genomic bins in close proximity to loop anchors. Although different prediction accuracies were achieved by the three algorithms, overall the sets of top important features they provided were similar. Since XGBoost yielded the best performance, we focused on the importances reported by this algorithm. We observed that different transcription factors govern the contribution of the two cell lines. While bins associated with REST and MAX were predominant among the top 10 features in K562 (Figure 6, top and right), this was not the case in GM12878, for which ATF3 and CEBPB (together with DNAse-seq and Pol II) were found to contribute most to the predictions (Figure 6, bottom and right). Given the role that chromatin interactions play in gene regulation, these results agree with distinct gene regulatory programs being maintained through cell-type specific binding of transcription factors [40,41], and highlights transcriptional features as important determinants of chromatin wiring mediated by RAD21.

Table 3. Machine learning performance of models trained without architectural factors information in K562 cell line.

Algorithm	Accuracy	Precision	Recall	F1-Score
Decision Trees	0.8257	0.8259	0.8257	0.8257
Random Forests	0.7846	0.7877	0.7846	0.7840
XGBoost	0.9467	0.9469	0.9467	0.9467
SVM	0.7264	0.7264	0.7237	0.7228
MLP	0.7168	0.7202	0.7169	0.7157
Deep learning ANN	0.6872	0.6873	0.6872	0.6871

Table 4. Machine learning performance of models trained without architectural factors information in GM12878 cell line.

Algorithm	Accuracy	Precision	Recall	F1-Score
Decision Trees	0.6806	0.6817	0.6806	0.6805
Random Forests	0.7626	0.7648	0.7627	0.7624
XGBoost	0.8327	0.8334	0.8327	0.8327
SVM	0.7046	0.7068	0.7046	0.7042
MLP	0.7018	0.7061	0.7018	0.7008
Deep learning ANN	0.6608	0.6613	0.6608	0.6608

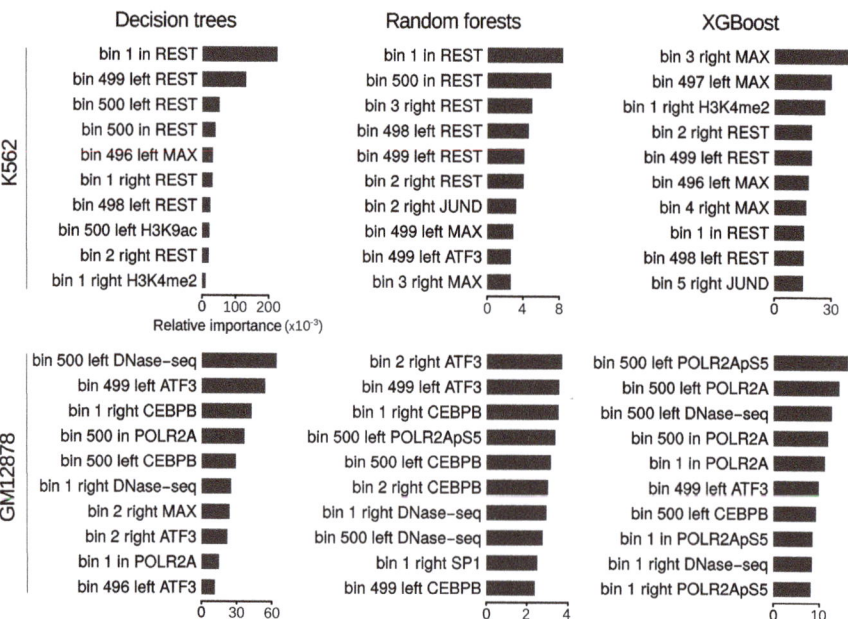

Figure 6. Ranking of top 10 important features for the prediction of RAD21 chromatin loops using only features associated with transcription. Horizontal bars represent relative importances as in Figure 3.

3.6. XGboost Models Achieve Accurate Predictions When Trained with Subsets of Chromatin Features

Since the removal of architectural components yielded different outcomes depending both on the algorithm type and the cell line, we next explored to what extent specific subsets of chromatin features provide different prediction abilities. To that aim, we trained and tested DT, RF and XGBoost models based on the following categories: *Architectural* (only bins associated with CTCF and RAD21), *TF* (bins associated with transcription factors ATF3, CEBPB, JUND, MAX, REST, SIN3A, SP1, SRF and YY1), *Architectural-anchors* (CTCF and RAD21 around loop anchors) and *TF-anchors* (TF around loop anchors). To only account for information around anchors, we restricted the model matrices to 100 bins centered at left and right anchors, respectively, obtaining 200 bins (out of the total 1500 bins; Figure 2b) for each chromatin feature belonging to the defined categories. As a matter of fact, we also included in the analysis the two categories explored in previous sections, which we named *All* (all bins, as in Sections 3.3 and 3.4) and *Transcription* (TF + DNase-seq + RNA-seq + histone marks, as in Section 3.5).

For all the evaluated subsets, XGBoost yielded the best performance in both cell lines (Figure 7 and Tables 1–4 and S2–S9), in agreement with our previous observations. We also observed that models trained with subsets restricted to bins around anchors achieved performance at least as accurate as those obtained using also bins within the loops, which confirms that genomic information away from the anchors poorly contributes to chromatin wiring prediction. Overall, different accuracies were observed for the grouped categories, with GM12878 models being more sensible to subset selection. In this sense, DT and XGBoost showed a similar behaviour (Figure 7, left and right panels and Tables 2, 4, S3, S5, S7 and S9). For both algorithms, performance of K562 models were found to be somehow stable across categories, achieving accuracies of 0.83–0.87 (DT) and 0.94–0.96 (XGBoost) (Figure 7, left and right panels and Tables 1, 3, S2, S4, S6 and S8). On the other hand, GM12878 models achieved greatly variable predictions for different subsets of features, with *TF* associated categories yielding the worst performance (0.660.68 and ~0.79 for DT and XGBoost, respectively). Conversely, *Architectural* categories were found among the most predictive ones, with accuracies of ~0.85 (DT) and ~0.93 (XGBoost) (Figure 7, left and right panels and Tables 2, 4, S3, S5, S7 and S9).

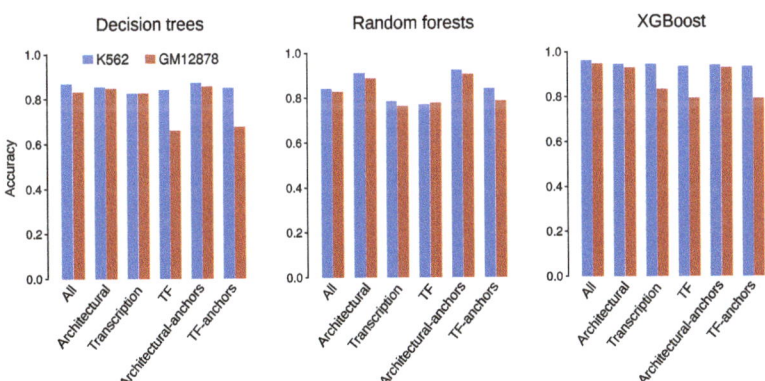

Figure 7. Accuracies of the Decision trees (DT), Random forests (RF) and XGBoost models trained with specific subset of chromatin features in K562 (blue) and GM12878 (red).

Unlike DT and XGBoost, RF performance seemed to be more consistent across cell lines and categories, with K562 achieving slightly better predictions (Figure 7, center panel and Tables 1–4 and S2–S9). *Architectural* associated categories yielded the best performance, with accuracies of 0.91–0.93 and 0.89–0.91 in K562 and GM12878, respectively. It is worth noting that *Architectural-anchors* not only outperformed *Architectural* category, but also models trained with all the datasets (*All*) in both cell lines. This is also true for DT (Figure 7, left panel), and highlights the importance of information around anchors for the prediction of long-range chromatin interactions.

As we mentioned before, XGBoost yielded the best predictions (Figure 7, right panel) in both cell lines. In the case of K562, high accuracies were achieved independently of the selected features, confirming our observation that, at least in this cell line, not only architectural but also transcription factors are important determinants of RAD21-associated chromatin wiring.

3.7. Prediction across Cell Types

We next asked to what extend our DT, RF and XGBoost models could be generalized from one cell line to another. Models trained on GM12878 and applied to K562 yielded overall good performance when using the whole set of chromatin features (Figure 8, right panel). Again, XGBoost outperformed the other two algorithms, obtaining an accuracy of 0.9. While DT showed a moderate accuracy of 0.75, RF seemed to be the worst suited method for cross cell line predictions, yielding an accuracy of 0.63. When evaluating the subsets of features described in the previous section, different predictive performance was observed for the grouped subsets. Since these differences were consistent across the three methods and XGBoost always obtained the best results, we focused our analysis on the accuracies provided by this algorithm (Figure 8, right panel, grey bar). While models trained with architectural factors achieved satisfactory accuracies (0.91–0.92), those trained with TF or transcription-associated features showed only modest prediction abilities (accuracies of 0.65–0.67). Given the overall high predictive power that transcriptional features showed when trained and applied on the same cell line (accuracies of 0.79–0.95), these observations highlight that, unlike architectural factors, transcriptional features are highly cell line specific in the context of chromatin wiring prediction.

Although a similar pattern of performance was observed for the different subsets of features when we trained models on K562 and applied to GM12878, this time prediction accuracies dramatically decreased to 0.53–0.64 (Figure 8, left panel). Since the remarkable performance obtained for models trained and tested on K562 were evaluated on data matrices that were not used for training, we discard a potential overfitting within this cell line. However, the significant differences observed in cross cell line applications of GM12878 and K562 models suggest that the latter might be overfitting the cell line specific chromatin feature associations with RAD21 chromatin wiring. Therefore, although the results derived from our K562 models are consistent with those obtained using GM12878 and with previous findings [22–25], we conclude that these models are not adequate for cross cell line predictions.

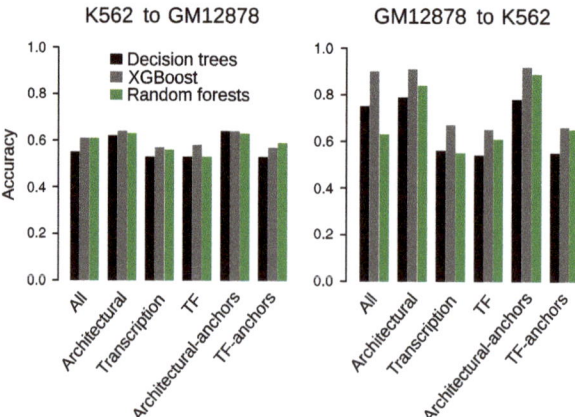

Figure 8. Cross cell lines accuracies of the DT, RF and XGBoost models trained with specific subset of chromatin features.

4. Conclusions

In light of our results, we propose XGBoost as the best suited algorithm for the prediction of long-range chromatin interactions. According to our data, XGBoost can be used to generate genome-wide maps of chromatin interactions, and information on a few chromatin features at the anchors may be enough to yield accurate predictions. For cross cell line application of the predictive models, architectural factors alone appear to be sufficient, while transcriptional features do not seem to have enough predictive ability, suggesting that they are highly cell line specific in the context of chromatin wiring. However, examination of other cell lines and tissues is needed to confirm these observations. Similarly, constructing generalizing models trained with datasets from several cell lines would overcome potential overfitting. In addition, analysis of interactions mediated by other proteins will help to clarify whether the observed performance for RAD21 mediated wiring in K562 can be generalized. Finally, prediction of de novo long-range chromatin maps genome-wide and subsequent comparisons with experimental data can be helpful to more comprehensively assess the predictive power of our strategy, as well as to exploit its full predictive potential.

Supplementary Materials: The following are available online at http://www.mdpi.com/2073-4425/11/9/985/s1. Figure S1: Top panels show heatmap representations of RAD21 and CTCF ChIP-seq reads enrichment within 10 kb around the anchors (0bp positions) of RAD21-associated chromatin loops. Bottom panels display average enrichment signals of the corresponding heatmaps. Plots were generated with seqplots [42], which extends or shrink regions within loops using linear approximation. Figure S2: Chromatin features associated with RAD21 loops in K562 cell line. Panels are those described in Figure 1. Figure S3: Ranking of top 30 important features for the prediction of RAD21 chromatin loops. Horizontal bars represent relative importances as in Figure 3. Figure S4: Position specific importances of the whole set of sequencing datasets in K562 (A–C) and GM12878 (D,E) cell lines for DT (A,D), RF (B,E) and XGBoost (C,F). Coordinates of the x-axis are similar to those described in Figure 3. Figure S5: Ranking of top 30 important features for models trained without architectural factors information. Figure S6: Position specific importances of the whole set of sequencing datasets in K562 (A–C) and GM12878 (D,E) cell lines for DT (A,D), RF (B,E) and XGBoost (C,F). Models were trained without architectural factors information. Figure S7: Ranking of top 30 important features for models corresponding to the described categories: *Architectural* (A), *TF* (B), *Architectural-anchors* (C) and *TF-anchors* (D). Table S1: Public data used in this study. Table S2: Performance of models trained with architectural factors binding information. K562 cell line. Table S3: Performance of models trained with architectural factors binding information. GM12878 cell line. Table S4: Performance of models trained with transcription factors binding information. K562 cell line. Table S5: Performance of models trained with transcription factors binding information. GM12878 cell line. Table S6: Performance of models trained with architectural factors binding information at loop anchors. K562 cell line. Table S7: Performance of models trained with architectural factors binding information at loop anchors. GM12878 cell line. Table S8: Performance of models trained with transcription factors binding information at loop anchors. K562 cell line. Table S9: Performance of models trained with transcription factors binding information at loop anchors. GM12878 cell line.

Author Contributions: P.M.M.-G., F.D. and W.V. supervised the project. P.M.M.-G. conceived the method and designed the data analysis. T.V., P.M.M.-G. and M.G.-T. wrote the code. T.V., P.M.M.-G., F.D., M.G.-T. and F.G.-V. analyzed the data. T.V., P.M.M.-G., F.D., M.G.-T. and W.V. interpreted the results. T.V., P.M.M.-G., F.D. and M.G.-T. wrote the paper. All authors have read and agreed to the published version of the manuscript.

Funding: This research was funded by grant TIN2015-64776-C3-2-R from the Spanish Government and the European Regional Development Fund.

Acknowledgments: We want to thank the Centro Informático Científico de Andalucía (CICA) for providing the high performance computing cluster, in which we performed all the analyses using custom scripts.

Conflicts of Interest: The authors declare no conflict of interest. The funders had no role in the design of the study; in the collection, analyses, or interpretation of data; in the writing of the manuscript, or in the decision to publish the results.

References

1. Bickmore, W.A.; Van Steensel, B. Genome architecture: Domain organization of interphase chromosomes. *Cell* **2013**, *152*, 1270–1284. [CrossRef] [PubMed]
2. Bonev, B.; Cavalli, G. Organization and function of the 3D genome. *Nat. Rev. Genet.* **2016**, *17*, 661–678. [CrossRef]

3. Rao, S.S.; Huntley, M.H.; Durand, N.C.; Stamenova, E.K.; Bochkov, I.D.; Robinson, J.T.; Sanborn, A.L.; Machol, I.; Omer, A.D.; Lander, E.S.; et al. A 3D map of the human genome at kilobase resolution reveals principles of chromatin looping. *Cell* **2014**, *159*, 1665–1680. [CrossRef] [PubMed]
4. Weintraub, A.S.; Li, C.H.; Zamudio, A.V.; Sigova, A.A.; Hannett, N.M.; Day, D.S.; Abraham, B.J.; Cohen, M.A.; Nabet, B.; Buckley, D.L.; et al. YY1 Is a Structural Regulator of Enhancer-Promoter Loops. *Cell* **2017**, *171*, 1573–1588. [CrossRef] [PubMed]
5. Dixon, J.R.; Selvaraj, S.; Yue, F.; Kim, A.; Li, Y.; Shen, Y.; Hu, M.; Liu, J.S.; Ren, B. Topological domains in mammalian genomes identified by analysis of chromatin interactions. *Nature* **2012**, *485*, 376–380. [CrossRef] [PubMed]
6. Nora, E.P.; Lajoie, B.R.; Schulz, E.G.; Giorgetti, L.; Okamoto, I.; Servant, N.; Piolot, T.; Van Berkum, N.L.; Meisig, J.; Sedat, J.; et al. Spatial partitioning of the regulatory landscape of the X-inactivation centre. *Nature* **2012**, *485*, 381–385. [CrossRef] [PubMed]
7. Lieberman-Aiden, E.; Van Berkum, N.L.; Williams, L.; Imakaev, M.; Ragoczy, T.; Telling, A.; Amit, I.; Lajoie, B.R.; Sabo, P.J.; Dorschner, M.O.; et al. Comprehensive mapping of long-range interactions reveals folding principles of the human genome. *Science* **2009**, *326*, 289–293. [CrossRef]
8. Zheng, H.; Xie, W. The role of 3D genome organization in development and cell differentiation. *Nat. Rev. Mol. Cell Biol.* **2019**, *20*, 535–550. [CrossRef]
9. Lupiáñez, D.G.; Kraft, K.; Heinrich, V.; Krawitz, P.; Brancati, F.; Klopocki, E.; Horn, D.; Kayserili, H.; Opitz, J.M.; Laxova, R.; et al. Disruptions of topological chromatin domains cause pathogenic rewiring of gene-enhancer interactions. *Cell* **2015**, *161*, 1012–1025. [CrossRef]
10. Kragesteen, B.K.; Spielmann, M.; Paliou, C.; Heinrich, V.; Schöpflin, R.; Esposito, A.; Annunziatella, C.; Bianco, S.; Chiariello, A.M.; Jerković, I.; et al. Dynamic 3D chromatin architecture contributes to enhancer specificity and limb morphogenesis. *Nat. Genet.* **2018**, *50*, 1463–1473. [CrossRef]
11. Li, Y.; Hu, M.; Shen, Y. Gene regulation in the 3D genome. *Hum. Mol. Genet.* **2018**, *27*, R228–R233. [CrossRef] [PubMed]
12. Schoenfelder, S.; Fraser, P. Long-range enhancer–promoter contacts in gene expression control. *Nat. Rev. Genet.* **2019**, *20*, 437–455. [CrossRef] [PubMed]
13. Sanborn, A.L.; Rao, S.S.P.; Huang, S.C.; Durand, N.C.; Huntley, M.H.; Jewett, A.I.; Bochkov, I.D.; Chinnappan, D.; Cutkosky, A.; Li, J.; et al. Chromatin extrusion explains key features of loop and domain formation in wild-type and engineered genomes. *Proc. Natl. Acad. Sci. USA* **2015**, *112*, E6456–E6465. [CrossRef] [PubMed]
14. Fudenberg, G.; Imakaev, M.; Lu, C.; Goloborodko, A.; Abdennur, N.; Mirny, L.A. Formation of Chromosomal Domains by Loop Extrusion. *Cell Rep.* **2016**, *15*, 2038–2049. [CrossRef] [PubMed]
15. Bouwman, B.A.; de Laat, W. Getting the genome in shape: The formation of loops, domains and compartments. *Genome Biol.* **2015**, *16*, 154. [CrossRef] [PubMed]
16. Nichols, M.H.; Corces, V.G. A CTCF Code for 3D Genome Architecture. *Cell* **2015**, *162*, 703–705. [CrossRef]
17. Busslinger, G.A.; Stocsits, R.R.; Van Der Lelij, P.; Axelsson, E.; Tedeschi, A.; Galjart, N.; Peters, J.M. Cohesin is positioned in mammalian genomes by transcription, CTCF and Wapl. *Nature* **2017**, *544*, 503–507. [CrossRef]
18. Dekker, J.; Marti-Renom, M.A.; Mirny, L.A. Exploring the three-dimensional organization of genomes: Interpreting chromatin interaction data. *Nat. Rev. Genet.* **2013**, *14*, 390–403. [CrossRef]
19. Vian, L.; Pękowska, A.; Rao, S.S.; Kieffer-Kwon, K.R.; Jung, S.; Baranello, L.; Huang, S.C.; El Khattabi, L.; Dose, M.; Pruett, N.; et al. The Energetics and Physiological Impact of Cohesin Extrusion. *Cell* **2018**, *73*, 1165–1178. [CrossRef]
20. Huang, J.; Marco, E.; Pinello, L.; Yuan, G.C. Predicting chromatin organization using histone marks. *Genome Biol.* **2015**, *16*, 162. [CrossRef]
21. Mourad, R.; Cuvier, O. Computational Identification of Genomic Features That Influence 3D Chromatin Domain Formation. *PLoS Comput. Biol.* **2016**, *12*, 1–24. [CrossRef] [PubMed]
22. Zhu, Y.; Chen, Z.; Zhang, K.; Wang, M.; Medovoy, D.; Whitaker, J.W.; Ding, B.; Li, N.; Zheng, L.; Wang, W. Constructing 3D interaction maps from 1D epigenomes. *Nat. Commun.* **2016**, *7*, 10812. [CrossRef] [PubMed]
23. Kai, Y.; Andricovich, J.; Zeng, Z.; Zhu, J.; Tzatsos, A.; Peng, W. Predicting CTCF-mediated chromatin interactions by integrating genomic and epigenomic features. *Nat. Commun.* **2018**, *9*, 4221. [CrossRef] [PubMed]
24. Al Bkhetan, Z.; Plewczynski, D. Three-dimensional Epigenome Statistical Model: Genome-wide Chromatin Looping Prediction. *Sci. Rep.* **2018**, *8*, 5217. [CrossRef] [PubMed]

25. Zhang, S.; Chasman, D.; Knaack, S.; Roy, S. In silico prediction of high-resolution Hi-C interaction matrices. *Nat. Commun.* **2019**, *10*, 5449. [CrossRef]
26. Consortium, E.P. An integrated encyclopedia of DNA elements in the human genome. *Nature* **2012**, *489*, 57–74. [CrossRef]
27. Handoko, L.; Xu, H.; Li, G.; Ngan, C.Y.; Chew, E.; Schnapp, M.; Lee, C.W.H.; Ye, C.; Ping, J.L.H.; Mulawadi, F.; et al. CTCF-mediated functional chromatin interactome in pluripotent cells. *Nat. Genet.* **2011**, *43*, 630–638. [CrossRef]
28. Pedregosa, F.; Varoquaux, G.; Gramfort, A.; Michel, V.; Thirion, B.; Grisel, O.; Blondel, M.; Prettenhofer, P.; Weiss, R.; Dubourg, V.; et al. Scikit-learn: Machine Learning in Python. *J. Mach. Learn. Res.* **2011**, *12*, 2825–2830.
29. Buitinck, L.; Louppe, G.; Blondel, M.; Pedregosa, F.; Mueller, A.; Grisel, O.; Niculae, V.; Prettenhofer, P.; Gramfort, A.; Grobler, J.; et al. API design for machine learning software: Experiences from the scikit-learn project. *arXiv* **2013**, arXiv:1309.0238.
30. Breiman, L. Random Forests. *Mach. Learn.* **2001**, *45*, 5–32. [CrossRef]
31. Chen, T.; Guestrin, C. XGBoost: A Scalable Tree Boosting System. In Proceedings of the 22nd ACM SIGKDD International Conference on Knowledge Discovery and Data Mining, San Francisco, CA, USA, 13–17 August 2016; pp. 785–794. [CrossRef]
32. Goodfellow, I.; Bengio, Y.; Courville, A. *Deep Learning*; MIT Press: Cambridge, MA, USA, 2016.
33. Haykin, S. *Neural Networks: A Comprehensive Foundation*, 2nd ed.; Prentice Hall PTR: Upper Saddle River, NJ, USA, 1998.
34. Chollet, F. *Keras: The Python Deep Learning Library*; Record ascl:1806.022; Astrophysics Source Code Library, 2018; p. 1806.
35. Hearst, M.A. Support Vector Machines. *IEEE Intell. Syst.* **1998**, *13*, 18–28. [CrossRef]
36. Chang, Y.W.; Hsieh, C.J.; Chang, K.W.; Ringgaard, M.; Lin, C.J. Training and Testing Low-degree Polynomial Data Mappings via Linear SVM. *J. Mach. Learn. Res.* **2010**, *11*, 1471–1490.
37. Powers, D.M.W. Evaluation: From precision, recall and f-measure to roc., informedness, markedness & correlation. *J. Mach. Learn. Technol.* **2011**, *2*, 37–63.
38. Haering, C.H.; Löwe, J.; Hochwagen, A.; Nasmyth, K. Molecular architecture of SMC proteins and the yeast cohesin complex. *Mol. Cell* **2002**, *9*, 773–788. [CrossRef]
39. Ivanov, D.; Nasmyth, K. A topological interaction between cohesin rings and a circular minichromosome. *Cell* **2005**, *122*, 849–860. [CrossRef]
40. Arvey, A.; Agius, P.; Noble, W.S.; Leslie, C. Sequence and chromatin determinants of cell-type-specific transcription factor binding. *Genome Res.* **2012**, *22*, 1723–1734. [CrossRef]
41. Rockowitz, S.; Lien, W.H.; Pedrosa, E.; Wei, G.; Lin, M.; Zhao, K.; Lachman, H.M.; Fuchs, E.; Zheng, D. Comparison of REST Cistromes across Human Cell Types Reveals Common and Context-Specific Functions. *PLoS Comput. Biol.* **2014**, *10*, 1–17. [CrossRef]
42. Stempor, P.; Ahringer, J. SeqPlots—Interactive software for exploratory data analyses, pattern discovery and visualization in genomics. *Wellcome Open Res.* **2016**, *1*, 14. [CrossRef]

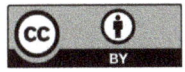

© 2020 by the authors. Licensee MDPI, Basel, Switzerland. This article is an open access article distributed under the terms and conditions of the Creative Commons Attribution (CC BY) license (http://creativecommons.org/licenses/by/4.0/).

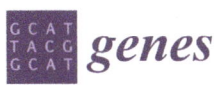

Article

metaRE R Package for Meta-Analysis of Transcriptome Data to Identify the *cis*-Regulatory Code behind the Transcriptional Reprogramming

Daria D. Novikova [1,2], Pavel A. Cherenkov [3], Yana G. Sizentsova [1] and Victoria V. Mironova [1,3,*]

[1] Institute of Cytology and Genetics, Lavrentyeva avenue 10, 630090 Novosibirsk, Russia; da6ik777@gmail.com (D.D.N.); sizentsova.yans@gmail.com (Y.G.S.)
[2] Laboratory of Biochemistry, Wageningen University, Stippeneng 4, 6708WE Wageningen, The Netherlands
[3] Novosibirsk State University, 2 Pirogova Street, 630090 Novosibirsk, Russia; cheburechko@gmail.com
[*] Correspondence: victoria.v.mironova@gmail.com

Received: 12 May 2020; Accepted: 5 June 2020; Published: 9 June 2020

Abstract: At the molecular level, response to an external factor or an internal condition causes reprogramming of temporal and spatial transcription. When an organism undergoes physiological and/or morphological changes, several signaling pathways are activated simultaneously. Examples of such complex reactions are the response to temperature changes, dehydration, various biologically active substances, and others. A significant part of the regulatory ensemble in such complex reactions remains unidentified. We developed *metaRE*, an R package for the systematic search for *cis*-regulatory elements enriched in the promoters of the genes significantly changed their transcription in a complex reaction. *metaRE* mines multiple expression profiling datasets generated to test the same organism's response and identifies simple and composite *cis*-regulatory elements systematically associated with differential expression of genes. Here, we showed *metaRE* performance for the identification of low-temperature-responsive *cis*-regulatory code in *Arabidopsis thaliana* and *Danio rerio*. MetaRE identified potential binding sites for known as well as unknown cold response regulators. A notable part of *cis*-elements was found in both searches discovering great conservation in low-temperature responses between plants and animals.

Keywords: meta-analysis; transcription factor; binding sites; genomics; transcriptomics; chilling stress; CBF; DREB; CAMTA1

1. Introduction

More than two decades have passed since the establishment of whole-genome expression profiling methods. Nowadays, thousands of transcriptomes are publicly available. Typically, several related experiments studying the same phenomenon can be found, thus, providing a rich set of material for analysis. Meta-analysis is applicable to sets of experiments testing the same hypotheses to extract robust signals and repetitive features that are impossible to derive from the individual experiments.

The typical example of meta-analysis is the definition of robust differentially expressed genes (DEGs) over many transcriptomic datasets. This approach is widely used in medical genomics to identify the gene signatures associated with a condition or disease, e.g., in [1–3]. To account for the most reliable and reproducible gene signatures, different authors applied such meta-analysis procedures as Fisher's methods, Stouffer's method, permutation, or machine-learning procedures. Recently, a ready-to-use framework GSMA has been developed to solve this task for any problem of interest [3].

Alternatively, a meta-analysis of transcriptome datasets can help to understand the *cis*-regulatory code behind the transcriptional response. The simplest way is to analyze the upstream regions of the robust DEGs for overrepresented sequences, e.g., as in [4,5]. However, the way to detect the robust gene sets might be comprehensive. He and coauthors (2016) analyzed DEGs in nine transcriptomic datasets on breast cancer: DEGs were identified by Fisher's method for *p*-values combination [6]. Subsequent enrichment analysis of motifs in promoters of DEGs was estimated by Fisher's exact test and allowed identifying transcription factors associated with breast cancer.

A better way to identify a full set of *cis*-elements, or a "cistrome", associated with a transcriptional response, is a meta-analysis of individual transcriptomes and not the robust DEGs. Authors of the cis-Metalysis program performed a meta-analysis of transcriptomics data on bee [7]. They revealed enrichment of transcription factors binding sites in the DEGs and their association with external factors that cause similar changes in the organism. An interesting approach has been applied to study the cistrome for iron deficiency response in Arabidopsis (*Arabidopsis thaliana*) roots [8]. Authors searched for the enrichment of *k*-mers in upstream regulatory regions of Fe-responsive genes taken from several experiments. They applied the machine learning algorithm, Random Forest, to identify enriched elements in different functional clusters of coexpressed genes revealed. However, on the different steps of their study, authors used separate tools and approaches aiming at a specific goal of identifying clusters of Fe-responsive genes regulated by the same pulls of *cis*-regulatory elements.

The methods for comprehensive meta-analysis of transcription profiles for *cis*-elements prediction described above have proven to be powerful in specific studies. However, they were not implemented in a ready-to-use package. Here, we developed a powerful but versatile pipeline for cistrome-wide meta-analysis, implemented as a *metaRE* R package. In this study, we show the performance of *metaRE* on cold-stress-responsive and hypothermia-responsive transcriptome datasets in Arabidopsis and zebrafish.

2. Materials and Methods

2.1. metaRE R Package Structure and Functionality

metaRE R package implements a pipeline to search for consensus sequences enriched in the promoters of DEGs. Its logic and methodology have been described in our earlier work [9], Here, we present the R package for the first time. We used C++ to speed up slow components and the *Rcpp* package to integrate the C++ code into R [10]. *metaRE* package performs a five-step analysis: (1) DEGs identification; (2) *cis*-regulatory consensus element search; (3) calculation of association between consensus presence and changes in gene expression; (4) meta-analysis over multiple datasets; (5) permutation test. The pipeline is detailed below and in Figure 1.

Software with source files, documentation, and example data files are freely available online at the repository (https://github.com/cheburechko/MetaRE).

2.1.1. DEGs Identification

As an input, *metaRE* uses transcriptome data. For users' convenience, we applied *GEOquery* [11], *limma* [12], and *edgeR* [13,14] packages to identify DEGs in the datasets from the GEO database [15]. *metaRE* function *prepareGEO* allows loading and adjusting the preprocessed GEO data frames. Functions *processMicroarray* and *processRNAcounts* could be used to identify DEGs in a single dataset using *limma* (microarray and RNA-seq, respectively), functions generate a new table for a particular experiment with user-defined expression classes. The function *preprocessGeneExpressionData* can perform the same analysis for multiple datasets at once, it generates the final data frame *GeneClassificationMatrix*, which combines information about DEGs from all experiments in the meta-analysis. Alternatively, the user can upload a data frame with already processed data on differentially expressed genes.

2.1.2. Cis-Regulatory Consensus Elements Search

Another input data for the *metaRE* package are the regulatory region sequences in *fasta* format. *MetaRE* uses the *Biostrings* R package [16] to upload the sequences from BioMart [17]. Next, *metaRE* annotates each sequence for the presence of a potential *cis*-element in the following format. Function *enumerateOligomers* searches for all possible *k*-mers without considering complementarity, e.g., in the case of hexamers, *metaRE* searches for 2080 nonredundant hexamers comprising 2016 complementary pairs and 64 palindromes instead of 4096 possible combinatorial variants. In addition to *k*-mers, it is possible to annotate systematically the regulatory regions with the information about all possible spaced repeats with the same *k*-mer as a core (*enumerateRepeats*), spaced bipartite elements with different *k*-mers as the cores (*enumerateDyadsWithCore*). It is also possible to search for a predetermined list of motifs described with 15 letters IUPAC ambiguity code (*enumeratePatterns*). For the *enumerateRepeats* and *enumerateDyadsWithCore* functions, it is possible to set maximum and minimum spacer length in both cases. *MetaRE* will search for *k*-mers' combinations with given spacer length diapason. For all the functions, the logic remains the same: reverse complement *k*-mers are considered to be the same element. Thus, the number of *k*-mers/bipartite elements/repeats/predetermined motifs in the analysis is reduced compared to the number of possible combinatorial variants.

The output of the second step of the procedure is a named list of integer vectors. Names are the consensus sequence; vectors are the indices of genes in which these sequences are present.

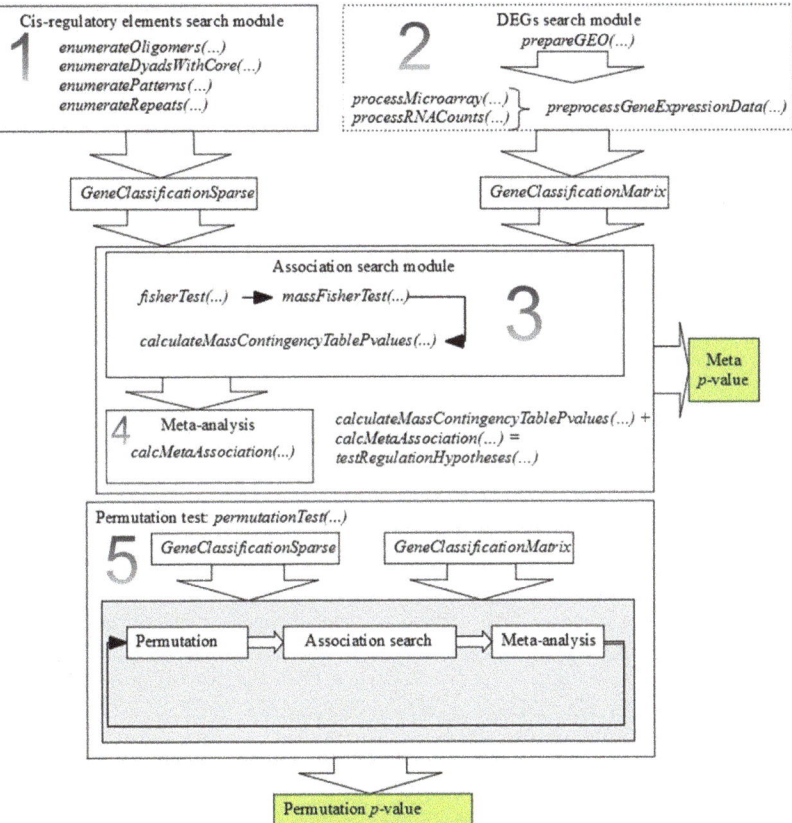

Figure 1. Scheme of *metaRE* modules that implement a five-step pipeline of the search for *cis*-elements significantly associated with differential gene expression over multiple datasets. DEGs—differentially expressed genes. Different modules are highlighted with squares; final sets of *p*-values are painted green. Described in the Methods steps are enumerated on the figure.

2.1.3. Calculation of Association Between Cis-Regulatory Element Presence and Changes in Gene Expression

At this step, for each *k*-mer and each experiment, an association with differentially expressed genes is estimated, separately for all regulation classes. A *p*-value for the association is calculated using a 2 × 2 contingency table by Fisher's exact test [9,18,19]. The test estimates the probability of getting such an association between two variables in the contingency table. In this case, the variables are "presence/absence of the *k*-mer" and "DEG/non-DEG". In *metaRE*, the procedure is implemented by a function *calculateMassContingencyTablePvalues*. The result is a float matrix of *p*-values for the association between the *k*-mer presence and up/downregulation, where, rows correspond to the *k*-mers, columns correspond to the datasets in which cells are calculated *p*-values.

2.1.4. Meta-Analysis

Function *calcMetaAssociation* used to combine the *p*-values calculated for a particular *k*-mer over many datasets. *MetaRE* uses Fisher's method to calculate meta-*p*-values (Figure 1, [9]). Due to multiple testing for many *k*-mers, *calcMetaAssociation* also estimates an adjusted *p*-value, for which the user can choose one of the following multiple correction methods: Bonferroni, Bonferroni–Holm [20,21], Benjamini–Hochberg [22], and Benjamini–Yakuteli [23]. Users also can set the cutoff threshold for adjusted meta-*p*-value—the *k*-mers which pass the cutoff are to be tested on Step (5).

2.1.5. Permutation Test

Finally, *metaRE* applies the permutation test to the *k*-mers with significantly adjusted meta-*p*-values. *MetaRE* uses the *foreach* package (CRAN project) for parallel permutation testing. *PermutationTest* function shuffles the regulatory regions between the genes and recalculates meta-*p*-value for each *k*-mer in the analysis. We optimized the procedure so that every iteration-run *permutationTest* stores the preliminary results in "outfile" and removes the *k*-mer that will not pass the cutoff threshold. After performing M permutations, *the function* computes the permutation *p*-value for *k*-mers left in the analysis as $p = (m + 1)/(M + 1)$, where m is a number of recorded *p*-values not greater than the meta-*p*-value. It also computes adjusted permutation-*p*-values to consider the multiple testing (for the amount of *k*-mers predetermined on Step (4)).

In the end, the *k*-mers with an adjusted permutation-*p*-value below the cutoff threshold are considered to be significantly associated with the differential expression.

2.2. Motifs Comparison

To annotate predicted *cis*-elements, we used the TOMTOM tool from Meme Suit [24] with the reference databases DAPv1, PBM, and Cis-BP. The best match with E-value < 0.05 was taken into the annotation.

2.3. Datasets

Arabidopsis and zebrafish transcriptome datasets on low positive temperature treatment were retrieved from the GEO database. 22 out of 40 datasets for *Arabidopsis thaliana* and 16 out of 24 datasets for *Danio rerio* passed the quality control for well-clustered replicas giving a sufficient number of DEGs (see Table S1). The identification of DEGs was made using the Benjamini–Hochberg method [22] to control the False Discovery Rate (FDR < 0.05).

3. Results

3.1. MetaRE R Package for Cistrome-Wide Association Study

We developed a *metaRE* R package which identifies the cistrome associated with the case of study via a meta-analysis of multiple transcriptomic experiments. *MetaRE* pipeline includes five steps: (1) DEGs identification in many transcriptomic datasets, (2) search for *cis*-regulatory elements in upstream gene sequences, (3) assessment of the association between *cis*-regulatory element presence and the changes in gene expression in each transcriptomic dataset, (4) meta-analysis over multiple datasets, and (5) permutation test to study the robustness of the prediction. The first step is performed in *metaRE* using standard R packages, or the user can upload processed data. At the second step, *metaRE* generates the information about the presence/absence of all combinatorially possible nucleotide sequences of a particular length and structure (encoded in the 15-nucleotide IUPAC alphabet) in a set of nucleotide sequences (for instance, promoter regions, transcription factors binding regions, etc.). We considered these short nucleotide sequences as potential regulatory elements of genes' expression. Since *metaRE* performs a search in the promoters which are located in *cis*-position relative to the genes, enriched in these promoters' sequences are predicted as potential *cis*-acting elements. The package allows the user to identify potential *cis*-regulatory elements of different lengths, which could consist of one element, repeats, or bipartite elements with a variable or fixed spacer and order of elements. In the third step, *metaRE* assesses the association between each *cis*-elements and differential gene expression in each of the datasets. At the fourth step, *metaRE* combines the *p*-values taken from the separate datasets and highlights which of the *cis*-elements are systematically overrepresented. In the last step, *metaRE* tests the independence of obtained results from external factors by the permutation test.

The main advantage of the *metaRE* package is that it identifies a reliable and reproducible set of potential *cis*-regulatory elements associated with the transcriptional response over many independent datasets, rather than in a single gene set. The R package can be used for the study cases on any organism with a sequenced genome. It is possible to adjust the procedure by changing the statistical tests, thresholds, *cis*-elements structure, promoters' length, etc. Other nucleotide sequences could be used instead of the promoters, e.g., 3′UTRs or ChIP-Seq profiles. Thus, *metaRE* gives the user freedom to adjust the package to the particular study, which is essential considering the differences and quality of raw data, annotation of the genome of different species, and knowledge on the location of *cis*-regulatory elements.

MetaRE was tested in several independent studies on different organisms, for instance, cold-induced zebrafish transcriptomes, dioxin-induced human and mouse transcriptomes, and auxin-induced Arabidopsis transcriptomes [9]. The application of *metaRE* was efficient for all of the cases. Here, we discuss *metaRE* performance to identify cold-responsive cistrome in Arabidopsis and zebrafish.

3.2. MetaRE for Identification of Cold-Responsive Cistrome

To demonstrate the utility of the *metaRE* package, we performed analysis on cold stress-induced transcriptomes in two model objects from animal and plant fields. All the datasets so far generated with good quality for *Arabidopsis thaliana* and *Danio rerio* (Table S1, [5,25–33]) have been processed independently using *metaRE*. On Step (1), *metaRE* identified DEGs (FDR < 0.05) lists for all of 22 and 16 transcriptomic datasets. We varied the threshold for fold-change from none to 1.5 and 2. As a result, three summary tables were generated for each organism summarizing information about the differential transcriptional response.

On Step (2), *metaRE* loaded Arabidopsis' and zebrafish' upstream regulatory regions [−1500; −1] of protein-coding genes from Ensemble BioMart Database (TAIR10 for *Arabidopsis thaliana* and GRCz11 for *Danio rerio*) [17,34]. *metaRE* annotated the upstream regions by the diversity of nonredundant *k*-mers. In this study, we searched for hexa-, hepta-, and octamers.

On Steps (3–5), *metaRE* identified all *k*-mers associated with the transcriptional cold stress response, separately for Arabidopsis and zebrafish. As the number of datasets for Arabidopsis allowed us to study time-resolved response, these cold-responsive transcriptome datasets were divided into two groups by the time of response: early response (up to six hours of cold exposure), and late response (12–24 h of cold exposure). We tried two multiple testing corrections (Bonferroni-Hochberg or Bonferroni) and set the stringent threshold for adjusted meta-p-value $< 1 \times 10^{-10}$ and adjusted permutation p-value $\leq 1 \times 10^{-3}$.

The summary tables for identified k-mers (Tables S2–S4) suggest that the cistrome size provided by *metaRE* depends on the parameter settings. However, the most significantly enriched cis-elements remain always the same. Noteworthy, to detect any motif associated with downregulation, we had to get rid of the threshold for fold-change to identify DEGs only by FDR. Despite a more stringent multiple testing correction applied for heptamers and octamers, *metaRE* found more of them in this study, compared to the number of significantly overrepresented hexamers (Tables S2–S4). This was not the case in another meta-analysis performed by *metaRE* [9]. We can explain this fact by significant enrichment of many degenerated A/T-rich motifs in the transcriptional response to cold for both Arabidopsis and zebrafish (Figure S1; discussed below). To sum up, we recommend performing a preliminary analysis under different settings to define the most appropriate one. Below we discuss only the results obtained under the stringent Bonferroni criterium for hexamers.

3.3. Analytics on Cold-Stress-Responsive Cistrome for Arabidopsis thaliana

We detected 95/43 and 10/26 hexamers associated with up- and downregulation in the early/late cold stress response (Table 1). A strong bias in a cistrome diversity was detected towards the early activatory response, but apparently, it correlates with many AT-rich elements found overrepresented in the upstream regions of early cold-responsive genes (even more AT-rich motifs were found in septamers and octamers; Figure S1; Tables S2 and S3). Another trend is that cold-responsive cistrome has fewer cis-elements associated with downregulation than with upregulation. With only one exception, E-box CACGTG, hexamers were explicitly associated with either up- or downregulation.

Table 1. Summary of predicted hexamers associated with cold stress response in Arabidopsis.

	Early Response (<6 h)	Late Response (>12 h)
Up	95	43
Down	10	26
Without A/T-rich hexamers		
Up	25	40
Down	10	26

Next, we applied the TOMTOM tool [24] to annotate the predicted cis-elements associated with early and late cold response. We were able to annotate more than 65% of detected cis-elements, however, many AT-rich elements and elements related to downregulation remained unidentified (Tables S2–S3). Many of the hexamers associated with the cold stress response significantly match the binding sites of known cold response regulators from CAMTA, AP2/ERF, bHLH, MYB, and bZIP families (Figure 2A) and this fitness confirms the adequacy of *metaRE* pipeline.

The binding sites for C-REPEAT BINDING FACTORs (CBFs) transcription factors from AP2/ERF family (CCGACA, ACCGAC; GCCGAC, CCGACC) were expected to be found as associated with the transcriptional cold response, as CBFs are the major regulator of cold acclimation [35–38]. However, CBF binding sites were not the most abundant and significant in early response (Table S2). The most significantly enriched in early response to cold stress motifs appeared to be: (1) ACGCGT (adjusted meta-p-value = 5.96×10^{-84}), the potential binding sites for CAMTA; (2) CACGTG ($p = 1.52 \times 10^{-54}$), the G-box bound by bHLH and bZIP transcription factors; (3) ACACGT ($p = 2.3 \times 10^{-53}$), the motif bound by NAC, BES, bZIP, and bHLH transcription factors; (4) ACGTGG ($p = 2.65 \times 10^{-52}$), potential binding site for bZIP and bHLH; and (5) a group of AT-rich elements ($3.47 \times 10^{-11} < p < 2.89 \times 10^{-50}$). The involvement of transcription factors bound to (1) – (4) with the cold response was known beforehand [28,39–44]. However, the fact that they are more relevant to early cold response comparing CBF binding sites is tempting, as CBF factors were recently shown to be involved in freezing not chilling resistance and may not be essential to survive in response to low positive temperatures [33,45]. Potential binding sites for CBFs were found the most significant for the late response to cold (Table S3).

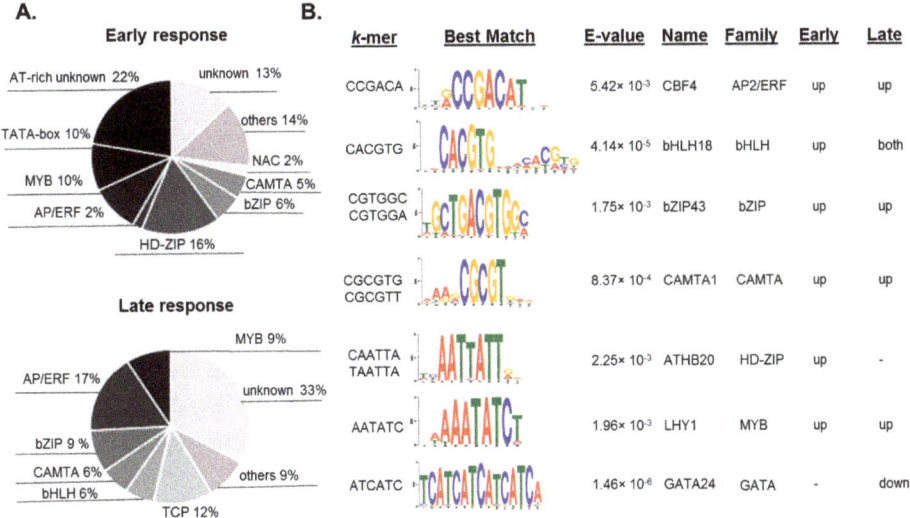

Figure 2. *Cis*-regulatory elements predicted with *metaRE* as systematically enriched in upstream regulatory regions of cold-induced genes in Arabidopsis. (**A**) Annotation of the hexamers to the known binding sites of *Arabidopsis thaliana* with the help of the TOMTOM tool [24]. Only significant best matches (E-value < 0.05, one per hexamer) were calculated to build the round diagram. (**B**) Annotation details for particular hexamers associated with early, late, or both early and late responses. The best significant matches of the hexamers with the known binding sites associated with downregulation in response to cold stress.

However, most of the detected AT-rich elements remain unknown; some of these sequences significantly match (TOMTOM, E-value < 0.05) the known binding sites for HD-ZIP and MYB families (Table S3, Figure 2B). Although it is not clear if the detected association with HD-ZIP transcription factors is relevant, the involvement of LHY1 and CCA1 MYB transcription factors into cold stress has been discussed in several works [39,46–48]. The motifs associated with downregulation were also poorly annotated. Among the rare examples of annotated motifs associated with downregulation are GATGAT/ATCATC, the potential binding site of GATA transcription factors (Figure 2B), and a family of potential TCP-binding motifs (Table S3). These results demonstrate the perspectives of *metaRE* usage in the study of the *cis*-regulatory code behind transcriptional reprogramming in complex reactions. It allows not only predicting the diversity of involved *cis*-elements and respective transcription factors but also ranking them and clarifying their role in certain phases of transcriptional response.

3.4. Analytics on Hypothermia-Related Cistrome for Danio rerio

A similar study for zebrafish yielded 67 hexamers enriched in promoters of hypothermia-induced genes. As for predicted cold-associated elements in Arabidopsis, most of the zebrafish ones are associated with upregulation and there are many A/T-rich hexamers (Table S4). The only motif associated with both upregulation and downregulation is CGGAAG, the potential binding site for ETS transcription factor Elk1 (E-value < 2.64×10^{-4}). In vertebrates, the role of Elk1 transcriptional activator was widely discussed in relation to many developmental processes [49,50], but not in the response to the low-temperature stress. In *Danio rerio*, it was only shown that Elk1 and its homologs express around the developing bone [51]. Unfortunately, *cis*-elements and transcription factors from *Danio rerio* genome are much less annotated comparing to Arabidopsis. We were not able to annotate overlapped hexamers (AAACGT, AACGTT, and ACGTTA), that show the greatest association with the hypothermia condition, using publicly available data. However, we assume that they compose the binding site for zebrafish' transcriptional regulator(s) that mediate the low-temperature responses.

One-third of hypothermia-related hexamers have been annotated using TOMTOM (E-value < 0.05). Among them: (1) two groups of AT-rich motifs resembling the binding sites for Dmrt2a (AATTTA, ATACAT, AATATA, ATAAAT, AATGTA, $2.61 \times 10^{-32} < p < 8.09 \times 10^{-22}$) and the binding sites for Homeobox transcription factors (CATAAA, AATTAA, ATAAAA, $p < 3.7 \times 10^{-11}$); (2) potential binding sites for bHLH transcription factors ACATAT ($p = 2.19 \times 10^{-22}$) and CACGTG ($p = 4.4 \times 10^{-17}$); (3) potential bZIPs binding sites (CGTCAC, CCGCCA, GACGTA, $p < 8.74 \times 10^{-14}$); (4) ACCAAT, the binding site for Nfya ($p = 5.28 \times 10^{-18}$), and many others (Table S4). E-box CACGTG, A/T-reach sequences, and Nfya binding sites have been associated with the cold stress response in zebrafish earlier [33,52]. Although we have not found in the literature strong evidence for the other hypothermia-related elements to mediate low-temperature response, this might be due to the fact that this topic is largely understudied in zebrafish [33].

Unexpectedly, but a notable part of hypothermia-related motifs (27 out of 67) identified by *metaRE* for *Danio rerio* matched those identified as cold-responsive for Arabidopsis. Among them E-box CACGTG and a group of A/T-rich elements. We discuss this finding further in Section 4.2.

4. Discussion

4.1. metaRE Tool for Identification of Cis-Regulatory Elements Repertoire

The main idea behind the method implemented in the *metaRE* R package is that if the *cis*-regulatory elements are involved in a transcriptional response, then they should be overrepresented in the promoters of differentially expressed genes. This idea is not new, and there are many approaches facilitating the analysis of *cis*-elements overrepresentation within upstream regions of pre-compiled gene sets, e.g., in [6,53–55]. The pipeline which analyzes *cis*-elements overrepresentation systematically and summarizes the output taken from many independent datasets has been still required, these tasks were solved in the *metaRE* R package.

The novelty of the *metaRE* method lies in: (1) taking into account a large number of comparable transcriptome experiments, and (2) the consideration of enrichment significance for an individual *cis*-element. Usually, authors evaluate the enrichment of *cis*-elements in one or more gene lists independently; the results of enrichment between the lists are not compared [4,5]. In this case, information about differences in the degree of enrichment of the same *cis*-element in different datasets is leveled, which can lead to over- and underpredictions. The method underlying *metaRE* solves this problem.

Separate studies showed that systematic analysis of transcriptome datasets is powerful in the identification of the cistrome behind a complex reaction [7,8,19]. The basic assumption in these studies, as well as in the *metaRE* algorithm, is that only robust and significant *cis*-element association with transcriptional response will be detected across multiple, diverse transcriptomic datasets that test similar experimental variables. This could be considered both as an advantage and as a disadvantage of the systematic analysis. On the one hand, analysis of several datasets excludes a bias that could be caused by separate experiments (tissue sampling, treatment duration, concentration, growth conditions, quality of data, etc.). Thus, meta analysis would detect the major *cis*-elements that operate under a variety of conditions. On the other hand, this approach will miss rare and condition-specific *cis*-elements. The latter could be solved by separate analysis of the datasets from experiments performed on different tissues, so one can have a tissue-specific cistrome. For example, in this study for cold-stress-responsive cistrome, as well as in [9] for auxin-regulated cistrome, we saw apparent differences in time-resolved results. If the number of transcriptomes allowed, these differences would be detected for tissue- and condition-specific reactions.

Cis-elements enrichment analysis is especially powerful when performed using the position weight matrices (PWM) for known transcription factors. E.g., using Homer [54], one can yield the list of exact regulators whose binding sites are overrepresented in the upstream regions of candidate genes. However, in *metaRE* we intentionally used a simpler consensus model for identification of overrepresented elements, making it more versatile and applicable for more organisms. First, for almost all organisms, including the model ones, the binding sites of most transcription factors remain unknown. Moreover, only very few organisms have PWMs for at least a hundred transcription factors (e.g., *Saccharomyces cerevisiae, Arabidopsis thaliana, Drosophila melanogaster, Caenorhabditis elegans, Mus musculus, Homo sapiens*) [56]. Second, *metaRE* could be applied not only to the upstream regions but to any sequences associated with the genes to find the signals unrelated to transcription factor DNA binding and not described by PWMs. For example, analyzing the 3′UTR *metaRE* could help identify the sites for the miRNA seeds binding. Third, in the present study of cold-responsive *cis*-elements, consensus search in *metaRE* with the subsequent analysis of identified sequences using PWMs for known transcription factors in TOMTOM [24] was shown to be very fruitful, with more than 65% of the elements annotated in Arabidopsis. We believe that the hybrid approaches with preliminary screening for enriched consensuses and subsequent annotation and reanalysis of the data using more powerful models are in need. Like an approach used in the study to annotate transcription factor binding sites in Nannochloropsis spp. microalgae [57].

4.2. Hypothermia-Related and Cold-Stress Responsive Cistromes in Zebrafish and Arabidopsis

Here, we employ *metaRE* in the investigation of widely studied processes, cold stress response, in which molecular mechanisms are still full of gaps. We performed an analysis using datasets generated for model objects in plant and animal fields, Arabidopsis, and zebrafish.

For plants, the cold stress response was studied in more detail, so that we were able to infer more data. Large-scale transcriptome studies showed that the CBF1-3, the major regulators of cold acclimation, in fact, regulate only a small portion of cold-responsive genes [27,30,45,58] which means that other regulators may exist. Here, we see that CBFs binding sites are, indeed, not overrepresented in early cold stress response as the potential binding sites for other transcription factors (Table S2). CBFs binding sites seemed to be the most overrepresented in the late response (Table S3), which explains why only a small portion of cold-responsive genes are CBF-regulated. The most significantly enriched *cis*-element in early cold stress response detected by *metaRE* was the potential binding site for CAMTA (Figure 1, Table S1). CAMTA1-3 are known upstream regulators of CBF1-3, they increase freezing tolerance via activation of ~15% cold-responsive genes [28,40].

Park et al. (2015) found that, in parallel with CBF genes, 27 other "first-wave" transcription factor genes were highly upregulated at an early stage of cold treatment. Analysis of gene expression in transgenic plants overexpressing 11 of these first-wave transcription factors identified four transcription factors from bZIP family (ZAT12, ZF, ZAT10, and CZF1) and heat-shock factor HSFC1 involved in the regulation of cold-stress-responsive genes [27,45,59]. *metaRE* identified bZIP transcription factors binding sites as one of the most significantly enriched in promoters of early responsive to cold genes (Figure 2; Table S2), however, their impact was not that big in the late response.

Another interesting result relates to the *cis*-elements overrepresented in the promoters of downregulated by cold genes, which regulatory mechanisms are completely unknown. Here, we found potential binding sites for GATA and TCP transcription factors, as well as many unknown motifs.

A further experimental study is required to clarify the role of predicted unknown *cis*-elements, they could be rare versions of transcription factors binding sites, or form the biochemical environment for transcription factors binding, or be involved in chromatin structure formation. Anyway, to study these hypotheses experimental investigations are required. The role of candidate genes like GATA, HD-Zip, TCP, and others in the cold stress response still lacks the total understanding and explanation which we need to search for with experimental approaches.

Although we found a great number of transcriptomes generated on zebrafish under suboptimal temperatures, the mechanisms of cold acclimation for this animal appeared to be largely unknown. In one of the few studies, a comprehensive analysis of the *cis*-regulatory code behind the low-temperature response has been performed [33]. In 16 RNA-Seq experiments, the authors inferred 33 gene clusters with common or tissue-specific expression patterns and then searched with the DREME tool [60] for *cis*-elements overrepresented in the clusters. As a result, they identified 17 octamers, overrepresented in one of the clusters, and experimentally verified two of them, AG(A/C)AACCA and (C/G)AGTCA. Here, we have applied an alternative strategy to search for the systematically enriched *cis*-elements over the same set of transcriptomes using *metaRE*. Notably, but not unexpectedly, that the *cis*-elements identified by [33] and in the present study were largely different; however, we both detected Nfya binding sites and a set of A/T-rich elements.

An exciting finding was that *cis*-elements detected in two separate *metaRE* studies for Arabidopsis and zebrafish significantly overlap by 27 hexamers. E-box motif CACGTG was highly overrepresented in promoters of both hypothermia-induced zebrafish' and cold-stress-induced Arabidopsis' genes. The E-box elements are known to be bound by bHLH transcription factors in many species including Arabidopsis and zebrafish [61]. In zebrafish, bHLH are involved in the control of developmental processes, one of which muscle development—is highly influenced by cold exposure [62]. The experimental study of E-box in the promoter of circadian clock gene Per4 showed that the amplitude of E-box-driven rhythmic expression response to temperature [52].

In both searches, *metaRE* detected the overrepresentation of A/T-rich sequences. Earlier, we got a similar result for auxin-regulated cistrome in Arabidopsis [9], but not in other studies (data not shown). The role of A/T-rich sequences can be different: they might be the parts of A/T-rich transcription factors binding sites (e.g., for Homeobox Factors), or they might be the TATA-box sequences, or they might be a part of chromatin landscape. The half of A/T-rich sequences identified for Arabidopsis were annotated by TOMTOM either as HD-ZIP binding sites or as TATA-boxes. As for *Danio rerio*, A/T-rich motifs were recognized as the potential binding sites of ZF (Zinc Finger) and Homeobox transcription factors. Homeobox transcription factors are known as development regulators [63]. Since exposure to low-temperatures crucially influences the developmental processes their involvement could be required. Unannotated AT-rich sequences still can predict a specific epigenetic landscape; in plants, cold-induced genes show enhanced chromatin accessibility, and a large number of active genes in cold-stored potato tubers are associated with a bivalent H3K4me3-H3K27me3 mark [64].

Temperature response is one of the basic stress responses with which primitive organisms had to cope millions of years before the separation of plant and animal kingdoms in evolution. Thus, we believe that comparative studies of the *cis*-elements conservation between plants and animals will help to clarify the mechanisms of low-temperature response. To do that, a more rigorous meta-analysis study on many organisms is in need. *metaRE* provides a framework of how this can be studied when a sufficient number of transcriptomes is generated.

Supplementary Materials: The following are available online at http://www.mdpi.com/2073-4425/11/6/634/s1, Figure S1: The percentage of A/T-rich motifs among predicted k-mers ($n = 6$–8) detected in promoters of differentially expressed genes with different settings (nFC - no threshold for fold-change; FC1.5 - the threshold is fold-change 1.5; FC2 is fold-change 2)., Table S1: The list of cold-stress-responsive transcriptome datasets taken for meta-analysis with metaRE, Table S2: *Cis*-elements associated with early cold stress response on Arabidopsis, Table S3: *Cis*-elements associated with late cold stress response on Arabidopsis, Table S4: *Cis*-elements associated with hypothermia on zebrafish.

Author Contributions: Methodology, V.V.M., D.D.N., and P.A.C.; software, P.A.C.; validation and investigation, V.V.M., D.D.N., P.A.C., and Y.G.S.; writing—original draft preparation, D.D.N. and V.V.M.; writing—review and editing, V.V.M., D.D.N., P.A.C., and Y.G.S.; visualization, D.D.N., P.A.C., and Y.G.S.; supervision, V.V.M.; funding acquisition, V.V.M. All authors have read and agreed to the published version of the manuscript.

Funding: *metaRE* development was funded by Russian Foundation for Basic Research, grant number 18-04-01130, and by Russian State Budget, project number 0259-2019-0008-C-01. D.D.N. was supported by a PhD sandwich fellowship from Wageningen Graduate School. The study of cold stress response was supported by Russian Science Foundation, grant number 18-74-10008.

Acknowledgments: We thank Ivo Grosse, Nadya Omelyanchuk, Jian Xu and Dolf Weijers for fruitful discussions and inspiration. We are grateful to Viktor Levitsky for consultations on the technical part of the algorithm. We acknowledge the Center of Shared Facilities "Bioinformatics" in IC&G for providing us an access to high performance computing facilities.

Conflicts of Interest: The authors declare no conflicts of interest. The funders had no role in the design of the study; in the collection, analyses, or interpretation of data; in the writing of the manuscript, or in the decision to publish the results.

References

1. Rhodes, D.R.; Yu, J.; Shanker, K.; Deshpande, N.; Varambally, R.; Ghosh, D.; Barrette, T.; Pandey, A.; Chinnaiyan, A.M. Large-scale meta-analysis of cancer microarray data identifies common transcriptional profiles of neoplastic transformation and progression. *Proc. Natl. Acad. Sci. USA* **2004**, *101*, 9309–9314. [CrossRef] [PubMed]
2. Phan, J.H.; Young, A.N.; Wang, M.D. Robust Microarray Meta-Analysis Identifies Differentially Expressed Genes for Clinical Prediction. *Sci. World J.* **2012**, *2012*, 1–9. [CrossRef] [PubMed]
3. Shafi, A.; Nguyen, T.; Peyvandipour, A.; Draghici, S. GSMA: An approach to identify robust global and test Gene Signatures using Meta-Analysis. *Bioinformatics* **2019**, btz561. [CrossRef] [PubMed]
4. Bargmann, B.O.R.; Vanneste, S.; Krouk, G.; Nawy, T.; Efroni, I.; Shani, E.; Choe, G.; Friml, J.; Bergmann, D.C.; Estelle, M.; et al. A map of cell type-specific auxin responses. *Mol. Syst. Biol.* **2013**, *9*, 688. [CrossRef]
5. Vogel, J.T.; Zarka, D.G.; Van Buskirk, H.A.; Fowler, S.G.; Thomashow, M.F. Roles of the CBF2 and ZAT12 transcription factors in configuring the low temperature transcriptome of Arabidopsis: Arabidopsis low temperature transcriptome. *Plant J.* **2004**, *41*, 195–211. [CrossRef]
6. He, H.; Cao, S.; Niu, T.; Zhou, Y.; Zhang, L.; Zeng, Y.; Zhu, W.; Wang, Y.; Deng, H. Network-Based Meta-Analyses of Associations of Multiple Gene Expression Profiles with Bone Mineral Density Variations in Women. *PLoS ONE* **2016**, *11*, e0147475. [CrossRef]
7. Ament, S.A.; Blatti, C.A.; Alaux, C.; Wheeler, M.M.; Toth, A.L.; Le Conte, Y.; Hunt, G.J.; Guzman-Novoa, E.; DeGrandi-Hoffman, G.; Uribe-Rubio, J.L.; et al. New meta-analysis tools reveal common transcriptional regulatory basis for multiple determinants of behavior. *Proc. Nat. Acad. Sci. USA* **2012**, *109*, E1801–E1810. [CrossRef]
8. Schwarz, B.; Azodi, C.B.; Shiu, S.-H.; Bauer, P. Putative *cis*-Regulatory Elements Predict Iron Deficiency Responses in Arabidopsis Roots. *Plant Physiol.* **2020**, *182*, 1420–1439. [CrossRef]
9. Cherenkov, P.; Novikova, D.; Omelyanchuk, N.; Levitsky, V.; Grosse, I.; Weijers, D.; Mironova, V. Diversity of *cis*-regulatory elements associated with auxin response in Arabidopsis thaliana. *J. Exp. Bot.* **2018**, *69*, 329–339. [CrossRef]
10. Eddelbuettel, D. *Seamless R and C++ Integration with Rcpp*; Springer: New York, NY, USA, 2013; ISBN 978-1-4614-6867-7.
11. Davis, S.; Meltzer, P.S. GEOquery: A bridge between the Gene Expression Omnibus (GEO) and BioConductor. *Bioinformatics* **2007**, *23*, 1846–1847. [CrossRef]
12. Ritchie, M.E.; Phipson, B.; Wu, D.; Hu, Y.; Law, C.W.; Shi, W.; Smyth, G.K. limma powers differential expression analyses for RNA-sequencing and microarray studies. *Nucleic Acids Res.* **2015**, *43*, 47. [CrossRef]
13. Robinson, M.D.; McCarthy, D.J.; Smyth, G.K. edgeR: A Bioconductor package for differential expression analysis of digital gene expression data. *Bioinformatics* **2010**, *26*, 139–140. [CrossRef]
14. McCarthy, D.J.; Chen, Y.; Smyth, G.K. Differential expression analysis of multifactor RNA-Seq experiments with respect to biological variation. *Nucleic Acids Res.* **2012**, *40*, 4288–4297. [CrossRef]
15. Edgar, R. Gene Expression Omnibus: NCBI gene expression and hybridization array data repository. *Nucleic Acids Res.* **2002**, *30*, 207–210. [CrossRef]
16. Pagès, H.; Aboyoun, P.; Gentleman, R.; DebRoy, S. Biostrings: Efficient Manipulation of Biological Strings. R Package Version 2.56.0. 2020. Available online: https://bioconductor.org/packages/release/bioc/html/Biostrings.html (accessed on 8 June 2020). [CrossRef]
17. Durinck, S.; Moreau, Y.; Kasprzyk, A.; Davis, S.; De Moor, B.; Brazma, A.; Huber, W. BioMart and Bioconductor: A powerful link between biological databases and microarray data analysis. *Bioinformatics* **2005**, *21*, 3439–3440. [CrossRef]

18. Mironova, V.V.; Omelyanchuk, N.A.; Wiebe, D.S.; Levitsky, V.G. Computational analysis of auxin responsive elements in the *Arabidopsis thaliana* L. genome. *BMC Genom.* **2014**, *15*, S4. [CrossRef]
19. Zemlyanskaya, E.V.; Wiebe, D.S.; Omelyanchuk, N.A.; Levitsky, V.G.; Mironova, V.V. Meta-analysis of transcriptome data identified TGTCNN motif variants associated with the response to plant hormone auxin in *Arabidopsis thaliana* L. *J. Bioinform. Comput. Biol.* **2016**, *14*, 1641009. [CrossRef]
20. Holm, S. A simple sequentially rejective multiple test procedure. *Scand. J. Stat.* **1979**, *6*, 65–70.
21. Hochberg, Y. A sharper Bonferroni procedure for multiple tests of significance. *Biometrika* **1988**, *75*, 800–802. [CrossRef]
22. Benjamini, Y.; Hochberg, Y. Controlling the false discovery rate: A practical and powerful approach to multiple testing. *J. R. Stat. Soc. Ser. B* **1995**, *57*, 289–300. [CrossRef]
23. Benjamini, Y.; Yekutieli, D. The Control of the False Discovery Rate in Multiple Testing under Dependency. *Ann. Stat.* **2001**, *29*, 1165–1188.
24. Gupta, S.; Stamatoyannopoulos, J.A.; Bailey, T.L.; Noble, W. Quantifying similarity between motifs. *Genome Biol.* **2007**, *8*, R24. [CrossRef]
25. Guan, Q.; Wu, J.; Zhang, Y.; Jiang, C.; Liu, R.; Chai, C.; Zhu, J. A DEAD Box RNA Helicase Is Critical for Pre-mRNA Splicing, Cold-Responsive Gene Regulation, and Cold Tolerance in *Arabidopsis*. *Plant Cell* **2013**, *25*, 342–356. [CrossRef]
26. Chiba, Y.; Mineta, K.; Hirai, M.Y.; Suzuki, Y.; Kanaya, S.; Takahashi, H.; Onouchi, H.; Yamaguchi, J.; Naito, S. Changes in mRNA Stability Associated with Cold Stress in Arabidopsis Cells. *Plant Cell Physiol.* **2013**, *54*, 180–194. [CrossRef]
27. Park, S.; Lee, C.-M.; Doherty, C.J.; Gilmour, S.J.; Kim, Y.; Thomashow, M.F. Regulation of the Arabidopsis CBF regulon by a complex low-temperature regulatory network. *Plant J.* **2015**, *82*, 193–207. [CrossRef]
28. Kim, Y.; Park, S.; Gilmour, S.J.; Thomashow, M.F. Roles of CAMTA transcription factors and salicylic acid in configuring the low-temperature transcriptome and freezing tolerance of Arabidopsis. *Plant J.* **2013**, *75*, 364–376. [CrossRef]
29. Lee, B.; Henderson, D.A.; Zhu, J.-K. The *Arabidopsis* Cold-Responsive Transcriptome and Its Regulation by ICE1. *Plant Cell* **2005**, *17*, 3155–3175. [CrossRef]
30. Jia, Y.; Ding, Y.; Shi, Y.; Zhang, X.; Gong, Z.; Yang, S. The *cbfs* triple mutants reveal the essential functions of *CBFs* in cold acclimation and allow the definition of CBF regulons in *Arabidopsis*. *New Phytol.* **2016**, *212*, 345–353. [CrossRef]
31. Kilian, J.; Whitehead, D.; Horak, J.; Wanke, D.; Weinl, S.; Batistic, O.; D'Angelo, C.; Bornberg-Bauer, E.; Kudla, J.; Harter, K. The AtGenExpress global stress expression data set: Protocols, evaluation and model data analysis of UV-B light, drought and cold stress responses: AtGenExpress global abiotic stress data set. *Plant J.* **2007**, *50*, 347–363. [CrossRef]
32. Schlaen, R.G.; Mancini, E.; Sanchez, S.E.; Perez-Santángelo, S.; Rugnone, M.L.; Simpson, C.G.; Brown, J.W.S.; Zhang, X.; Chernomoretz, A.; Yanovsky, M.J. The spliceosome assembly factor GEMIN2 attenuates the effects of temperature on alternative splicing and circadian rhythms. *Proc. Natl. Acad. Sci. USA* **2015**, *112*, 9382–9387. [CrossRef] [PubMed]
33. Hu, P.; Liu, M.; Zhang, D.; Wang, J.; Niu, H.; Liu, Y.; Wu, Z.; Han, B.; Zhai, W.; Shen, Y.; et al. Global identification of the genetic networks and cis-regulatory elements of the cold response in zebrafish. *Nucleic Acids Res.* **2015**, *43*, 9198–9213. [CrossRef] [PubMed]
34. Durinck, S.; Spellman, P.T.; Birney, E.; Huber, W. Mapping identifiers for the integration of genomic datasets with the R/Bioconductor package biomaRt. *Nat. Protoc.* **2009**, *4*, 1184–1191. [CrossRef]
35. Thomashow, M.F. PLANT COLD ACCLIMATION: Freezing Tolerance Genes and Regulatory Mechanisms. *Annu. Rev. Plant. Physiol. Plant. Mol. Biol.* **1999**, *50*, 571–599. [CrossRef]
36. Gilmour, S.J.; Zarka, D.G.; Stockinger, E.J.; Salazar, M.P.; Houghton, J.M.; Thomashow, M.F. Low temperature regulation of theArabidopsisCBF family of AP2 transcriptional activators as an early step in cold-inducedCORgene expression. *Plant J.* **1998**, *16*, 433–442. [CrossRef]
37. Zarka, D.G.; Vogel, J.T.; Cook, D.; Thomashow, M.F. Cold Induction of Arabidopsis *CBF* Genes Involves Multiple ICE (Inducer of *CBF* Expression) Promoter Elements and a Cold-Regulatory Circuit That Is Desensitized by Low Temperature. *Plant Physiol.* **2003**, *133*, 910–918. [CrossRef]

38. Novillo, F.; Alonso, J.M.; Ecker, J.R.; Salinas, J. CBF2/DREB1C is a negative regulator of CBF1/DREB1B and CBF3/DREB1A expression and plays a central role in stress tolerance in Arabidopsis. *Proc. Natl. Acad. Sci. USA* **2004**, *101*, 3985–3990. [CrossRef]
39. Yamaguchi-Shinozaki, K.; Shinozaki, K. Organization of *cis*-acting regulatory elements in osmotic- and cold-stress-responsive promoters. *Trends Plant Sci.* **2005**, *10*, 88–94. [CrossRef]
40. Doherty, C.J.; Van Buskirk, H.A.; Myers, S.J.; Thomashow, M.F. Roles for *Arabidopsis* CAMTA Transcription Factors in Cold-Regulated Gene Expression and Freezing Tolerance. *Plant Cell* **2009**, *21*, 972–984. [CrossRef]
41. Kidokoro, S.; Maruyama, K.; Nakashima, K.; Imura, Y.; Narusaka, Y.; Shinwari, Z.K.; Osakabe, Y.; Fujita, Y.; Mizoi, J.; Shinozaki, K.; et al. The Phytochrome-Interacting Factor PIF7 Negatively Regulates *DREB1* Expression under Circadian Control in Arabidopsis. *Plant Physiol.* **2009**, *151*, 2046–2057. [CrossRef]
42. Lee, C.-M.; Thomashow, M.F. Photoperiodic regulation of the C-repeat binding factor (CBF) cold acclimation pathway and freezing tolerance in Arabidopsis thaliana. *Proc. Natl. Acad. Sci. USA* **2012**, *109*, 15054–15059. [CrossRef]
43. Maruyama, K.; Todaka, D.; Mizoi, J.; Yoshida, T.; Kidokoro, S.; Matsukura, S.; Takasaki, H.; Sakurai, T.; Yamamoto, Y.Y.; Yoshiwara, K.; et al. Identification of *Cis*-Acting Promoter Elements in Cold- and Dehydration-Induced Transcriptional Pathways in Arabidopsis, Rice, and Soybean. *DNA Res.* **2012**, *19*, 37–49. [CrossRef] [PubMed]
44. Jiang, B.; Shi, Y.; Zhang, X.; Xin, X.; Qi, L.; Guo, H.; Li, J.; Yang, S. PIF3 is a negative regulator of the *CBF* pathway and freezing tolerance in *Arabidopsis*. *Proc. Natl. Acad. Sci. USA* **2017**, *114*, E6695–E6702. [CrossRef]
45. Zhao, C.; Zhang, Z.; Xie, S.; Si, T.; Li, Y.; Zhu, J.-K. Mutational Evidence for the Critical Role of CBF Genes in Cold Acclimation in Arabidopsis. *Plant Physiol.* **2016**, *533*. [CrossRef]
46. Agarwal, M.; Hao, Y.; Kapoor, A.; Dong, C.-H.; Fujii, H.; Zheng, X.; Zhu, J.-K. A R2R3 Type MYB Transcription Factor Is Involved in the Cold Regulation of CBF Genes and in Acquired Freezing Tolerance. *J. Biol. Chem.* **2006**, *281*, 37636–37645. [CrossRef]
47. Dong, M.A.; Farre, E.M.; Thomashow, M.F. CIRCADIAN CLOCK-ASSOCIATED 1 and LATE ELONGATED HYPOCOTYL regulate expression of the C-REPEAT BINDING FACTOR (CBF) pathway in Arabidopsis. *Proc. Natl. Acad. Sci. USA* **2011**, *108*, 7241–7246. [CrossRef]
48. Kidokoro, S.; Yoneda, K.; Takasaki, H.; Takahashi, F.; Shinozaki, K.; Yamaguchi-Shinozaki, K. Different Cold-Signaling Pathways Function in the Responses to Rapid and Gradual Decreases in Temperature. *Plant Cell* **2017**, *29*, 760–774. [CrossRef]
49. Yang, S.-H.; Sharrocks, A.D. Convergence of the SUMO and MAPK pathways on the ETS-domain transcription factor Elk-1. *Biochem. Soc. Symp.* **2006**, *73*, 121–129. [CrossRef]
50. Ducker, C.; Chow, L.K.Y.; Saxton, J.; Handwerger, J.; McGregor, A.; Strahl, T.; Layfield, R.; Shaw, P.E. De-ubiquitination of ELK-1 by USP17 potentiates mitogenic gene expression and cell proliferation. *Nucleic Acids Res.* **2019**, *47*, 4495–4508. [CrossRef]
51. Felber, K.; Elks, P.M.; Lecca, M.; Roehl, H.H. Expression of osterix Is Regulated by FGF and Wnt/β-Catenin Signalling during Osteoblast Differentiation. *PLoS ONE* **2015**, *10*, e0144982. [CrossRef]
52. Lahiri, K.; Vallone, D.; Gondi, S.B.; Santoriello, C.; Dickmeis, T.; Foulkes, N.S. Temperature Regulates Transcription in the Zebrafish Circadian Clock. *PLoS Biol.* **2005**, *3*, e351. [CrossRef]
53. van Helden, J.; André, B.; Collado-Vides, J. A web site for the computational analysis of yeast regulatory sequences. *Yeast* **2000**, *16*, 177–187. [CrossRef]
54. Heinz, S.; Benner, C.; Spann, N.; Bertolino, E.; Lin, Y.C.; Laslo, P.; Cheng, J.X.; Murre, C.; Singh, H.; Glass, C.K. Simple Combinations of Lineage-Determining Transcription Factors Prime *cis*-Regulatory Elements Required for Macrophage and B Cell Identities. *Mol. Cell* **2010**, *38*, 576–589. [CrossRef] [PubMed]
55. Liu, T.; Ortiz, J.A.; Taing, L.; Meyer, C.A.; Lee, B.; Zhang, Y.; Shin, H.; Wong, S.S.; Ma, J.; Lei, Y.; et al. Cistrome: An integrative platform for transcriptional regulation studies. *Genome Biol.* **2011**, *12*, R83. [CrossRef]
56. Khan, A.; Fornes, O.; Stigliani, A.; Gheorghe, M.; Castro-Mondragon, J.A.; van der Lee, R.; Bessy, A.; Chèneby, J.; Kulkarni, S.R.; Tan, G.; et al. JASPAR 2018: Update of the open-access database of transcription factor binding profiles and its web framework. *Nucleic Acids Res.* **2018**, *46*, D260–D266. [CrossRef] [PubMed]
57. Hu, J.; Wang, D.; Li, J.; Jing, G.; Ning, K.; Xu, J. Genome-wide identification of transcription factors and transcription-factor binding sites in oleaginous microalgae Nannochloropsis. *Sci. Rep.* **2015**, *4*, 5454. [CrossRef]

58. Chinnusamy, V.; Zhu, J.; Zhu, J.-K. Cold stress regulation of gene expression in plants. *Trends Plant Sci.* **2007**, *12*, 444–451. [CrossRef]
59. Zhao, C.; Lang, Z.; Zhu, J.-K. Cold responsive gene transcription becomes more complex. *Trends Plant Sci.* **2015**, *20*, 466–468. [CrossRef] [PubMed]
60. Bailey, T.L. DREME: Motif discovery in transcription factor ChIP-seq data. *Bioinformatics* **2011**, *27*, 1653–1659. [CrossRef]
61. Chen, Y.-H.; Lee, W.-C.; Cheng, C.-H.; Tsai, H.-J. Muscle regulatory factor gene: Zebrafish (*Danio rerio*) myogenin cDNA. *Comp. Biochem. Physiol. Part B Biochem. Mol. Biol.* **2000**, *127*, 97–103. [CrossRef]
62. Campos, C.; Valente, L.; Conceição, L.; Engrola, S.; Fernandes, J. Temperature affects methylation of the myogenin putative promoter, its expression and muscle cellularity in Senegalese sole larvae. *Epigenetics* **2013**, *8*, 389–397. [CrossRef] [PubMed]
63. Goulding, M.D.; Gruss, P. The homeobox in vertebrate development. *Curr. Opin. Cell Biol.* **1989**, *1*, 1088–1093. [CrossRef]
64. Zeng, Z.; Zhang, W.; Marand, A.P.; Zhu, B.; Buell, C.R.; Jiang, J. Cold stress induces enhanced chromatin accessibility and bivalent histone modifications H3K4me3 and H3K27me3 of active genes in potato. *Genome Biol.* **2019**, *20*, 123. [CrossRef] [PubMed]

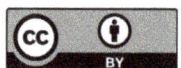 © 2020 by the authors. Licensee MDPI, Basel, Switzerland. This article is an open access article distributed under the terms and conditions of the Creative Commons Attribution (CC BY) license (http://creativecommons.org/licenses/by/4.0/).

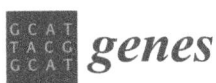

Article

Computational Analysis of Transcriptomic and Proteomic Data for Deciphering Molecular Heterogeneity and Drug Responsiveness in Model Human Hepatocellular Carcinoma Cell Lines

Panagiotis C. Agioutantis [1,2], Heleni Loutrari [2,*] and Fragiskos N. Kolisis [1,*]

1. Biotechnology Laboratory, School of Chemical Engineering, National Technical University of Athens, 5 Iroon Polytechniou Str., Zografou Campus, 15780 Athens, Greece; panagiout@mail.ntua.gr
2. G.P. Livanos and M. Simou Laboratories, 1st Department of Critical Care Medicine & Pulmonary Services, Evangelismos Hospital, Medical School, National Kapodistrian University of Athens, 3 Ploutarchou Str., 10675 Athens, Greece
* Correspondence: elloutrar@med.uoa.gr (H.L.); kolisis@chemeng.ntua.gr (F.N.K.)

Received: 6 April 2020; Accepted: 2 June 2020; Published: 5 June 2020

Abstract: Hepatocellular carcinoma (HCC) is associated with high mortality due to its inherent heterogeneity, aggressiveness, and limited therapeutic regimes. Herein, we analyzed 21 human HCC cell lines (HCC lines) to explore intertumor molecular diversity and pertinent drug sensitivity. We used an integrative computational approach based on exploratory and single-sample gene-set enrichment analysis of transcriptome and proteome data from the Cancer Cell Line Encyclopedia, followed by correlation analysis of drug-screening data from the Cancer Therapeutics Response Portal with curated gene-set enrichment scores. Acquired results classified HCC lines into two groups, a poorly and a well-differentiated group, displaying lower/higher enrichment scores in a "Specifically Upregulated in Liver" gene-set, respectively. Hierarchical clustering based on a published epithelial–mesenchymal transition gene expression signature further supported this stratification. Between-group comparisons of gene and protein expression unveiled distinctive patterns, whereas downstream functional analysis significantly associated differentially expressed genes with crucial cancer-related biological processes/pathways and revealed concrete driver-gene signatures. Finally, correlation analysis highlighted a diverse effectiveness of specific drugs against poorly compared to well-differentiated HCC lines, possibly applicable in clinical research with patients with analogous characteristics. Overall, this study expanded the knowledge on the molecular profiles, differentiation status, and drug responsiveness of HCC lines, and proposes a cost-effective computational approach to precision anti-HCC therapies.

Keywords: hepatocellular carcinoma; transcriptomics; proteomics; bioinformatics analysis; differentiation; Gene Ontology; Reactome Pathways; gene-set enrichment

1. Introduction

Liver cancer is one of the most frequently occurring life-threatening neoplasms worldwide. Hepatocellular carcinoma (HCC)—the most predominant type of primary liver cancer (85% to 90%)—usually arises in the context of inflammatory-induced stress and chronically progressing liver cirrhosis. Depending on the region of incidence, a wide range of risk factors have been implicated in the development of HCC. Hepatitis B and aflatoxin B1 exposure are widely associated with HCC cases occurring in eastern Asia and Sub-Saharan Africa, while hepatitis C, alcohol consumption, and non-alcoholic fatty liver disease prevail as leading causative factors in the Western world and Japan [1]. Regardless of the potentially implicated risk factors, HCC incidence constitutes a remarkably complex multistep process, involving various genomic and epigenomic aberrations leading to an inevitable molecular heterogeneity [2,3]. Deregulated cell proliferation, increased inflammatory and oxidative stress, enriched tumor microenvironment, and abnormally active angiogenic switches characterize the progression of HCC, through the early stage of initiation up to the point of invasion and metastasis [4].

Despite existing surveillance protocols for cirrhotic patients, HCC is often diagnosed in advanced stages, resulting in limited applicable treatments or effective therapies. Moreover, HCC chemopreventive strategies are additionally hampered by the aforementioned innate molecular heterogeneity of the disease. To date, only a handful of available treatment regimens have been proven effective (first-line options sorafenib and lenvatinib, along with second-line options regorafenib, cabozantinib, and ramucirumab), and only to some extent [4]. Therefore, it is of the utmost importance to identify novel biomarkers and potent drug agents to address the miscellaneous characteristics of HCC cases. Cancer cell lines have been extensively used during the last decades as valuable research model systems. Although not ideal in portraying the physiological and molecular traits of patients' malignancies, they have enabled a plethora of low-cost experiments towards the genomic and functional characterization of cancers [5]. Furthermore, diverse well-characterized cell lines could provide a convenient platform for pharmacogenomic studies deciphering the molecular complexity of tumors in association with drug-specific sensitivity [6,7].

To this end, in the present work, we aimed to shed light on the distinct/shared molecular features of 21 widely used human HCC cell lines (HCC lines), and to investigate their potential connection to drug efficiency. Our strategy implemented a thorough bioinformatics exploratory and functional enrichment analysis of publicly available transcriptomic and proteomic data from HCC lines, along with a correlation analysis of existing drug-response data to defined molecular signatures. Furthermore, tumors from HCC patients were characterized accordingly by analyzing gene expression data from the Cancer Genome Atlas (TCGA). Acquired results provided information on (a) potentially discrete subtypes amongst the investigated HCC lines, mainly dictated by their molecular resemblance (or not) to normal hepatocytes; (b) differentially expressed genes (DEGs) and differentially expressed proteins (DEPs) representative of inherent cancer heterogeneity; (c) biological processes and pathways significantly related to DEGs; and (d) HCC-subtype-specific sensitivity/resistance to drugs. Overall, the present work sets the basis of a computational platform for the integration and analysis of publicly accessible -omics and drug-screening data from tumor cell lines—and eventually tissue specimens—enabling the development of patient-tailored anti-cancer medications.

2. Materials and Methods

2.1. Data Acquisition and Pre-Processing

Publicly available transcriptomic and proteomic data were obtained from the Cancer Cell Line Encyclopedia (CCLE) database [7] (https://portals.broadinstitute.org/ccle/data). Gene-centric RMA-normalized mRNA expression (CCLE_Expression_Entrez_2012-09-29.gct), reverse-phase protein array (RPPA-CCLE_RPPA_20181003.csv), and HCC line annotation (CCLE_sample_info_file_2012-10-18.txt) data were downloaded. The RPPA data file contained median-centered log_2-normalized relative protein expression values as previously described [8]. Out of all the total cancer cell line entries in the CCLE database, 23 liver cancer cell lines with available microarray gene expression data and RPPA protein expression data were extracted. Two cell lines—namely SNU398 and NCIH684—were excluded from subsequent analyses, the former due to the highly anaplastic nature of the cells [9], and the latter because it originates from primary colon cancer metastasized to the liver. Remaining liver cancer cell lines included 20 HCC lines and SKHEP1, a widely used liver adenocarcinoma cell line of endothelial origin [10]. SKHEP1 has been sporadically used in HCC-associated studies, despite recent recommendations [11].

Drug-screening data containing area under concentration–response curve (AUC) sensitivity measurements for 481 drugs, regarding 15 of the extracted cell lines, were obtained from the Cancer

Therapeutics Response Portal (CTRPv2, https://portals.broadinstitute.org/ctrp.v2.1/) [12]. AUCs are based on percentage viability scores compared to dimethyl sulfoxide (DMSO)-treated cells [13]. Drugs with missing values for three or more cell lines were subsequently discarded. To conclude, 21 HCC lines (Table 1) with corresponding gene expression (18,900 genes) and protein/phosphoprotein expression (214 proteins/phosphoproteins) data were studied. For the vast majority of cell lines, additional drug-screening sensitivity data for 344 compounds were investigated.

Table 1. HCC lines with available gene and protein/phosphoprotein expression data used in data analysis.

Cell Line Name	Cancer Type	Cell Line Name	Cancer Type	Cell Line Name	Cancer Type
HEP3B217	HCC	JHH4	HCC	SNU387	HCC
HEPG2	HCC	JHH5	HCC	SNU423	HCC
HLF	HCC	JHH6	HCC	SNU449	HCC
HUH1	HCC	JHH7	HCC	SNU475	HCC
HUH7	HCC	LI7	HCC	SNU761	HCC
JHH1	HCC	PLCPRF5	HCC	SNU878	HCC
JHH2	HCC	SKHEP1	Adenocarcinoma	SNU886	HCC

Blue font indicates cell lines with drug sensitivity data available from the Cancer Therapeutics Response Portal (CTRPv2) and used in pharmacogenomic analysis. HCC: Hepatocellular carcinoma

Finally, gene-expression RNA-seq data from the TCGA HCC cohort [14] were downloaded as gene-level raw expression values produced by *RSEM* [15] (LIHC.uncv2.mRNAseq_raw_counts.txt) from the Broad Institute portal (https://gdac.broadinstitute.org/) along with corresponding clinical information. Raw gene expression values were appropriately normalized using the TMM (trimmed mean of M values) normalization method [16] and transformed in $\log_2$ scale.

2.2. Exploratory Analysis of Transcriptomic and Proteomic Data

Pairwise Pearson's correlation coefficients were computed between each pair of HCC lines, based on the expression of the 500 genes with the largest cross-sample variation (median absolute deviation) and the expression of 214 available proteins/phosphoproteins, respectively. Graphical displays of correlation matrices were produced using the *corrplot* package in R.

Principal component analysis (PCA) was performed using the dedicated PCA function from the *mixomics* R package [17]. Optimal univariate *k*-means clustering was conducted by implementing the *Ckmeans.1d.dp* package in R [18]. The core function of this package performs one-dimensional (1D), weighted or unweighted, *k*-means clustering and provides the optimal number of clusters using the Bayesian information criterion (BIC) [19]. HCC line weights were considered equal (weight = 1.0).

Single-sample gene-set enrichment analysis (ssGSEA) scores were computed against curated gene-sets (C2) from MSigDB by implementing the *GSVA* package in the R environment [20]. ssGSEA defines an enrichment score that represents the degree of absolute enrichment of a gene-set in each sample within a given dataset [21]. Essentially, ssGSEA enrichment scores signify the degree to which genes in a particular gene-set are coordinately up- or downregulated within a given sample.

A recently published epithelial-to-mesenchymal transition (EMT) gene expression signature [22] consisting of 239 genes —215 epithelial and 24 mesenchymal markers— was further used to enhance the exploratory data-analysis process. More specifically, hierarchical clustering (average linkage, Euclidean distance) was performed based on the EMT signature, to support/supplement PCA-identified clusters.

2.3. Between-Group Differential Gene and Protein Expression Analysis

Between-group gene and protein differential expression analyses were conducted by implementing the *limma* package in R [23]. Genes with overall very low expression were filtered out, while the full set of available proteins/phosphoproteins was used. Regarding the identification of DEGs, the *treat* function [24], which tests for significance relative to fold-change thresholds, was implemented. Genes with an adjusted p-value < 0.1 (Benjamini–Hochberg correction) and |fold-change| > 1.2 were considered DEGs. Proteins/phosphoproteins with an adjusted p-value < 0.1 (Benjamini–Hochberg correction) after moderated t-tests implemented through the *eBayes* function, were considered differentially expressed as well. Volcano plots illustrating identified DEGs and DEPs were created using the *EnhancedVolcano* package in R [25]. Scaled gene/protein expression values were used in heatmap illustrations for individual HCC lines regarding identified DEGs and DEPs.

2.4. Functional Enrichment Analysis of Differentially Expressed Genes

Reactome Pathway and Gene Ontology (GO) enrichment analysis of DEGs was conducted using *Bioinfominer* [26,27], a bioinformatics tool that delivers unsupervised, fast, and integrative interpretation of -omics experiments. This tool accepts lists of genes and performs enrichment analysis along with prioritization of detected systemic processes, ultimately resulting in a compact signature consisting of systemic processes and their hub driver-genes. This signature constitutes a deconvoluted projection onto biological networks of hierarchical structure (ontologies, Reactome Pathway database), corrected for biases as well as other inconsistencies. The significance threshold for altered biological processes/pathways was set at a corrected hypergeometric p-value of 0.05.

Testing for enrichment of curated gene-sets (C2) from MSigDB amongst the between-group differential gene expression data was performed using the *camera* function [28] in the *limma* package, a competitive gene-set test procedure based on the idea of taking into account the intergene correlation to adjust the gene-set test statistic. Statistically significant enriched gene-sets were controlled at an adjusted FDR = 0.05 threshold, after Benjamini–Hochberg correction for multiple testing.

2.5. Drug-Specific Sensitivity in Association with Differentiation Status of HCC lines

Drug-sensitivity AUC measurements available for 15 of the HCC lines (Table 1, blue font) were correlated with their enrichment scores for a specific/selected (SU_LIVER) gene-set, in an attempt to elucidate differentiation-status-associated drug-sensitivity. Lower AUC sensitivity measurements corresponded to an enhanced drug effect against cell line viability. Liver-like well-differentiated cell lines were characterized by higher enrichment scores than the poorly differentiated ones; therefore, positive correlations highlighted drugs more effective against poorly differentiated cell lines, while negative correlations drugs more effective against well-differentiated ones. Drugs with a p-value < 0.05, an adjusted p-value < 0.3 (after Benjamini–Hochberg correction), and |Spearman's ρ| > 0.5 were considered to be significantly correlated with the investigated enrichment score.

2.6. HCC Tumor Clustering Based on SU_LIVER Gene-Set Expression Data From TCGA

HCC patients (n = 354) with available gene-expression data and documented histological grades were extracted from the downloaded TCGA RNA-seq dataset. A total 224 samples have been characterized as well/moderately differentiated tumors of Grade 1 and Grade 2 (G1+G2), while 130 samples have been characterized as poorly/undifferentiated tumors of Grade 3 and Grade 4 (G3+G4). Hierarchical clustering (Ward linkage, Euclidean distance) of the 354 patients was conducted based on the scaled expression of all 58 genes involved in the SU_LIVER gene-set. Subsequently, a χ^2 test in the R environment was conducted to test for a possible association between the formed clusters and histological grading.

3. Results

3.1. HCC Lines Clustered into Two Distinct Differentiation Subtypes

The present study focused on the global comparison of 21 patient-derived HCC lines for which gene and protein/phosphoprotein expression data are publicly available (Table 1). An initial correlation matrix analysis based on (i) the expression of 500 genes exhibiting the largest cross-sample variation

(Figure S1) and (ii) the abundance of all 214 proteins/phosphoproteins offered from the RPPA dataset (Figure S2) notably showed that some of the examined cell lines shared a higher similarity compared to others. Further investigation of these results by PCA, using the same subset of 500 genes, revealed a clear spread of HCC lines across PC1, explaining 33% of variance amongst samples (Figure 1A). Subsequent 1D *k*-means clustering performed on the PC1 scores of HCC lines indicated two optimal discrete clusters across PC1 (Figure 1B, Figure S3) which notably corresponded to a "high PC1 score" cluster and a "low PC1 score" cluster, respectively.

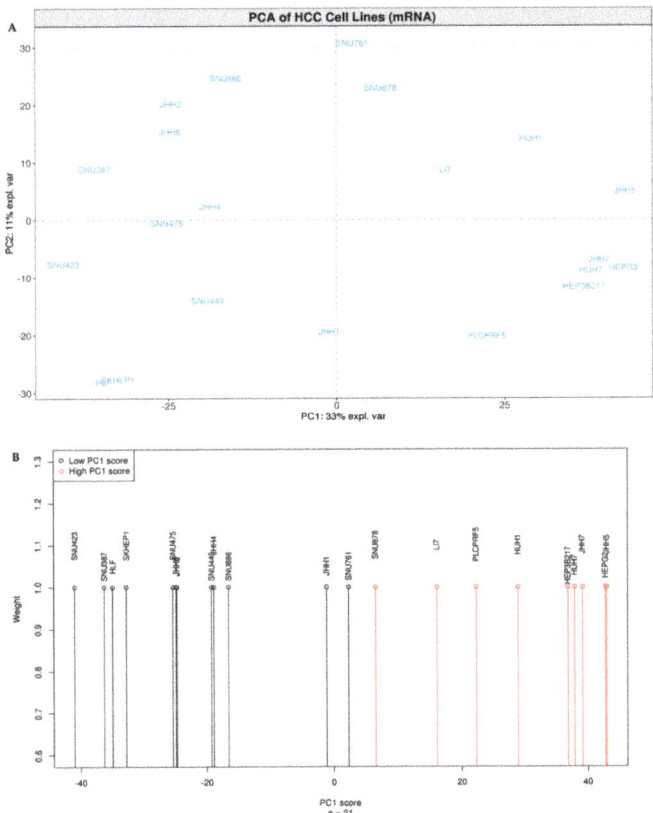

Figure 1. Gene-based principal component analysis (PCA) and clustering of HCC lines (**A**) PCA on 500 genes with the largest cross-sample variation. PC1 (x-axis) versus PC2 (y-axis) for 21 HCC lines indicated by blue color. Dashed horizontal and vertical lines mark zero values of PC1 and PC2, respectively. (**B**) The two optimal *k*-means clusters based on PC1 scores as identified by the Bayesian information criterion (BIC). All HCC lines were treated as equally weighted.

Compared to the microarray gene expression data, RNA-seq data retrieved from CCLE provided almost identical results for the examined HCC lines in gene-based PCA (Figure S4). Most importantly, a high cross-platform Pearson correlation (mean value 0.85 ± 0.01 standard deviation) was found for all 21 same-cell-line pairs (e.g., $HEPG2_{RNAseq} - HEPG2_{microarray}$), based on the expression of 16,667 genes found to be shared within the two datasets.

In order to highlight the biological background underlying this discrete cell-line grouping across PC1, we subsequently computed the ssGSEA scores against curated gene-sets from MSigDB, based on calculated PC1 loadings (Table S1). Interestingly, a "Specifically Upregulated in Liver" gene-set (SU_LIVER), containing genes upregulated specifically in human liver tissue [29], was identified as one of the top gene-sets with positive enrichment scores. Additionally, individual cell-line enrichment scores for each particular gene-set were computed by ssGSEA (Table S2). After examining and evaluating many HCC-related top enriched gene-sets regarding their ability to predict PC1 scores, we focused on SU_LIVER, as this gene-set exhibited the best predictive performance. We performed 1D *k*-means clustering, which again highlighted two optimal clusters (Figure 2A, Figure S5), a "high SU_LIVER score" and a "low SU_LIVER score" cluster, respectively. Subsequent correlation of PC1 scores with the individual cell-line SU_LIVER enrichment scores revealed that 86% of observed PC1 variance was explained by that term (Pearson's $r = 0.93$, $R^2 = 0.86$, p-value $= 1.874 \times 10^{-9}$). Cell lines included in both the "high SU_LIVER score" and "high PC1 score" clusters were therefore considered to be liver-like and well-differentiated, while the ones belonging in both the "low SU_LIVER score" and "low PC1 score" clusters were characterized as poorly differentiated (Figure 2B).

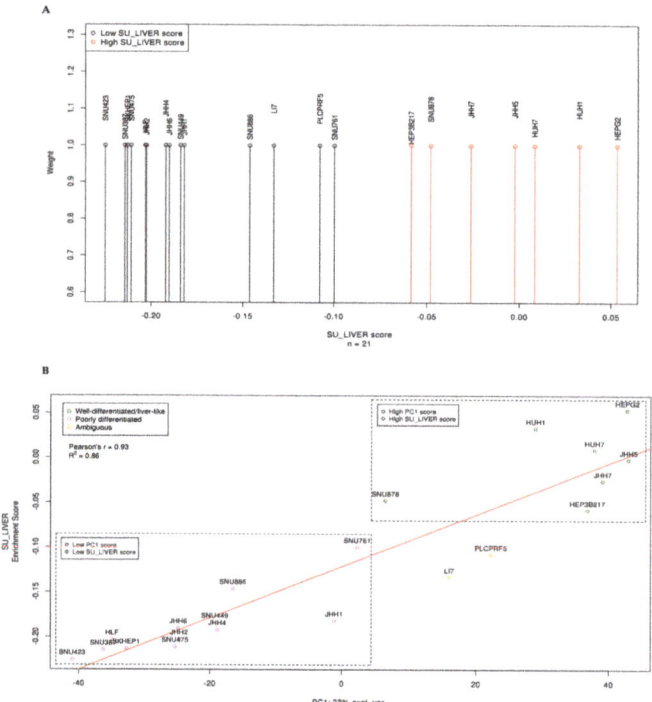

Figure 2. Specifically Upregulated in Liver (SU_LIVER) clustering of HCC lines and PC1-SU_LIVER correlation. (**A**) The two optimal *k*-means clusters based on computed cell line ssGSEA SU_LIVER enrichment scores as identified by the BIC. All HCC lines were treated as equally weighted. (**B**) PC1 score correlation (Pearson's) with individual cell-line enrichment scores for the SU_LIVER gene-set. Cell lines included in the "high SU_LIVER score"/"high PC1 score" clusters were identified as liver-like and well-differentiated (green circles), while the ones in the "low SU_LIVER score"/"low PC1 score" clusters were characterized as poorly differentiated (purple circles). Yellow circles indicate ambiguous cell lines.

Results for only two cell lines, namely LI7 and PLCPRF5, were conflicting, because their PC1 score clustering opposed their SU_LIVER enrichment score clustering; therefore, these cell lines were characterized as ambiguous.

We subsequently used a recently published EMT gene expression signature to further challenge the proposed differentiation-associated stratification of test HCC lines, since EMT is a process highly related to the differentiation/de-differentiation status of cancer cells [29]. Notably, the hierarchical clustering of

HCC lines —as depicted in the corresponding heatmap— unveiled again their classification into two main groups, based on the EMT gene expression signature pattern, while additionally identified JHH1 as a rather ambiguous cell line of discrete nature (Figure 3). This clustering generally corroborated the differentiation groups demonstrated in Figure 2B.

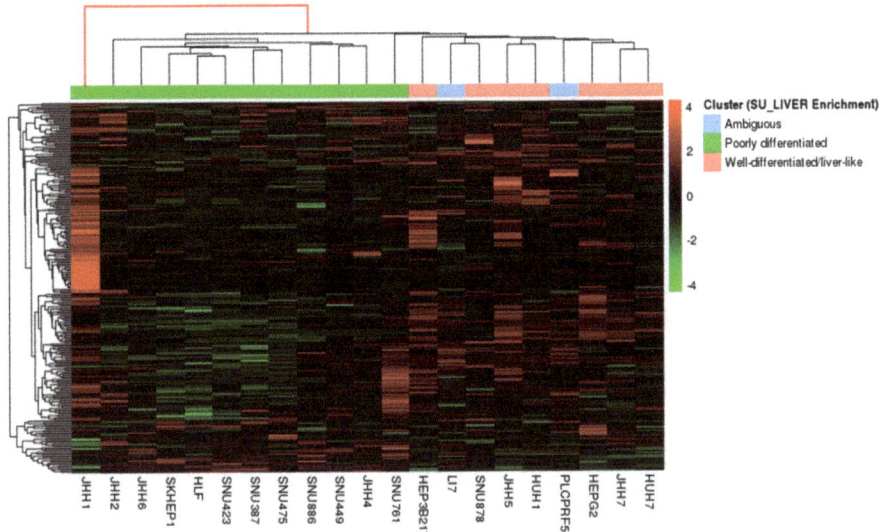

Figure 3. Heatmap illustrating the hierarchical clustering of cancer cell lines (columns) based on the epithelial-to-mesenchymal transition (EMT) signature of 239 genes (rows). Scaled values indicate relative downregulation (green color) or upregulation (red color) of gene expression. Cell lines are annotated by color, based on the clusters that were predicted by the SU_LIVER enrichment scores shown in Figure 2B.

Finally, PCA based on protein/phosphoprotein RPPA expression data showed that the clustering of HCC lines was widely consistent, not only at the gene but also at the protein expression level (Figure 4) and further confirmed the discrete/ambiguous nature of the JHH1 cell line. Based on these findings, JHH1 along with LI7 and PLCPRF5 were considered to be ambiguously characterized in the context of this study and were therefore excluded from downstream analyses, in order to get a more straightforward and comprehensive grasp of distinct differentiation-associated molecular characteristics amongst the remaining HCC lines.

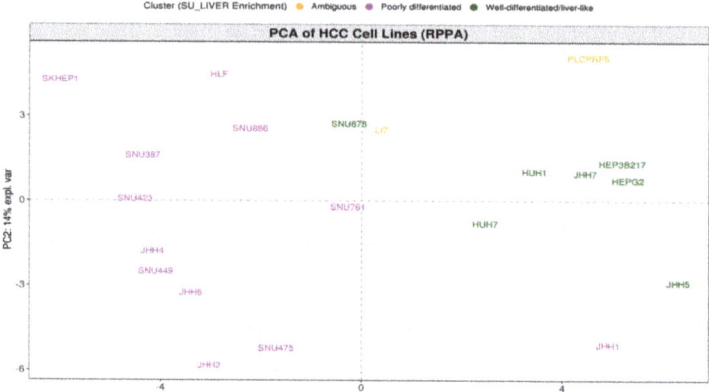

Figure 4. PCA based on all 214 protein/phosphoprotein reverse-phase protein array (RPPA) expression data. PC1 (x-axis) versus PC2 (y-axis). Cell lines are annotated by color, based on the gene-expression-derived clusters that are predicted by the SU_LIVER enrichment scores shown in Figure 2B.

3.2. Differential Gene and Protein Expression between Poorly and Well-Differentiated HCC Lines

Between-group differential gene and protein expression analysis was subsequently carried out to investigate the molecular basis underlying the distinct classification of the examined HCC lines. The volcano plots shown in Figure 5A,B depict the number of DEGs and DEPs respectively, between poorly and well-differentiated liver-like HCC lines. Considering the latter as controls, since they undoubtedly uphold molecular features closer to functional normal hepatocytes, we accordingly identified a significant differential expression of 935 genes (462 upregulated and 473 downregulated) and 16 proteins (10 upregulated and 6 downregulated). Full lists of DEGs and DEPs are provided in Tables S3 and S4. Additionally, heatmaps illustrating the scaled expression values of HCC lines regarding identified DEGs and DEPs are provided in Figures S6 and S7, respectively, offering a comprehensive representation of individual cell-line expression patterns irrespective of assigned control group.

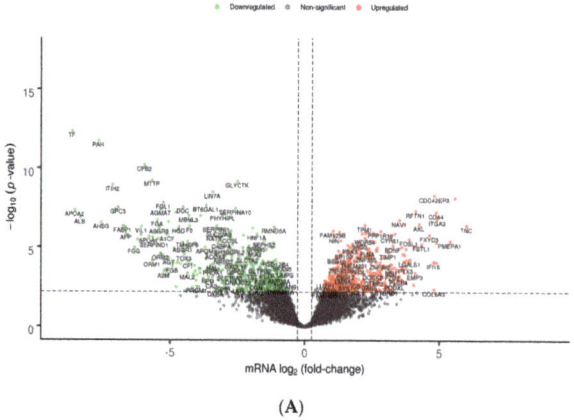

(A)

Figure 5. *Cont.*

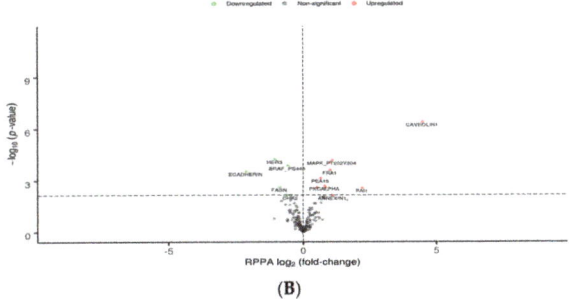

(B)

Figure 5. Volcano plots illustrating differentially expressed genes (DEGs) (**A**) and differentially expressed proteins (DEPs) (**B**) in poorly differentiated versus well-differentiated HCC lines. Red and green dots represent up- and downregulated genes/proteins, respectively; grey dots represent non-statistically-significant altered genes/proteins. Horizontal dashed lines indicate a statistical threshold corresponding to an adjusted p-value of < 0.1; x-axis: mRNA $\log_2$ fold-change (**A**) or RPPA $\log_2$ fold-change (**B**), y-axis: p-value in negative $\log_{10}$ scale.

Identified DEPs included downregulated proteins ECADHERIN, HER3, FASN, BRAF, CHK2, and phospho-BRAF, along with upregulated proteins CAVEOLIN1, PAI1, PAXILLIN, PEA15, PKCALPHA, AKT, NF2, FRA1, ANNEXIN1, and phospho-MAPK1/MAPK3. Pairwise total protein–mRNA relationships were investigated, excluding only for this analysis the two phosphorylated DEPs (MAPK_PT202Y204 and BRAF_PS445). For the majority of observed DEPs (HER3, ECADHERIN, BRAF, NF2, PAXILLIN, AKT, ANNEXIN1, PEA15, PAI1, FRA1, CAVEOLIN1) corresponding genes (*ERBB3, CDH1, BRAF, NF2, PXN, AKT3, ANXA1, PEA15, SERPINE1, FOSL1, CAV1*) were also found to be differentially expressed. A noteworthy observation was made concerning AKT: out of the three genes encoding for the corresponding isoforms—namely *AKT1, AKT2,* and *AKT3* (all detected by a single antibody in applied RPPA procedures [8])—only the expression of *AKT3* was significantly upregulated. Furthermore, mRNA expression fold-changes positively correlated with the respective total protein expression changes (Figure 6, Pearson's $r = 0.78$, $R^2 = 0.61$, p-value $= 0.00458$). The genes encoding the remaining DEPs (*FASN, CHK2,* and *PKCALPHA*) were either not identified as DEGs based on the predefined criteria, or were not included in the starting list of available genes.

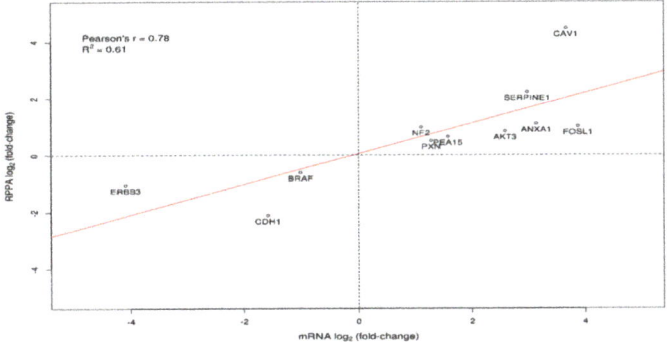

Figure 6. Pairwise Pearson correlation between identified DEPs (total proteins) and their corresponding DEGs. x-axis: mRNA $\log_2$(fold-change) of DEGs, y-axis: RPPA $\log_2$(fold-change) of DEPs. Protein–gene pairs are represented by their corresponding HGNC gene symbol.

3.3. Differentially Enriched Biological Processes/Pathways and Hub Driver-Gene Signatures between Poorly and Well-Differentiated HCC Lines

To better comprehend the molecular basis underlying the classification of the examined HCC lines into two distinct differentiation subtypes, DEGs were next subjected to downstream functional GO and Reactome Pathway enrichment analysis to reveal potentially implicated biological processes/pathways. By implementing the *Bioinfominer* software, a total of 114 significantly enriched GO biological processes and 28 additional biological Reactome pathways were identified (Tables S5 and S6). Figure 7 depicts the top 30 enriched GO terms, ranked by their corrected hypergeometric *p*-values, while Figure 8 shows all Reactome-Pathway-enriched terms. Recurring biological features were easily identifiable in both enrichment datasets, as in fact terms associated to wound healing, blood coagulation and hemostasis, fibrinolysis and clotting cascades, extracellular matrix (ECM) organization, platelet activation, and cell migration and motility were commonly observed. Furthermore, terms related to altered metabolism along with lipid/cholesterol homeostasis were assertively present.

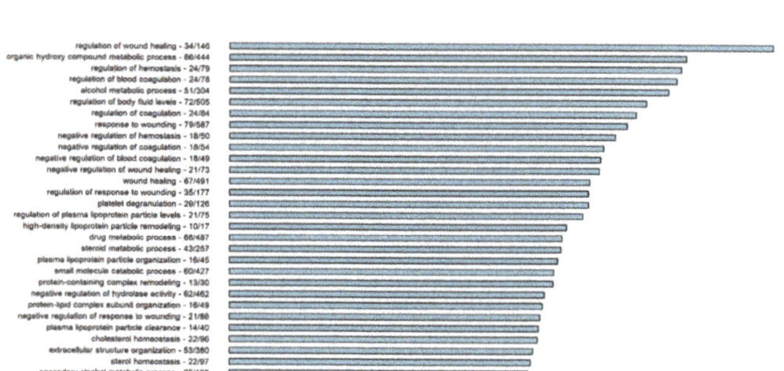

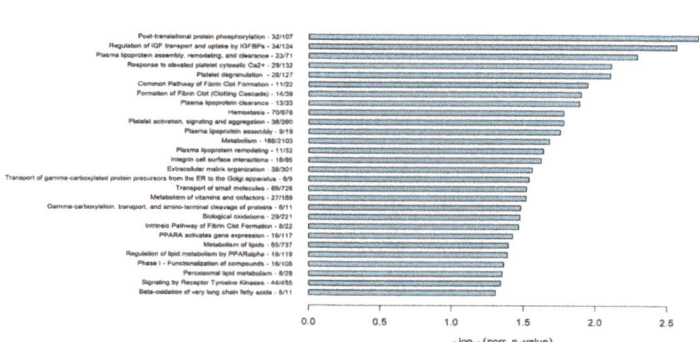

Figure 7. Top 30 significantly enriched Gene Ontology (GO) biological process terms, ranked by their hypergeometric corrected *p*-value in negative $\log_{10}$ scale (x-axis). Gene enrichment is also presented in total gene numbers, right after each GO term.

Figure 8. Significantly enriched Reactome Pathway terms ranked by their hypergeometric corrected *p*-value in negative $\log_{10}$ scale (x-axis). Gene enrichment is also presented in total gene numbers, right after each Reactome Pathway term.

Apart from the typical enrichment analysis, we exploited the *Bioinfominer's* ability to aggregate ontologically similar/interconnected enriched terms and prioritize them in the context of systemic processes for both GO and Reactome Pathway database vocabularies. A compact signature of hub driver-genes implicated in these prioritized systemic processes was produced in each case. As a result, systemic processes derived from the GO biological process and Reactome Pathway enrichment analyses were inferred and are presented in Figures S8 and S9, respectively. Prioritized systemic processes, as expected, included biological terms commonly encountered in both enrichment analyses, highlighting aforementioned recurring features such as fibrinolysis, hemostasis, platelet activation, wounding, ECM structure, and metabolism as core affected systemic processes, amongst others. Derived signatures of driver-genes associated with the recorded systemic processes are presented in Table 2 (41 hub genes, GO-based gene signature) and Table 3 (21 hub genes, Reactome-Pathway-based gene signature).

Table 2. Bioinfominer gene signature (poorly versus well-differentiated cell lines) based on implicated GO systemic processes. The signature consisted of 41 hub driver-genes, which are presented along with their corresponding number of implicated systemic processes and $\log_2$(fold-changes).

Gene Symbol	Gene Name	Systemic Processes	$\log_2$ (Fold-Change)
APOA1	apolipoprotein A1	19	−5.81
APOE	apolipoprotein E	14	−4.11
APOA2	apolipoprotein A2	12	−8.62
CAV1	caveolin 1	12	3.67
SERPINF2	serpin family F member 2	12	−2.43
TGFB2	transforming growth factor beta 2	11	2.84
AGTR1	angiotensin II receptor type 1	11	−2.95
ANXA1	annexin A1	11	3.14
AGT	angiotensinogen	10	−5.06
APOH	apolipoprotein H	10	−7.09
FGF2	fibroblast growth factor 2	10	2.84
SCARB1	scavenger receptor class B member 1	10	−1.57
APOC3	apolipoprotein C3	10	−4.89
APOC1	apolipoprotein C1	10	−5.47
THBS1	thrombospondin 1	10	2.21
APOB	apolipoprotein B	9	−6.71
NRP1	neuropilin 1	9	1.80
FGG	fibrinogen gamma chain	9	−6.37
FGA	fibrinogen alpha chain	9	−5.49
FGB	fibrinogen beta chain	9	−4.93
SERPINE1	serpin family E member 1	9	2.98
CEACAM1	carcinoembryonic antigen related cell adhesion molecule 1	8	−2.67
DYSF	dysferlin	8	1.76
NR1H4	nuclear receptor subfamily 1 group H member 4	8	−4.08
TSPO	translocator protein	8	2.48
CPB2	carboxypeptidase B2	8	−5.98
HNF4A	hepatocyte nuclear factor 4 alpha	8	−1.24
XBP1	X-box binding protein 1	8	−1.38
ANGPTL3	angiopoietin like 3	7	−3.90
NR1H3	nuclear receptor subfamily 1 group H member 3	7	−1.42
FLNA	filamin A	7	2.32
F2	coagulation factor II, thrombin	7	−5.12
BAD	BCL2 associated agonist of cell death	7	0.96

Table 2. Cont.

Gene Symbol	Gene Name	Systemic Processes	log₂ (Fold-Change)
LIPC	lipase C, hepatic type	7	−4.24
GAS6	growth arrest specific 6	7	2.39
VTN	vitronectin	7	−5.08
FGFR1	fibroblast growth factor receptor 1	7	1.49
ARG1	arginase 1	7	−2.79
CYBA	cytochrome b-245 alpha chain	7	−3.33
SULT1E1	sulfotransferase family 1E member 1	4	−2.07
ACOX1	acyl-CoA oxidase 1	4	−1.10

Table 3. Bioinfominer gene signature (poorly versus well-differentiated cell lines) based on implicated Reactome Pathway systemic processes. The signature consisted of 21 hub driver-genes, which are presented along with their corresponding number of implicated systemic processes and $\log_2$ (fold-changes).

Gene Symbol	Gene Name	Systemic Processes	log₂ (Fold- Change)
APOA1	apolipoprotein A1	5	−5.81
APOA2	apolipoprotein A2	4	−8.62
APOB	apolipoprotein B	4	−6.71
ALB	albumin	4	−8.42
SERPINC1	serpin family C member 1	3	−2.66
GNG11	G protein subunit gamma 11	3	3.24
GNG12	G protein subunit gamma 12	3	2.41
FGG	fibrinogen gamma chain	3	−6.37
FGA	fibrinogen alpha chain	3	−5.49
F2	coagulation factor II, thrombin	3	−5.12
KNG1	kininogen 1	3	−1.82
APOE	apolipoprotein E	3	−4.11
NR1H3	nuclear receptor subfamily 1 group H member 3	3	−1.42
GAS6	growth arrest specific 6	3	2.39
PROC	protein C, inactivator of coagulation factors Va and VIIIa	3	−3.25
A2M	alpha-2-macroglobulin	3	−5.26
SERPIND1	serpin family D member 1	3	−5.60
F5	coagulation factor V	3	−4.30
ACOX1	acyl-CoA oxidase 1	3	−1.10
PRKACB	protein kinase cAMP-activated catalytic subunit beta	3	1.11
TF	transferrin	3	−8.73

Additional gene-set enrichment analysis using the R function *camera* [28] provided further complementary information about the differentiation-associated characteristics beyond the obtained GO and Reactome Pathway results, based on the differential expression analysis data between the two identified groups of HCC lines and against curated (C2) gene-sets from MSigDB. Complete gene-set enrichment results are provided in Table S7, and included an important number of statistically significant enriched gene-sets, along with the projected enrichment direction in each set (genes either up- or downregulated in poorly differentiated cell lines). Poorly differentiated HCC lines were characterized by downregulation of gene expression associated with epithelial liver-like traits

(HSIAO_LIVER_SPECIFIC_GENES, SU_LIVER) [30,31] and various metabolic processes. In contrast, these HCC lines significantly overexpressed genes associated with Slug-related EMT initiation (ANASTASSIOU_CANCER_MESENCHYMAL_TRANSITION_SIGNATURE) [32], along with hypoxia (ELVIDGE_HYPOXIA_UP) [33] and migration (WU_CELL_MIGRATION) [34]. In addition, *camera* results unveiled a connection amongst HCC line subtypes and the three distinct molecular subclasses identified by Hoshida et al. [35] in HCC tissues (Subclasses S1, S2 and S3). The top 35 statistically significant gene-sets, ranked by their *p*-value, are illustrated in Figure 9.

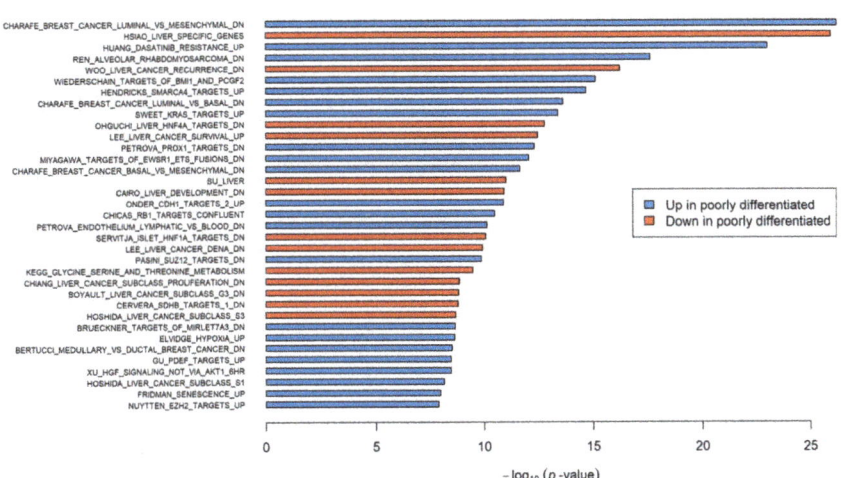

Figure 9. Top 35 gene-set enrichment terms as identified by *camera* testing, ranked by their *p*-value in negative $\log_{10}$ scale (x-axis).

3.4. Cell Line Differentiation Status Correlated with Drug-Specific Sensitivity

We next attempted to associate the drug-specific response of examined HCC lines with their differentiation status by correlating available drug-sensitivity AUC measurements with SU_LIVER enrichment scores. The volcano plot illustrated in Figure 10 demonstrates significant correlations (either positive or negative) between AUC measurements and SU_LIVER enrichment scores for 34 out of the 344 investigated drugs. Poorly differentiated cell lines were significantly more sensitive compared to well-differentiated ones against 11 investigated drugs, while, conversely, well-differentiated cell lines were relatively more sensitive against a panel of 23 investigated drugs, including but not limited to various tyrosine kinase inhibitors (TKIs). Table S8 provides a full listing of the correlation analysis results for all 344 studied drugs.

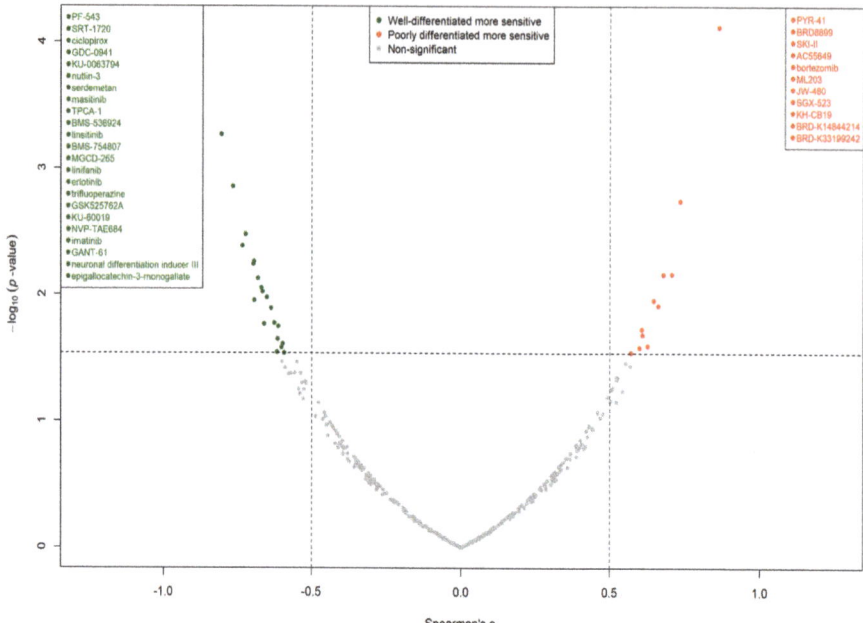

Figure 10. Volcano plot depicting drugs characterized by a statistically significant correlation between area under concentration–response curve (AUC) response measurements and SU_LIVER enrichment scores. Green dots represent drugs that were more effective against well-differentiated cell lines compared to poorly differentiated ones, while red dots mark drugs that were relatively more effective against poorly differentiated HCC lines. Grey dots indicate drugs without a significant correlation between their effect and the differentiation status of cell lines. The horizontal dashed line marks the highest p-value corresponding to an adjusted p-value < 0.3, whereas the two vertical dashed lines mark Spearman's ρ values equal to –0.5 and 0.5; x-axis: Spearman's ρ, y-axis: p-value in negative $\log_{10}$ scale.

3.5. SU_LIVER-Based Clustering of HCC Patients Associated with the Assigned Tumor Grade

In order to explore the potential connection between acquired results from examined HCC lines and HCC patients' data, we next tried to compare the differentiation characteristics of 354 tumors from the HCC TCGA cohort by hierarchical clustering based on the expression of SU_LIVER gene-set, as this was the main gene-set applied throughout the exploratory, ssGSEA, and drug screening analyses in HCC lines. Heatmap representation of the results (Figure 11) revealed two main obvious clusters. One major cluster consisted of 237 mostly well/moderately differentiated tumors (n_{G1+G2} = 172, n_{G3+G4} = 65) that generally overexpressed SU_LIVER genes, and a second smaller cluster contained 117 mostly poorly/undifferentiated tumors (n_{G1+G2} = 52, n_{G3+G4} = 65) that overall exhibited lower gene expression levels. Notably, as shown by the χ^2- test, there was a statistically significant association (p-value = 2.41 × 10^{-7}) between the formed clusters and the assigned tumor histological grading, a clear indicator of the degree of tumor differentiation.

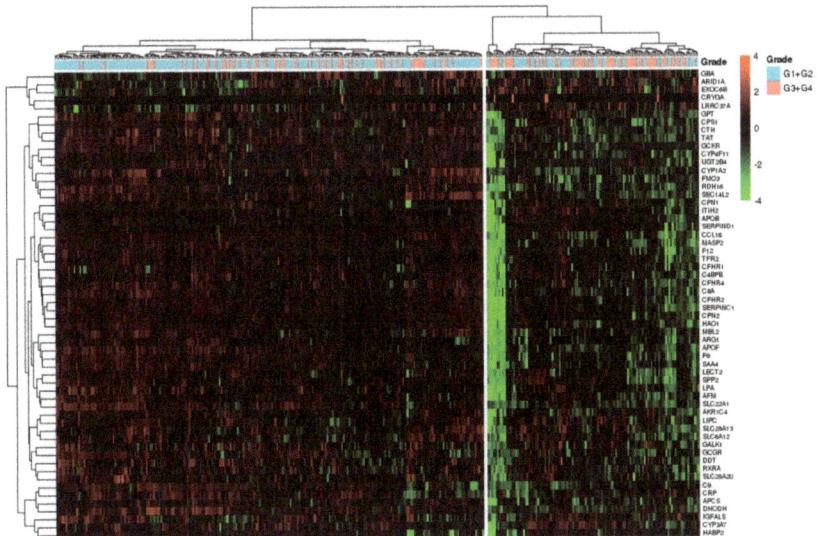

Figure 11. Heatmap illustrating the hierarchical clustering of HCC tumors (columns) based on the full set of SU_LIVER genes (rows). Scaled values indicate relative downregulation (green color) or upregulation (red color) of gene expression. HCC tumors are annotated by color according to their documented histological grade (G1+G2 versus G3+G4).

4. Discussion

The use of current systems biology methodologies has greatly advanced the global investigation of intertumor heterogeneity in connection to drug-specific sensitivity/resistance, paving the way for the evolution of future therapeutic breakthroughs, including biomarker-driven treatments and precision medicine [6,22,36,37]. To this end, we applied an entirely computational approach implementing a multi-level bioinformatics analysis of publicly available transcriptomic, proteomic, and drug-screening datasets which enabled us to explore the molecular diversity of a large panel of established HCC lines and its association to drug responsiveness.

Exploratory data analysis and a subsequent ssGSEA approach on DNA microarray data led to the classification of investigated cell lines into two main subgroups mainly defined by their respective differentiation status: a group of poorly and a group of well-differentiated cell lines overexpressing genes that are specifically upregulated in normal human liver tissues, and therefore were considered to retain a liver-like epithelial molecular profile. Notably, this subgrouping of HCC lines proved to be highly consistent at the proteome level and was further supported by hierarchical clustering based on an EMT gene signature. As EMT is a process highly implicated in tumor cell de-differentiation [29,38], this result provided complementary information to the differentiation profiling of HCC lines. It is recognized that high-grade poorly differentiated tumors are characterized by increased aggressiveness and poor prognosis [39]; consequently, histological grading of HCC presents an important prognostic marker along with various other molecular traits [40]. Although epithelial and/or mixed epithelial–mesenchymal characteristics are no longer considered to be completely disentangled from aggressive phenotypes [41], there is strong evidence that EMT is tightly associated with increased HCC growth and metastasis [42]. For this reason, several recent endeavors have generated and/or surveyed transcriptome and proteome data in various cancer cell line models —including HCC— in order to identify expression patterns connected to differentiation/EMT-related characteristics [6,22,36]; hence, the present work aspired to contribute accordingly. As a matter of fact, the differential gene and protein expression analysis conducted in order to explore the distinctive molecular background of poorly versus well-differentiated HCC lines highlighted 935 DEGs and 16 DEPs. Notably, the expression of almost all the genes encoding the identified DEPs was also accordingly modified, thus indicating that the observed changes in protein levels were attributed to a diverse transcriptional regulation of the corresponding genes. The most outstanding DEP findings included downregulation of the important epithelial/EMT marker ECADHERIN (*CDH1*) [43] and upregulation of CAVEOLIN1 (*CAV1*) [44] and PAI1 (*SERPINE1*) [45], both associated with increased aggressiveness, invasion, and metastasis.

Subsequent functional enrichment analyses of identified DEGs against GO and Reactome Pathway databases were performed to efficiently elucidate significantly associated biological processes and pathways, while acquired enrichment data were further aggregated by *Bioinfominer* to identify core systemic biological processes/pathways and hub driver-gene signatures. Results from both ontological databases commonly revealed a specific pattern of differentially regulated processes and pathways involved in wound healing, hemostasis, coagulation, platelet dynamics, fibrinolysis, ECM remodeling, and cell migration/motility, as indicated by the high recurrence of relevant terminologies in the lists of the top 30 significantly enriched GO biological processes, and of 28 Reactome Pathway terms. Notably, the majority of these processes/pathways are biologically inter-connected and are either directly or indirectly associated with cancer progression, invasive/metastatic potential and overall aggressiveness. Tumors are often characterized as wounds that do not heal, constantly remodeling the stroma cells' microenvironment and reorganizing ECM. This complex procedure involves provisional biological mechanisms that include inflammatory responses, clotting cascade activation, fibrin formation and fibrinolysis, angiogenesis, and enhanced vasculature [46,47]. Therefore, the attained deregulation of relevant processes/pathways in poorly compared to well-differentiated HCC lines is highly indicative of their augmented malignant capacity and offers useful information about the roles of implicated genes. Moreover, terms related to altered/impaired metabolism (especially of lipids, cholesterol/steroids, and lipoproteins)—a well-established cancer hallmark sustaining cancer cell growth and proliferation [48]—were evidently present in both functional enrichment lists, pointing out the significant role of metabolism-related genes and functions in defining the differential characteristics of HCC subtypes, in agreement with a recent metabolism-focused study on liver cancer [49]. *Bioinfominer* analysis proposed two distinct hub driver-gene signatures (each based on GO and Reactome Pathway results, respectively) involving molecular agents playing major roles in multiple underlying biological mechanisms. A number of genes, including several metabolism-related apolipoproteins and fibrinogens, commonly appeared in both signatures (*APOA1, APOA2, APOB, FGG, FGA, F2, APOE, NR1H3, GAS6, ACOX1*). Interestingly, *GAS6* upregulation emerged as a prominent factor in poorly differentiated HCC lines, implicated in a variety of systemic ontological terms. This finding, along with the observed overexpression of *AXL* and *SNAI2* (Slug), points to a key role for Gas6/Axl pathway, known to promote invasion and migration in HCC through Slug activation [50]. Moreover, AXL acts as a crucial regulator of cancer-related EMT [51]; particularly in HCC, the cooperation between Gas6/Axl and TGF-β signaling pathways appears to be crucial in differentiation, EMT, and the advancement of invasion [52]. Suitably, the TGF-β pathway was represented in the respective GO-derived hub gene signature by upregulated *TGFB2* gene, while other TGF-β signaling-associated genes were identified as DEGs as well, including overexpressed *TGFB1*. Both *TGFB1* and *TGFB2* are recognized as being heavily linked to EMT and tumor progression [38,53]. Additional noteworthy driver DEGs included in hub gene signatures were those known to be involved in fibrinolysis and platelet degranulation, such as *SERPINE1* (upregulated) and *A2M* (downregulated). *SERPINE1*, along with the identified (overexpressed) DEGs *PLAU* and *PLAUR*, is centrally implicated in cancer angiogenesis [54], while *A2M* possesses antitumorigenic properties [55]. Furthermore, *FGF2* along and its corresponding receptor *FGFR1* (both upregulated) were also found in the identified hub driver-gene signatures. It is well established that FGF2/FGFR signaling deregulation is associated with aggressive tumor phenotypes and drug resistance [56], features recurrently linked to the poorly differentiated HCC subtypes. Additionally, *HNF4A*'s (downregulated) characterization as a distinctive molecular player between differentiation states of examined HCC lines was in fact anticipated, due to the pivotal role of this transcription factor in liver function and hepatocyte differentiation [57]. Finally, the ontological term "biological oxidations"—widely associated with oxidative stress and fatty acid metabolism in HCC [58]—was also demonstrated as systemic core process in the Reactome Pathway data, represented by *GNG11*, *GNG12*, *ACOX1*, and multiple apolipoprotein genes.

Complementary information regarding potentially implicated biological mechanisms was subsequently gathered by performing supplementary gene-set enrichment analysis against curated datasets from MSigDB based on differential expression analysis data. Results once again highlighted a more aggressive phenotype for poorly differentiated HCC lines. It is worth noting that this group of HCC lines shared common upregulated genes with the S1 HCC subtype identified by Hoshida et al. in primary HCC—characterized by mesenchymal characteristics/active TGF-β signaling—while the group of better-differentiated ones resembled subtypes S2 and S3, retaining a more hepatocyte-like phenotype while overexpressing certain hepatoblast markers like *AFP* and *EPCAM* [35].

Lastly, the association of HCC differentiation status with drug sensitivity/resistance—explored by correlating cell line SU_LIVER enrichment scores with drug efficacy measurements for a panel of compounds—resulted in the identification of drugs that were more effective against poorly than well-differentiated cell lines, and vice versa. HCC lines in the well-differentiated group proved to be more sensitive than their counterparts against a larger number of investigated drugs/agents, including several TKIs such as those targeting EGFR (erlotinib), IGF1R (linsitinib, BMS-536924, BMS-754807), or other kinases (linifanib, masitinib, imatinib). EMT has been identified as a major contributor of acquired resistance against EGFR-TKIs in non-small-cell lung cancers [59], while protein-level pan-cancer studies have highlighted an EMT-status-dependent efficacy of several EGFR inhibitors and other targeted therapies [37]. Interestingly, as both genes were overexpressed in poorly differentiated cell lines, FGF2/FGFR1 activation in non-small-cell lung cancer has been proposed as an important EGFR-TKI-resistance-acquisition mechanism [60]. Furthermore, the present results for IGF1R and MDM2 inhibitors corroborated those of a recent study on numerous cancer liver cell lines providing experimental evidence of an augmented efficacy of IGF1R inhibitor linsitinib as well as of MDM2 inhibitor nutlin-3 against liver cancer lines with prominent hepatoblast/hepatocyte-like characteristics [36], thus supporting the validity of our approach. Additionally, the natural compound epigallocatechin-3-monogallate was identified as being comparatively more effective against well-differentiated HCC lines, in full agreement with previous studies highlighting HEP3B and HEPG2 cell lines as particularly responsive against that nutraceutical [61,62].

On the other hand, a smaller portion of examined drugs displayed an enhanced efficacy against the poorly differentiated group in comparison to well-differentiated HCC lines. Among them, it is worth discussing the role of three compounds, namely the retinoic acid receptor β (RARB) agonist AC55649, the SPHK1 inhibitor SKI-II, and the PKM2 activator ML203. All-trans retinoic acid (ATRA), a known pan-retinoic receptor agonist, has been found to regulate EMT and inhibit migration in breast cancer via the TGF-β pathway [63], a notion that might support the use of RARB agonists against poorly differentiated HCC with TGF-β-dependent EMT features. As for SPHK1, it is known to induce EMT in hepatoma cells through the promotion of *CDH1*/ECADHERIN degradation [64], and thus, SPHK1-inhibitors could be a reasonable option against mesenchymal-like HCC. Finally, PKM2 activation through ML203 presents an interesting prospect, since PKM2—a metabolic enzyme in glycolysis—is attracting growing attention due to a manifold possible involvement in cancer progression [65]. It has been shown that PKM2 activity is negatively regulated by the increased presence of CD44 (a known cancer biomarker), and this effect mediates the aggressive glycolytic phenotype of colon cancer cells [66]. Notably, the *CD44* gene was one of the most significantly upregulated DEGs in poorly differentiated HCC lines. It is thus possible that the compound ML203 could counteract the hampered PKM2 activation by overexpressed *CD44*, and therefore inhibit the glycolytic phenotype of poorly differentiated HCC.

Although our analysis was entirely based on data from HCC lines, the acquired information of drug sensitivity in poorly and well-differentiated cell lines might be of clinical relevance for HCC patients with characterized tumor differentiation profiles. To this end, tumors from 354 patients from the HCC TCGA cohort were stratified on the basis of SU_LIVER gene-set expression data into two clusters statistically significant for tumor grade, one with samples generally displaying high/moderate differentiation and overexpression of SU_LIVER genes, and one with overall poorly/undifferentiated tumors and lower SU_LIVER gene expression levels. Since HCC patient clustering corroborated with the corresponding stratification of HCC lines into poorly and well-differentiated groups, the present TCGA investigation (a) broadened the reliability of SU_LIVER genes-based clustering as an informative analysis that significantly correlates gene expression pattern with the differentiation status of HCC lines and—very importantly—of patient tumors as well, and (b) in conjunction with the aforementioned drug-sensitivity data for HCC lines (also based on SU_LIVER enrichment scores), may offer preliminary clues in future clinical research for predicting drug efficiency in HCC patients possessing analogous gene expression characteristics and histological grade. However, it should be noted that cell-line models—lacking crucial interactions with immune/stromal cells and surrounding ECM—are not perfect representations of in vivo tumors and thus, cannot fully recapitulate the wide spectrum of tumor heterogeneity and consequently their response to drugs.

Certainly, the availability and the constantly growing volume of several types of -omics and drug-screening data in multiple public resources make their computational integration and investigation of their biological/clinical relevance a real challenge in ongoing cancer research. Focusing on HCC—in addition to the currently presented analysis of transcriptomic and proteomic data—future studies exploiting available genomics data, including DNA alterations, especially in genes and gene-expression-regulatory elements, as well as evaluating metabolome variations, are required in order to provide further insights into the mechanisms underlying HCC heterogeneity. Preliminary bioinformatics analysis by our group, which was based on accessible data for coding-gene mutations and copy-number variations (deletions/amplifications) in HCC lines provided some interesting initial observations that merit further investigation.

5. Conclusions

The present work, by using a thorough in silico analysis of publicly available transcriptomic, proteomic, and drug-screening data, classified a large panel of HCC lines into two representative differentiation subtypes of either higher or lower differentiation status, each exhibiting a discrete sensitivity pattern against numerous evaluated drugs. Furthermore, the identification of two hub driver DEGs signatures across informative ontology/pathway databases provided evidence on functionally significant biomarkers, thus offering a starting basis for mechanistic and pharmacogenomic studies. Overall, the described methodologies provide a comprehensive cost-effective computational framework, able to be applied in any model cancer cell lines as long as relevant -omics and drug-screening data are accessible in dedicated repositories, which allows the investigation of inherent tumor molecular diversity and the design of therapeutic regimes effective for each cancer subtype.

Supplementary Materials: The following are available online at http://www.mdpi.com/2073-4425/11/6/623/s1, Figure S1: Correlation matrix for HCC line pairs based on the expression of the 500 genes with the largest cross-sample variation, Figure S2: Correlation matrix for HCC line pairs based on the expression of 214 proteins/phosphoproteins, Figure S3: BIC results for optimal number of k-means clusters based on PC1 scores, Figure S4: PCA of HCC lines based on CCLE RNA-seq gene expression data, Figure S5: BIC results for optimal number of k-means clusters based on computed cell-line ssGSEA SU_LIVER enrichment scores, Figure S6: Heatmap illustrating the scaled expression values of HCC lines regarding identified DEGs, Figure S7: Heatmap illustrating the scaled expression values of HCC lines regarding identified DEPs, Figure S8: GO systemic processes and involved hub genes, Figure S9: Reactome Pathway systemic processes and involved hub genes, Table S1: ssGSEA scores based on PC1 loadings, Table S2: ssGSEA scores for individual cell lines, Table S3: List of DEGs, Table S4: List of DEPs, Table S5: GO enrichment results, Table S6: Reactome Pathway enrichment results, Table S7: Gene-set enrichment results from *camera*, Table S8: Drug-response correlation with SU_LIVER enrichment score results.

Author Contributions: Conceptualization, H.L. and F.N.K.; methodology, P.C.A., H.L. and F.N.K.; software, P.C.A.; validation, P.C.A., H.L. and F.N.K.; formal analysis, P.C.A., H.L. and F.N.K.; investigation, P.C.A; resources, H.L. and F.N.K.; data curation, P.C.A., H.L. and F.N.K.; writing-original draft preparation, P.C.A., H.L. and F.N.K.; writing-review and editing, P.C.A., H.L. and F.N.K.; visualization, P.C.A. and H.L.; supervision, H.L. and F.N.K.; project administration, H.L. and F.N.K.; funding acquisition, H.L. and F.N.K. All authors have read and agreed to the published version of the manuscript.

Funding: We acknowledge support of this work by the project "Synthetic Biology: from omics technologies to genomic engineering (OMIC-ENGINE)" (MIS 5002636) which is implemented under the Action Reinforcement of the Research and Innovation Infrastructure, funded by the Operational Programme "Competitiveness, Entrepreneurship and Innovation" (NSRF 2014-2020) and co-financed by Greece and the European Union (European Regional Development Fund).

Conflicts of Interest: The authors declare no conflict of interest. The funders had no role in the design of the study; in the collection, analyses, or interpretation of data; in the writing of the manuscript, or in the decision to publish the results.

References

1. Forner, A.; Reig, M.; Bruix, J. Hepatocellular carcinoma. *Lancet* **2018**, *391*, 1301–1314. [CrossRef]
2. Fujiwara, N.; Friedman, S.L.; Goossens, N.; Hoshida, Y. Risk factors and prevention of hepatocellular carcinoma in the era of precision medicine. *J. Hepatol.* **2018**, *68*, 526–549. [CrossRef]
3. Aravalli, R.N.; Cressman, E.N.K.; Steer, C.J. Cellular and molecular mechanisms of hepatocellular carcinoma: An update. *Arch. Toxicol.* **2013**, *87*, 227–247. [CrossRef] [PubMed]
4. Llovet, J.M.; Montal, R.; Sia, D.; Finn, R.S. Molecular therapies and precision medicine for hepatocellular carcinoma. *Nat. Rev. Clin. Oncol.* **2018**, *15*, 599–616. [CrossRef] [PubMed]
5. Katt, M.E.; Placone, A.L.; Wong, A.D.; Xu, Z.S.; Searson, P.C. In vitro tumor models: Advantages, disadvantages, variables, and selecting the right platform. *Front. Bioeng. Biotechnol.* **2016**, *4*, 12. [CrossRef] [PubMed]
6. Berg, K.C.G.; Eide, P.W.; Eilertsen, I.A.; Johannessen, B.; Bruun, J.; Danielsen, S.A.; Bjørnslett, M.; Meza-Zepeda, L.A.; Eknæs, M.; Lind, G.E.; et al. Multi-omics of 34 colorectal cancer cell lines—A resource for biomedical studies. *Mol. Cancer* **2017**, *16*, 1–16. [CrossRef]
7. Barretina, J.; Caponigro, G.; Stransky, N.; Venkatesan, K.; Margolin, A.A.; Kim, S.; Wilson, C.J.; Lehár, J.; Gregory, V.; Sonkin, D.; et al. The Cancer Cell Line Encyclopedia enables predictive modeling of anticancer drug sensitivity. *Nature* **2012**, *483*, 603–607. [CrossRef]
8. Ghandi, M.; Huang, F.W.; Jané-Valbuena, J.; Kryukov, G.V.; Lo, C.C.; McDonald, E.R.; Barretina, J.; Gelfand, E.T.; Bielski, C.M.; Li, H.; et al. Next-generation characterization of the Cancer Cell Line Encyclopedia. *Nature* **2019**, *569*, 503–508. [CrossRef]
9. Park, J.; Lee, J.; Kang, M.; Park, K.; Jeon, Y.; Lee, H.; Kwon, H.; Park, H.; Yeo, K.; Lee, K.; et al. Characterization of cell lines established from human hepatocellular carcinoma. *Int. J. Cancer* **1995**, *62*, 276–282. [CrossRef]
10. Heffelfinger, S.C.; Hawkins, H.H.; Barrish, J.; Taylor, L.; Darlington, G.J. SK HEP-1: A human cell line of endothelial origin. *Cell. Dev. Biol. Anim.* **1992**, *28*, 136–142. [CrossRef]
11. Rebouissou, S.; Zucman-Rossi, J.; Moreau, R.; Qiu, Z.; Hui, L. Note of caution: Contaminations of hepatocellular cell lines. *J. Hepatol.* **2017**, *67*, 896–897. [CrossRef] [PubMed]
12. Seashore-Ludlow, B.; Rees, M.G.; Cheah, J.H.; Coko, M.; Price, E.V.; Coletti, M.E.; Jones, V.; Bodycombe, N.E.; Soule, C.K.; Gould, J.; et al. Harnessing connectivity in a large-scale small-molecule sensitivity dataset. *Cancer Discov.* **2015**, *5*, 1210–1223. [CrossRef] [PubMed]
13. Basu, A.; Bodycombe, N.E.; Cheah, J.H.; Price, E.V.; Liu, K.; Schaefer, G.I.; Ebright, R.Y.; Stewart, M.L.; Ito, D.; Wang, S.; et al. An interactive resource to identify cancer genetic and lineage dependencies targeted by small molecules. *Cell* **2013**, *154*, 1151–1161. [CrossRef] [PubMed]
14. Ally, A.; Balasundaram, M.; Carlsen, R.; Chuah, E.; Clarke, A.; Dhalla, N.; Holt, R.A.; Jones, S.J.M.; Lee, D.; Ma, Y.; et al. Comprehensive and integrative genomic characterization of hepatocellular carcinoma. *Cell* **2017**, *169*, 1327–1341.e23. [CrossRef]
15. Li, B.; Dewey, C.N. RSEM: Accurate transcript quantification from RNA-Seq data with or without a reference genome. *BMC Bioinform.* **2011**, *12*, 323. [CrossRef]
16. Robinson, M.D.; Oshlack, A. A scaling normalization method for differential expression analysis of RNA-seq data. *Genome Biol.* **2010**, *11*, R25. [CrossRef]

17. Rohart, F.; Gautier, B.; Singh, A.; Lê Cao, K.A. mixOmics: An R package for 'omics feature selection and multiple data integration. *PLoS Comput. Biol.* **2017**, *13*, 1–19. [CrossRef]
18. Wang, H.; Song, M. Ckmeans.1d.dp: Optimal k-means clustering in one dimension by dynamic programming. *R Journal* **2011**, *3*, 29–33. [CrossRef]
19. Schwarz, G. Estimating the dimension of a model. *Ann. Stat.* **1978**, *6*, 461–464. [CrossRef]
20. Hänzelmann, S.; Castelo, R.; Guinney, J. GSVA: Gene set variation analysis for microarray and RNA-Seq data. *BMC Bioinform.* **2013**, *14*, 7. [CrossRef]
21. Barbie, D.A.; Tamayo, P.; Boehm, J.S.; Kim, S.Y.; Moody, S.E.; Dunn, I.F.; Schinzel, A.C.; Sandy, P.; Meylan, E.; Scholl, C.; et al. Systematic RNA interference reveals that oncogenic KRAS-driven cancers require TBK1. *Nature* **2009**, *462*, 108–112. [CrossRef] [PubMed]
22. Koplev, S.; Lin, K.; Dohlman, A.B.; Ma'ayan, A. Integration of pan-cancer transcriptomics with RPPA proteomics reveals mechanisms of epithelial-mesenchymal transition. *PLoS Comput. Biol.* **2018**, *14*, 1–19. [CrossRef] [PubMed]
23. Ritchie, M.E.; Phipson, B.; Wu, D.; Hu, Y.; Law, C.W.; Shi, W.; Smyth, G.K. Limma powers differential expression analyses for RNA-sequencing and microarray studies. *Nucleic Acids Res.* **2015**, *43*, e47. [CrossRef] [PubMed]
24. Mccarthy, D.J.; Smyth, G.K. Testing significance relative to a fold-change threshold is a TREAT. *Bioinformatics* **2009**, *25*, 765–771. [CrossRef]
25. Blighe, K. Publication-ready volcano plots with enhanced colouring and labeling. Available online: https://github.com/kevinblighe/EnhancedVolcano (accessed on 5 June 2020). (R-Package Version 1.0.1).
26. Koutsandreas, T.; Binenbaum, I.; Pilalis, E.; Valavanis, I.; Papadodima, O.; Chatziioannou, A. Analyzing and visualizing genomic complexity for the derivation of the emergent molecular networks. *Int. J. Monit. Surveill. Technol. Res.* **2016**, *4*, 30–49. [CrossRef]
27. Lhomond, S.; Avril, T.; Dejeans, N.; Voutetakis, K.; Doultsinos, D.; McMahon, M.; Pineau, R.; Obacz, J.; Papadodima, O.; Jouan, F.; et al. Dual IRE1 RNase functions dictate glioblastoma development. *EMBO Mol. Med.* **2018**, *10*, 1–19. [CrossRef]
28. Wu, D.; Smyth, G.K. Camera: A competitive gene set test accounting for inter-gene correlation. *Nucleic Acids Res.* **2012**, *40*, 1–12. [CrossRef]
29. Wang, H.; Unternaehrer, J.J. Epithelial-mesenchymal transition and cancer stem cells: At the crossroads of differentiation and dedifferentiation. *Dev. Dyn.* **2019**, *248*, 10–20. [CrossRef]
30. Su, A.I.; Cooke, M.P.; Ching, K.A.; Hakak, Y.; Walker, J.R.; Wiltshire, T.; Orth, A.P.; Vega, R.G.; Sapinoso, L.M.; Moqrich, A.; et al. Large-scale analysis of the human and mouse transcriptomes. *Proc. Natl. Acad. Sci. USA* **2002**, *99*, 4465–4470. [CrossRef]
31. Hsiao, L.L.; Dangond, F.; Yoshida, T.; Hong, R.; Jensen, R.V.; Misra, J.; Dillon, W.; Lee, K.F.; Clark, K.E.; Haverty, P.; et al. A compendium of gene expression in normal human tissues. *Physiol. Genom.* **2002**, *2002*, 97–104. [CrossRef]
32. Anastassiou, D.; Rumjantseva, V.; Cheng, W.; Huang, J.; Canoll, P.D.; Yamashiro, D.J.; Kandel, J.J. Human cancer cells express Slug-based epithelial-mesenchymal transition gene expression signature obtained in vivo. *BMC Cancer* **2011**, *11*, 529. [CrossRef] [PubMed]
33. Elvidge, G.P.; Glenny, L.; Appelhoff, R.J.; Ratcliffe, P.J.; Ragoussis, J.; Gleadle, J.M. Concordant regulation of gene expression by hypoxia and 2-oxoglutarate-dependent dioxygenase inhibition: The role of HIF-1α, HIF-2α, and other pathways. *J. Biol. Chem.* **2006**, *281*, 15215–15226. [CrossRef] [PubMed]
34. Wu, Y.; Siadaty, M.S.; Berens, M.E.; Hampton, G.M.; Theodorescu, D. Overlapping gene expression profiles of cell migration and tumor invasion in human bladder cancer identify metallothionein 1E and nicotinamide N-methyltransferase as novel regulators of cell migration. *Oncogene* **2008**, *27*, 6679–6689. [CrossRef] [PubMed]
35. Hoshida, Y.; Nijman, S.M.B.; Kobayashi, M.; Chan, J.A.; Brunet, J.P.; Chiang, D.Y.; Villanueva, A.; Newell, P.; Ikeda, K.; Hashimoto, M.; et al. Integrative transcriptome analysis reveals common molecular subclasses of human hepatocellular carcinoma. *Cancer Res.* **2009**, *69*, 7385–7392. [CrossRef] [PubMed]
36. Caruso, S.; Calatayud, A.L.; Pilet, J.; La Bella, T.; Rekik, S.; Imbeaud, S.; Letouzé, E.; Meunier, L.; Bayard, Q.; Rohr-Udilova, N.; et al. Analysis of liver cancer cell lines identifies agents with likely efficacy against hepatocellular carcinoma and markers of response. *Gastroenterology* **2019**, *157*, 760–776. [CrossRef] [PubMed]

37. Li, J.; Zhao, W.; Akbani, R.; Liu, W.; Ju, Z.; Ling, S.; Vellano, C.P.; Roebuck, P.; Yu, Q.; Eterovic, A.K.; et al. Characterization of human cancer cell lines by reverse-phase protein arrays. *Cancer Cell* **2017**, *31*, 225–239. [CrossRef]
38. Nieto, M.A.; Huang, R.Y.-J.; Jackson, R.A.; Thiery, J.P. EMT: 2016. *Cell* **2016**, *166*, 21–45. [CrossRef]
39. Dongre, A.; Weinberg, R.A. New insights into the mechanisms of epithelial–mesenchymal transition and implications for cancer. *Nat. Rev. Mol. Cell Biol.* **2019**, *20*, 69–84. [CrossRef]
40. Martins-Filho, S.N.; Paiva, C.; Azevedo, R.S.; Alves, V.A.F. Histological grading of hepatocellular carcinoma-a systematic review of literature. *Front. Med.* **2017**, *4*, 1–9. [CrossRef]
41. Williams, E.D.; Gao, D.; Redfern, A.; Thompson, E.W. Controversies around epithelial–mesenchymal plasticity in cancer metastasis. *Nat. Rev. Cancer* **2019**. [CrossRef]
42. Giannelli, G.; Koudelkova, P.; Dituri, F.; Mikulits, W. Role of epithelial to mesenchymal transition in hepatocellular carcinoma. *J. Hepatol.* **2016**, *65*, 798–808. [CrossRef] [PubMed]
43. Schmalhofer, O.; Brabletz, S.; Brabletz, T. E-cadherin, β-catenin, and ZEB1 in malignant progression of cancer. *Cancer Metastasis Rev.* **2009**, *28*, 151–166. [CrossRef] [PubMed]
44. Ting Tse, E.Y.; Fat Ko, F.C.; Kwan Tung, E.K.; Chan, L.K.; Wah Lee, T.K.; Wai Ngan, E.S.; Man, K.; Tsai Wong, A.S.; Ng, I.O.L.; Ping Yam, J.W. Caveolin-1 overexpression is associated with hepatocellular carcinoma tumourigenesis and metastasis. *J. Pathol.* **2012**, *226*, 645–653. [CrossRef] [PubMed]
45. Li, S.; Wei, X.; He, J.; Tian, X.; Yuan, S.; Sun, L. Plasminogen activator inhibitor-1 in cancer research. *Biomed. Pharmacother.* **2018**, *105*, 83–94. [CrossRef] [PubMed]
46. Dvorak, H.F. Tumors: Wounds that do not heal-redux. *Cancer Immunol. Res.* **2015**, *3*, 1–11. [CrossRef] [PubMed]
47. Foster, D.S.; Jones, R.E.; Ransom, R.C.; Longaker, M.T.; Norton, J.A. The evolving relationship of wound healing and tumor stroma. *JCI Insight* **2018**, *3*, 1–17. [CrossRef]
48. Hanahan, D.; Weinberg, R.A. Hallmarks of cancer: The next generation. *Cell* **2011**, *144*, 646–674. [CrossRef]
49. Nwosu, Z.C.; Battello, N.; Rothley, M.; Piorońska, W.; Sitek, B.; Ebert, M.P.; Hofmann, U.; Sleeman, J.; Wölfl, S.; Meyer, C.; et al. Liver cancer cell lines distinctly mimic the metabolic gene expression pattern of the corresponding human tumours. *J. Exp. Clin. Cancer Res.* **2018**, *37*, 211. [CrossRef]
50. Lee, H.J.; Jeng, Y.M.; Chen, Y.L.; Chung, L.; Yuan, R.H. Gas6/Axl pathway promotes tumor invasion through the transcriptional activation of slug in hepatocellular carcinoma. *Carcinogenesis* **2014**, *35*, 769–775. [CrossRef]
51. Antony, J.; Huang, R.Y.J. AXL-driven EMT state as a targetable conduit in cancer. *Cancer Res.* **2017**, *77*, 3725–3732. [CrossRef]
52. Reichl, P.; Dengler, M.; van Zijl, F.; Huber, H.; Führlinger, G.; Reichel, C.; Sieghart, W.; Peck-Radosavljevic, M.; Grubinger, M.; Mikulits, W. Axl activates autocrine transforming growth factor-β signaling in hepatocellular carcinoma. *Hepatology* **2015**, *61*, 930–941. [CrossRef] [PubMed]
53. Ikushima, H.; Miyazono, K. TGFB 2 signalling: A complex web in cancer progression. *Nat. Rev. Cancer* **2010**, *10*, 415–424. [CrossRef] [PubMed]
54. Kwaan, H.C.; Lindholm, P.F. Fibrin and fibrinolysis in cancer. *Semin. Thromb. Hemost.* **2019**, *45*, 413–422. [CrossRef] [PubMed]
55. Kurz, S.; Thieme, R.; Amberg, R.; Groth, M.; Jahnke, H.G.; Pieroh, P.; Horn, L.C.; Kolb, M.; Huse, K.; Platzer, M.; et al. The anti-tumorigenic activity of A2M—A lesson from the naked mole-rat. *PLoS ONE* **2017**, *12*, 1–24. [CrossRef] [PubMed]
56. Akl, M.R.; Nagpal, P.; Ayoub, N.M.; Tai, B.; Prabhu, S.A.; Capac, C.M.; Gliksman, M.; Goy, A.; Suh, K.S. Molecular and clinical significance of fibroblast growth factor 2 (FGF2/bFGF) in malignancies of solid and hematological cancers for personalized therapies. *Oncotarget* **2016**, *7*, 44735–44762. [CrossRef]
57. Ning, B.F.; Ding, J.; Yin, C.; Zhong, W.; Wu, K.; Zeng, X.; Yang, W.; Chen, Y.X.; Zhang, J.P.; Zhang, X.; et al. Hepatocyte nuclear factor 4α suppresses the development of hepatocellular carcinoma. *Cancer Res.* **2010**, *70*, 7640–7651. [CrossRef]
58. Wang, M.; Han, J.; Xing, H.; Zhang, H.; Li, Z.; Liang, L.; Li, C.; Dai, S.; Wu, M.; Shen, F.; et al. Dysregulated fatty acid metabolism in hepatocellular carcinoma. *Hepatic Oncol.* **2016**, *3*, 241–251. [CrossRef]
59. Zhu, X.; Chen, L.; Liu, L.; Niu, X. EMT-Mediated Acquired EGFR-TKI Resistance in NSCLC: Mechanisms and Strategies. *Front. Oncol.* **2019**, *9*, 1–15. [CrossRef]

60. Terai, H.; Soejima, K.; Yasuda, H.; Nakayama, S.; Hamamoto, J.; Arai, D. Activation of the FGF2-FGFR1 autocrine pathway: A novel mechanism of acquired resistance to gefitinib in NSCLC. *Mol. Cancer Res.* **2013**, *1*, 759–768. [CrossRef]
61. Michailidou, M.; Melas, I.; Messinis, D.; Klamt, S.; Alexopoulos, L.; Kolisis, F.; Loutrari, H. Network-based analysis of nutraceuticals in human hepatocellular carcinomas reveals mechanisms of chemopreventive action. *CPT Pharmacomet. Syst. Pharmacol.* **2015**, *4*, 350–361. [CrossRef]
62. Agioutantis, P.C.; Kotsikoris, V.; Kolisis, F.N.; Loutrari, H. RNA-seq data analysis of stimulated hepatocellular carcinoma cells treated with epigallocatechin gallate and fisetin reveals target genes and action mechanisms. *Comput. Struct. Biotechnol. J.* **2020**, *18*, 686–695. [CrossRef] [PubMed]
63. Zanetti, A.; Affatato, R.; Centritto, F.; Fratelli, M.; Kurosaki, M.; Barzago, M.M.; Bolis, M.; Terao, M.; Garattini, E.; Paroni, G. All-trans-retinoic acid modulates the plasticity and inhibits the motility of breast cancer cells role of notch1 and transforming growth factor (TGF β). *J. Biol. Chem.* **2015**, *290*, 17690–17709. [CrossRef] [PubMed]
64. Liu, H.; Ma, Y.; He, H.W.; Zhao, W.L.; Shao, R.G. SPHK1 (sphingosine kinase 1) induces epithelial-mesenchymal transition by promoting the autophagy-linked lysosomal degradation of CDH1/E-cadherin in hepatoma cells. *Autophagy* **2017**, *13*, 900–913. [CrossRef] [PubMed]
65. Hsu, M.C.; Hung, W.C. Pyruvate kinase M2 fuels multiple aspects of cancer cells: From cellular metabolism, transcriptional regulation to extracellular signaling. *Mol. Cancer* **2018**, *17*, 1–9. [CrossRef]
66. Tamada, M.; Nagano, O.; Tateyama, S.; Ohmura, M.; Yae, T.; Ishimoto, T.; Sugihara, E.; Onishi, N.; Yamamoto, T.; Yanagawa, H.; et al. Modulation of glucose metabolism by CD44 contributes to antioxidant status and drug resistance in cancer cells. *Cancer Res.* **2012**, *72*, 1438–1448. [CrossRef] [PubMed]

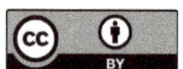

© 2020 by the authors. Licensee MDPI, Basel, Switzerland. This article is an open access article distributed under the terms and conditions of the Creative Commons Attribution (CC BY) license (http://creativecommons.org/licenses/by/4.0/).

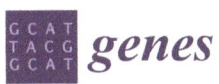

Article

Computational Analysis of the Global Effects of *Ly6E* in the Immune Response to Coronavirus Infection Using Gene Networks

Fernando M. Delgado-Chaves *,[†], Francisco Gómez-Vela [†], Federico Divina, Miguel García-Torres and Domingo S. Rodriguez-Baena

Pablo de Olavide University, Carretera de Utrera km 1, ES-41013 Seville, Spain; fgomez@upo.es (F.G.-V.); fdiv@upo.es (F.D.); mgarciat@upo.es (M.G.-T.); dsrodbae@upo.es (D.S.R.-B.)
* Correspondence: fmdelcha@upo.es
† These authors contributed equally to this work.

Received: 23 May 2020; Accepted: 13 July 2020 ; Published: 21 July 2020

Abstract: Gene networks have arisen as a promising tool in the comprehensive modeling and analysis of complex diseases. Particularly in viral infections, the understanding of the host-pathogen mechanisms, and the immune response to these, is considered a major goal for the rational design of appropriate therapies. For this reason, the use of gene networks may well encourage therapy-associated research in the context of the coronavirus pandemic, orchestrating experimental scrutiny and reducing costs. In this work, gene co-expression networks were reconstructed from RNA-Seq expression data with the aim of analyzing the time-resolved effects of gene *Ly6E* in the immune response against the coronavirus responsible for murine hepatitis (MHV). Through the integration of differential expression analyses and reconstructed networks exploration, significant differences in the immune response to virus were observed in $Ly6E^{\Delta HSC}$ compared to *wild type* animals. Results show that *Ly6E* ablation at hematopoietic stem cells (HSCs) leads to a progressive impaired immune response in both liver and spleen. Specifically, depletion of the normal leukocyte mediated immunity and chemokine signaling is observed in the liver of $Ly6E^{\Delta HSC}$ mice. On the other hand, the immune response in the spleen, which seemed to be mediated by an intense chromatin activity in the normal situation, is replaced by ECM remodeling in $Ly6E^{\Delta HSC}$ mice. These findings, which require further experimental characterization, could be extrapolated to other coronaviruses and motivate the efforts towards novel antiviral approaches.

Keywords: gene co-expression network; murine coronavirus; viral infection; immune response; data mining; systems biology

---

1. Introduction

The recent SARS-CoV-2 pandemic has exerted an unprecedented pressure on the scientific community in the quest for novel antiviral approaches. A major concern regarding SARS-CoV-2 is the capability of the *coronaviridae* family to cross the species barrier and infect humans [1]. This, along with the tendency of coronaviruses to mutate and recombine, represents a significant threat to global health, which ultimately has put interdisciplinary research on the warpath towards the development of a vaccine or antiviral treatments.

Given the similarities found amongst the members of the *coronaviridae* family [2,3], analyzing the global immune response to coronaviruses may shed some light on the natural control of viral infection, and inspire prospective treatments. This may well be achieved from the perspective of systems biology, in which the interactions between the biological entities involved in a certain process are represented by means of a mathematical system [4]. Within this framework, gene networks (GN) have become an important tool in the modeling and analysis of biological processes from gene expression data [5]. GNs constitute an abstraction of a given biological reality by means of a graph composed by nodes and edges. In such a graph, nodes represent the biological elements involved (i.e., genes, proteins or RNAs) and edges represent the relationships between the nodes. In addition, GNs are also useful to identify genes of interest in biological processes, as well as to discover relationships among these. Thus, they provide a comprehensive picture of the studied processes [6,7].

Among the different types of GNs, gene co-expression networks (GCNs) are widely used in the literature due to their computational simplicity and good performance in order to study biological processes or diseases [8–10]. GCNs usually compute pairwise co-expression indices for all genes. Then, the level of interaction between two genes is considered significant if its score is higher than a certain threshold, which is set *ad hoc*. Traditionally, statistical-based co-expression indices have been used to calculate the dependencies between genes [5,7]. Some of the most popular correlation coefficients are Pearson, Kendall or Spearman [11–13]. Despite their popularity, statistical-based measures present some limitations [14]. For instance, they are not capable of identifying non-linear interactions and the dependence on the data distribution in the case of parametric correlation coefficients. In order to overcome some of these limitations, new approaches, e.g., the use of information theory-based measures or ensemble approaches, are receiving much attention [15–17].

Gene Co-expression Networks (GCNs) have already been applied to the study of dramatic impact diseases, such as cancer [18], diabetes [19] or viral infections (e.g., HIV) in order to study the role of immune response to these illnesses [20,21]. Genetic approaches are expected to be the best strategy to understand viral infection and the immune response to it, potentially identifying the mechanisms of infection and assisting the design of strategies to combat infection [22,23]. The current gene expression profiling platforms, in combination with high-throughput sequencing, can provide time-resolved transcriptomic data, which can be related to the infection process. The main objective of this approach is to generate knowledge on the immune functioning upon viral entry into the organism, which means mean a perturbation to the system.

In the context of viral infection, a first defense line is the innate response mediated by interferons, a type of cytokines which eventually leads to the activation of several genes of antiviral function [24]. Globally, these genes are termed interferon-stimulated genes (ISGs), and regulate processes like inflammation, chemotaxis or macrophage activation among others. Furthermore, ISGs are also involved in the subsequent acquired immune response, specific for the viral pathogen detected [25]. Gene *Ly6E* (lymphocyte antigen 6 family member e), which has been related to T cell maturation and tumorogenesis, is amongst the ISGs [26]. This gene is transcriptionally active in a variety of tissues, including liver, spleen, lung, brain, uterus and ovary. Its role in viral infection has been elusive due to contradictory findings [27]. For example, in Liu et al. [28], *Ly6E* was associated with the resistance to Marek's disease virus (MDV) in chickens. Moreover, differences in the immune response to mouse adenovirus type 1 (MAV-1) have been attributed to *Ly6E* variants [29]. Conversely, *Ly6E* has also been related to an enhancement of human immunodeficiency viruses (HIV-1) pathogenesis, by promoting HIV-1 entry through virus–cell fusion processes [30]. Also in the work by Mar et al. [31], the loss of function of *Ly6E* due to gene *knockout* reduced the infectivity of Influenza A virus (IAV) and yellow fever virus (YFV). This enhancing effect of *Ly6E* on viral infection has also been observed in other enveloped RNA viruses such as in West Nile virus (WNV), dengue virus (DEN), Zika virus (ZIKV), O'nyong nyong virus (ONNV) and Chikungunya virus (CHIKV) among others [32]. Nevertheless, the exact mechanisms through which *Ly6E* modulates viral infection virus-wise, and sometimes even cell type-dependently, require further characterization.

In this work we present a time-resolved study of the immune response of mice to a coronavirus, the murine hepatitis virus (MHV), in order to analyze the implications of gene *Ly6E*. To do so, we have applied a GCN reconstruction method called *EnGNet* [33], which is able to perform an ensemble strategy to combine three different co-expression measures, and a topology optimization of the final network. *EnGNet* has outscored other methods in terms of network precision and reduced network size, and has been proven useful in the modeling of disease, as in the case of Human post-traumatic stress disorder.

The rest of the paper is organized as follows. In the next section, we propose a description of related works. In Section 3, we first describe the dataset used in this paper, and then we introduce the *EnGNet* algorithm and the different methods used to infer and analyze the generated networks. The results obtained are detailed in Section 4, while, in Section 5, we propose a discussion of the results presented in the previous section. Finally, in Section 6, we draw the main conclusions of our work.

2. Related Works

As already mentioned, gene co-expression networks have been extensively applied in the literature for the understanding of the mechanisms underlying complex diseases like cancer, diabetes or Alzheimer [34–36]. Globally, GCN serve as an *in silico* genetic model of these pathologies, highlighting the main genes involved in these at the same time [37]. Besides, the identification of modules in the inferred GCNs, may lead to the discovery of novel biomarkers for the disease under study, following the 'guilt by association' principle. Along these lines, GCNs are also considered suitable for the study of infectious diseases, as those caused by viruses to the matter at hand [38]. To do so, multiple studies have analyzed the effects of viral infection over the organism, focusing on immune response or tissue damage [39,40].

For instance, the analysis of gene expression using co-expression networks is shown in the work by Pedragosa et al. [41], where the infection caused by Lymphocytic Choriomeningitis Virus (LCMV) is studied over time in mice spleen using GCNs. In Ray et al. [42], GCNs are reconstructed from different microarray expression data in order to study HIV-1 progression, revealing important changes across the different infection stages. Similarly, in the work presented by McDermott et al. [43], the over- and under-stimulation of the innate immune response to severe acute respiratory syndrome coronavirus (SARS-CoV) infection is studied. Using several network-based approaches on multiple *knockout* mouse strains, authors found that ranking genes based on their network topology made accurate predictions of the pathogenic state, thus solving a classification problem. In [39], co-expression networks were generated by microarray analysis of pediatric influenza-infected samples. Thanks to this study, genes involved in the innate immune system and defense to virus were revealed. Finally, in the work by Pan et al. [44], a co-expression network is constructed based on differentially-expressed microRNAs and genes identified in liver tissues from patients with hepatitis B virus (HBV). This study provides new insights on how microRNAs take part in the molecular mechanism underlying HBV-associated acute liver failure.

The alarm posed by the COVID-19 pandemic has fueled the development of effective prevention and treatment protocols for 2019-nCoV/SARS-CoV-2 outbreak [45]. Due to the novelty of SARS-CoV-2, recent research takes similar viruses, such as SARS-CoV and Middle East Respiratory Syndrome coronavirus (MERS-CoV), as a starting point. Other coronaviruses, like Mouse Hepatitis Virus (MHV), are also considered appropriate for comparative studies in animal models, as demonstrated in the work by De Albuquerque et al. [46] and Ding et al. [47]. MHV is a murine coronavirus (M-CoV) that causes an epidemic illness with high mortality, and has been widely used for experimentation purposes. Works like the ones by Case et al. [48] and Gorman et al. [49], study the innate immune response against MHV arbitrated by interferons, and those interferon-stimulated genes with potential antiviral function. This is the case of gene *Ly6E*, which has been shown to play an important role in viral infection, as well as various orthologs of the same gene [50,51]. Mechanistic approaches often involved the ablation of the gene under study, like in the work by Mar et al. [31], where gene *knockout* was used to characterize the implications of *Ly6E* in Influenza A infection. As it is the case of Giotis et al. [52], these studies often involve global transcriptome analyses, via RNA-seq or microarrays, together with computational efforts, which intend to screen the key elements of the immune system that are required for the appropriate response. This approach ultimately leads experimental research through predictive analyses, as in the case of co-expression gene networks [53].

3. Materials and Methods

In the following subsections, the main methods and GCN reconstruction steps are addressed. First, in Section 3.1, the original dataset used in the present work is described, together with the experimental design. Then, in Section 4.1, the data preprocessing steps are described. Subsequently in Section 3.3, key genes controlling the infection progression are extracted through differential expression analyses. Finally, the inference of GCNs and their analysis are detailed in Sections 3.4 and 3.5, respectively.

3.1. Original Dataset Description

The original experimental design can be described as follows. The progression of the MHV infection at genetic level was evaluated in two genetic backgrounds: wild type (*wt*, Ly6Efl/fl) and Ly6E *knockout* mutants (*ko*, $Ly6E^{\Delta HSC}$). The ablation of gene *Ly6E* in all cell types is lethal, hence the $Ly6E^{\Delta HSC}$ strain contains a disrupted version of gene Ly6E only in hematopoietic stem cells (HSC), which give rise to myeloid and lymphoid progenitors of all blood cells. *Wild type* and $Ly6E^{\Delta HSC}$ mice were injected intraperitoneally with 5000 PFU MHV-A59. At 3 and 5 days post-injection (d p.i.), mice were euthanized and biological samples for RNA-Seq were extracted. The overall effects of MHV infection in both *wt* and *ko* strains was assessed in liver and spleen.

In total 36 samples were analyzed, half of these corresponding to liver and spleen, respectively. From the 18 organ-specific samples, 6 samples correspond to mock infection (negative control), 6 to MHV-infected samples at 3 d p.i. and 6 to MHV-infected samples at 5 d p.i. For each sample, two technical replicates were obtained. Libraries of cDNA generated from the samples were sequenced using Illumina NovaSeq 6000. Further details on sample preparation can be found in the original article by Pfaender et al. [54]. For the sake of simplicity, MHV-infected samples at 3 and 5 d p.i. will be termed 'cases', whereas mock-infection samples will be termed 'controls'.

The original dataset consists of 72 files, one per sample replicate, obtained upon the mapping of the transcript reads to the reference genome. Reads were recorded in three different ways, considering whether these mapped introns, exons or total genes. Then, a count table was retrieved from these files by selecting only the total gene counts of each sample replicate file.

3.2. Data Pre-Processing

Pre-processing was performed using the *EdgeR* [55] R package. The original dataset by Pfaender et al. [54] was retrieved from GEO (accession ID: GSE146074) using the *GEOquery* [56] package. Additional files on sample information and treatment were also used to assist the modeling process.

By convention, a sequencing depth per gene below 10 is considered neglectable [57,58]. Genes meeting this criterion are known as low expression genes, and are often removed since they add noise and computational burden to the following analyses [59]. In order to remove genes showing less than 10 reads across all conditions, counts per million (CPM) normalization was performed, so possible differences between library sizes for both replicates would not affect the result.

Afterwards, Principal Components Analyses (PCA) were performed over the data in order to detect the main sources of variability across samples. PCA were accompanied by unsupervised k-medoid clustering analyses, in order to identify different groups of samples. In addition, multidimensional scaling plots (MDS) were applied to further separate samples according to their features. Last, between-sample similarities were assessed through hierarchical clustering.

3.3. Differential Expression Analyses

The analyses of differential expression served a two-way purpose, (i) the exploration of the directionality in the gene expression changes upon viral infection, and (ii) the identification of key regulatory elements for the subsequent network reconstruction. In the present application, differentially-expressed genes (DEG) were filtered from the original dataset and proceeded to the reconstruction process. This approximation enabled the modeling of the genetic relationships that are considered of relevance in the presented comparison [60–62]. In the present work mice samples were compared organ-wise depending on whether these corresponded to control, 3 d p.i. and 5 d p.i.

The identification of DEG was performed using the *Limma* [63] R package, which provides non-parametric robust estimation of the gene expression variance. This package includes *Voom*, a method that incorporates RNA-Seq count data into the *Limma* workbench, originally designed for microarrays [64]. In this case, a minimum log2-fold-change (log2FC) of 2 was chosen, which corresponds to four fold changes in the gene expression level. P-value was adjusted by Benjamini-Hochberg [65] and the selected adjusted p-value cutoff was 0.05.

3.4. Inference of the Gene Networks: EnGNet

In order to generate gene networks the *EnGNet* algorithm was used. This technique, presented in Gómez-Vela et al. [33], is able to compute gene co-expression networks with a competitive performance compared other approaches from the literature. *EnGNet* performs a two-step process to infer gene networks: (a) an ensemble strategy for a reliable co-expression networks generation, and (b) a greedy algorithm that optimizes both the size and the topological features of the network. These two features of *EnGNet* offer a reliable solution for generating gene networks. In fact, *EnGNet* relies on three statistical measures in order to obtain networks. In particular, the measures used are the Spearman, Kendall and normalized mutual information (NMI), which are widely used in the literature for inferring gene networks. *EnGNet* uses these measures simultaneously by applying an ensemble strategy based on major voting, i.e., a relationship will be considered correct if at least 2 of the 3 measures evaluate the relationship as correct. The evaluation is based on different independent thresholds. In this work, the different thresholds were set to the values originally used in [33]: 0.9, 0.8 and 0.7 for Spearman, Kendall and NMI, respectively.

In addition, as mentioned above, *EnGNet* performs an optimization of the topological structure of the networks obtained. This reduction is based on two steps: (i) the pruning of the relations considered of least interest in the initial network, and (ii) the analysis of the hubs present in the network. For this second step of the final network reconstruction, we have selected the same threshold that was used in [33], i.e., 0.7. Through this optimization, the final network produced by *EnGNet* results easier to analyze computationally, due to its reduced size.

3.5. Networks Analyses

Networks were imported to R for the estimation of topology parameters and the addition of network features that are of interest for the latter network analysis and interpretation. These attributes were added to the reconstructed networks to enrich the modeling using the *igraph* [66] R package. The networks were then imported into *Cytoscape* [67] through RCy3 [68] for examination and analyses purposes. In this case, two kind of analyses were performed: (i) a topological analysis and (ii) an enrichment analysis.

Regarding the topological analysis, clustering evaluation was performed in order to identify densely connected nodes, which, according to the literature, are often involved in a same biological process [69]. The chosen clustering method was community clustering (GLay) [70], implemented via *Cytoscape's ClusterMaker* app [71], which has yielded significant results in the identification of densely connected modules [72,73]. Among the topology parameters, *degree* and *edge betweenness* were estimated. The *degree* of a node refers to the number of its linking nodes. On the other hand, the *betweenness* of an edge refers to the number of shortest paths which go through that edge. Both parameters are considered as a measure of the implications of respectively nodes and edges in a certain network. Particularly, nodes whose *degree* exceeds the average network node *degree*, the so called *hubs*, are considered key elements of the biological processes modeled by the network. In this particular case, the distribution of nodes' degree network was analyzed so those nodes whose degree exceeded a threshold were selected as hubs. This threshold is defined as $Q3 + 1.5 \times IQR$, where $Q3$ is the third quartile and IQR the interquartile range of the degree distribution. This method has been widely used for the detection of upper outliers in non-parametric distributions [74,75], as it is the case. However, the outlier definition does not apply to this distribution since those nodes whose degree are far above the median degree are considered hubs.

On the other hand, Gene Ontology (GO) Enrichment Analysis provides valuable insights on the biological reality modeled by the reconstructed networks. The Gene Ontology Consortium [76] is a data base that seeks for a unified nomenclature for biological entities. GO has developed three different ontologies, which describe gene products in terms of the biological processes, cell components or molecular functions in which these are involved. Ontologies are built out of GO terms or annotations, which provide biological information of gene products. In this case, the *ClusterProfiler* [77] R package, allowed the identification of the statistically over-represented GO terms in the gene sets of interest. Additional enrichment analyses were performed using *DAVID* [78]. For both analyses, the complete genome of *Mus musculus* was selected as background. Finally, further details on the interplay of the genes under study was examined using the *STRING* database [79].

4. Results

The reconstruction of gene networks that adequately model viral infection involves multiple steps, which ultimately shape the final outcome. First, in Section 4.1, exploratory analyses and data preprocessing are detailed, which prompted the modeling rationale. Then, in Section 4.2, differential expression is evaluated for the samples of interest. Finally, networks reconstruction and analysis are addressed in Section 4.3. At the end, four networks were generated, both in an organ- and genotype-wise manner. A schematic representation of the GCN reconstruction approach is shown in Figure 1.

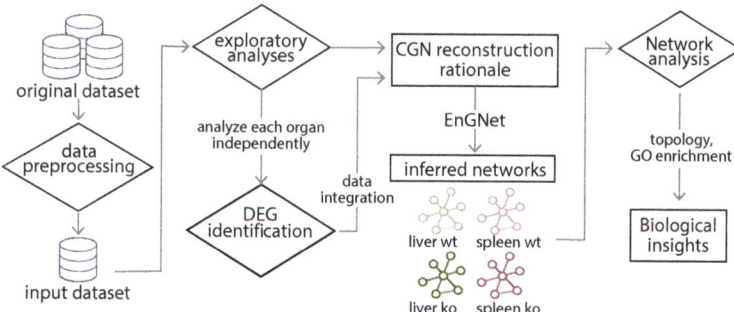

Figure 1. General scheme for the reconstruction method. The preprocessed data was subjected to exploratory and differential expression analyses, which imposed the reconstruction rationale. Four groups of samples were used to generate four independent networks, respectively modeling the immune response in the liver, both in the *wt* and the *ko* situations; and in the spleen, also in the *wt* and the *ko* scenarios.

4.1. Data Pre-Processing and Exploratory Analyses

In order to remove low expression genes, a sequencing depth of 10 was found to correspond to an average CPM of 0.5, which was selected as threshold. Hence, genes whose expression was found over 0.5 CPM in at least two samples of the dataset were maintained, ensuring that only genes which are truly being expressed in the tissue will be studied. The dataset was Log2-normalized with priority to the following analyses, in accordance to the recommendations posed in Law et al. [64].

The results of both PCA and k-medoid clustering are shown in Figure 2a. Clustering of the Log2-normalized samples revealed clear differences between liver and spleen samples. Also, for each organ, three subgroups of analogous samples that cluster together are identified. These groups correspond to mock infection, MHV-infected mice at 3 d p.i. and MHV-infected mice at 5 d p.i. (dashed lines in Figure 2a). Finally, subtle differences were observed in homologous samples of different genotypes (Figure A1).

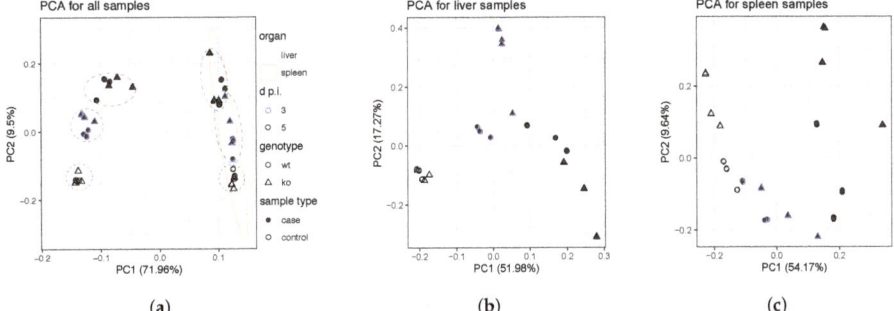

(a)   (b)   (c)

Figure 2. (a) PCA plot of the Log2-normalized counts for the exploratory analysis of all samples under study. The metric used for k-medoid partitioning was the Euclidean distance. Both replicates are included. Two groups, respectively corresponding to liver and spleen samples, are clearly differentiated. Dashed lines were added for improved visualization of the different groups that are distinguished within each organ. Organ-specific PCA for (b) liver and (c) spleen samples. Both replicates are included. PCA suggests the progressive nature of the MHV infection, where groups corresponding to mock infections, 3 d p.i. and 5 d p.i. are distinguished in varying degrees. Differences between controls and cases are more evident in liver samples. Figure 2a legend is the same for Figure 2b,c.

Organ-specific PCA revealed major differences between MHV-infected samples for $Ly6E^{\Delta HSC}$ and wt genotypes, at both 3 and 5 d p.i. These differences were not observed in the mock infection (control situation). Organ-wise PCA are shown in Figure 2b,c. The distances between same-genotype samples illustrate the infection-prompted genetic perturbation from the uninfected status (control) to 5 d p.i., where clear signs of hepatitis were observed according to the original physiopathology studies [54]. On the other hand, the differences observed between both genotypes are indicative of the role of gene $Ly6E$ in the appropriate response to viral infection. These differences are subtle in control samples, but in case samples, some composition biass is observed depending on whether these are ko or wt, especially in spleen samples. The comparative analysis of the top 500 most variable genes confirmed the differences observed in the PCA, as shown in Figure A2. Among the four different features of the samples under study: organ, genotype, sample type (case or control) and days post injection; the dissimilarities in terms of genotype were the subtlest.

In the light of these exploratory findings, the network reconstruction approach was performed as follows. Networks were reconstructed organ-wise, as these exhibit notable differences in gene expression. Additionally, a main objective of the present work is to evaluate the differences in the genetic response in the wt situation compared to the $Ly6E^{\Delta HSC}$ ko background, upon the viral infection onset in the two mentioned tissues.

For each organ, Log2-normalized samples were coerced to generate time-series-like data, i.e., for each genotype, 9 samples will be considered as a set, namely 3 control samples, 3 case samples at 3 d p.i. and 3 case samples at 5 d p.i. Both technical replicates were included. This rational design seeks for a gene expression span representative of the infection progress. Thereby, control samples may well be considered as a time zero for the viral infection, followed by the corresponding samples at 3 and 5 d p.i. The proposed rationale is supported by the exploratory findings, which position 3 d p.i. samples between control and 5 d p.i. samples. At the same time, the reconstruction of gene expression becomes robuster with increasing number of samples. In this particular case, 18 measuring points are attained for the reconstruction of each one of the four intended networks, since two technical replicates were obtained per sample [80].

4.2. Identification of Differentially-Expressed Genes Between Wild Type and Ly6E$^{\Delta HSC}$ Samples

The differential expression analyses were performed over the four groups of 9 samples explained above, with the aim of examining the differences in the immune response between Ly6E$^{\Delta HSC}$ and *wt* samples. Limma - Voom differential expression analyses were performed over the Log2-normalized counts, in order to evaluate the different genotypes whilst contrasting the three infection stages: control vs. cases at 3 d p.i., control vs. cases at 5 d p.i. and cases at 3 vs. 5 d p.i. The choice of a minimum absolute log2FC ≥ 2, enabled considering only those genes that truly effect changes between *wt* and Ly6E$^{\Delta HSC}$ samples, whilst maintaining a relatively computer-manageable number of DEG for network reconstruction. The latter is essential for the yield of accurate network sparseness values, as this is a main feature of gene networks [5].

For both genotypes and organs, the results of the differential expression analyses reveal that MHV injection triggers a progressive genetic program from the control situation to the MHV-infected scenario at 5 d p.i., as shown in Figure 3a. The absolute number of DEG between control vs. cases at 5 d p.i. was considerably larger than in the comparison between control vs. cases at 3 d p.i. Furthermore, in all cases, most of the DEG in control vs. cases at 3 d p.i. are also differentially-expressed in the control vs. cases at 5 d p.i. comparison, as shown in Figure 4.

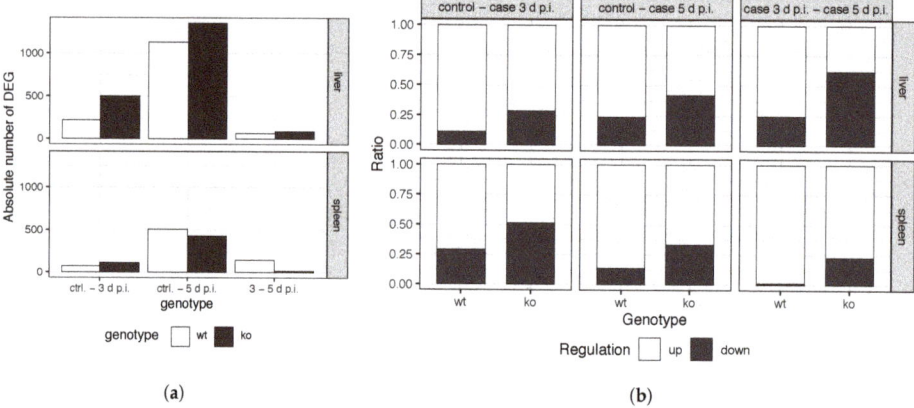

Figure 3. (a) Absolute numbers of DEG in the different comparisons (b) Ratio of up- and downregulated DEG in the different performed comparisons. Three comparisons were performed: control vs. case samples at 3 d p.i., control vs. case samples at 5 d p.i. and case samples at 3 vs. 5 d p.i. *ko* refers to Ly6E$^{\Delta HSC}$ samples.

Regarding genes fold change, an overall genetic up-regulation is observed upon infection. Around 70% of DEG are upregulated for all the comparisons performed for *wt* samples, as shown in Figure 3b. Nonetheless, a dramatic reduce in this genetic up-regulation is observed, by contrast, in *knockout* samples, even limiting upregulated genes to nearly 50% in the control vs. cases at 3 d p.i. comparison of liver Ly6E$^{\Delta HSC}$ samples. The largest differences are observed in the comparison of controls vs. cases at 5 d p.i (Figures A3 and A4). These DEG are of great interest for the understanding of the immune response of both *wt* and *ko* mice to viral infection. These genes were selected to filter the original dataset for latter network reconstruction.

The commonalities between *wt* and *ko* control samples for both organs were also verified through differential expression analysis following the same criteria (Log2FC > 2, p value < 0.05). The number of DEG between *wt* and *ko* liver control samples (2) and between *wt* and *ko* spleen control samples (20) were not considered significant, so samples were taken as analogous starting points for infection.

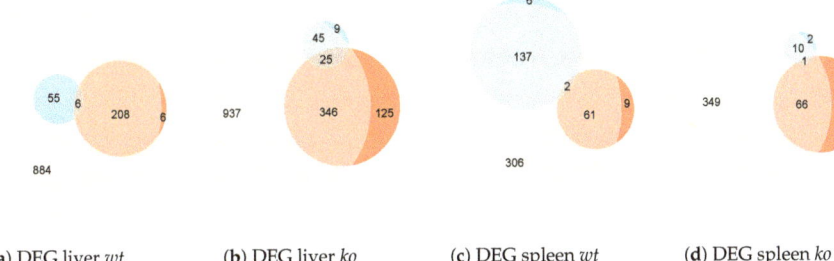

(a) DEG liver *wt*   (b) DEG liver *ko*   (c) DEG spleen *wt*   (d) DEG spleen *ko*

Figure 4. Euler diagrams showing the overlapping of DEG between the three possible contrast situations: control vs. cases at 3 d p.i. (red), control vs. cases at 5 d p.i. (yellow) and cases at 3 d p.i. vs. cases at 5 d p.i. (blue) *ko* refers to $Ly6E^{\Delta HSC}$ samples. These comparisons were performed both organ and genotype-wise considering four groups of samples: (a) liver *wt*, (b) liver $Ly6E^{\Delta HSC}$, (c) spleen *wt*, (d) spleen $Ly6E^{\Delta HSC}$.

4.3. Reconstruction and Analysis of Gene Networks

As stated above, the samples were arranged both organ and genotype-wise in order to generate networks which would model the progress of the disease in each scenario. GCNs were inferred from Log2-normalized expression datasets. A count of 1 was added at log2 normalization so the problem with remaining zero values was avoided. Each network was generated exclusively taking into consideration their corresponding DEG at control vs. cases at 5 d p.i., where larger differences were observed. Four networks were then reconstructed from these previously-identified DEG for liver *wt* samples (1133 genes), liver *ko* samples (1153 genes), spleen *wt* samples (506 genes) and spleen *ko* samples (426 genes). This approach results in the modeling of only those relationships that are related to the viral infection. Each sample set was then fed to *EnGNet* for the reconstruction of the subsequent network. Genes that remained unconnected due to weak relationships, which do not overcome the set threshold, were removed from the networks. Furthermore, the goodness of *EnGNet*-generated models outperformed other well-known inference approaches, as detailed in Appendix B.

Topological parameters were estimated and added as node attributes using *igraph*, together with Log2FC, prior to Cytoscape import. Specifically, networks were simplified by removing potential loops and multiple edges. The clustering topological scrutiny of the reconstructed networks revealed neat modules in all cases, as shown in Figure A5. The number of clusters identified in each network, as well as the number of genes harbored in the clusters is shown in Table A1.

As already mentioned, according to gene networks theory, nodes contained within the same cluster are often involved in the same biological process [5,81]. In this context, the GO-based enrichment analyses over the identified clusters may well provide an idea of the affected functions. Only clusters containing more than 10 genes were considered, since this is the minimum number of elements required by the enrichment tool *ClusterProfiler*. The results of the enrichment analyses revealed that most GO terms were not shared between *wt* and *ko* homologous samples, as shown in Figure 5.

In order to further explore the reconstructed networks, the intersection of *ko* and *wt* networks of a same organ was computed. This refers to the genes and relationships that are shared between both genotypes for a specific organ. Additionally, the genes and relationships that were exclusively present at the *wt* and *ko* samples were also estimated, as shown in Figure A6. The enrichment analyses over the nodes, separated using this criterion, would reveal the biological processes that make the difference between in $Ly6E^{\Delta HSC}$ mice compared to *wt* ones. The results of such analyses are shown in Figure A7.

Finally, the exploration of nodes' *degree* distribution would reveal those genes that can be considered hubs. Those nodes comprised within the top genes with highest degree (degree > Q3 + 1.5 × IQ), also known as upper outliers in the nodes distribution, were considered hubs. A representation of nodes' degree distribution throughout the four reconstructed networks is shown in Figure 6.

These distributions are detailed in Figure A8. This method provided four cutoff values for the degree, 24, 39, 21 and 21, respectively for liver *wt* and *ko*, spleen *wt* and *ko* networks. Above these thresholds, nodes would be considered as hubs in each network. These hubs are shown in Tables A2–A5.

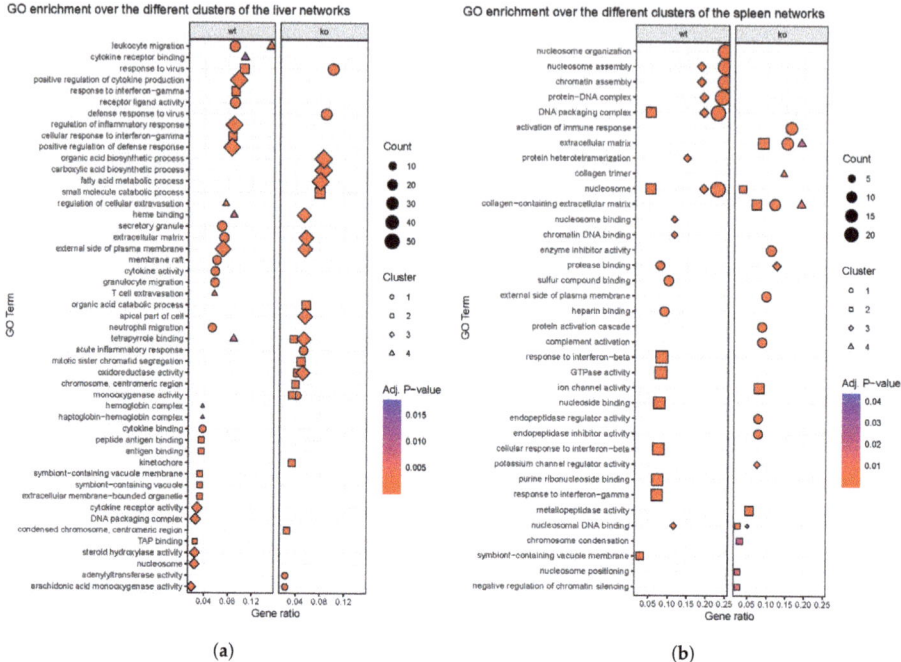

(a)   (b)

Figure 5. Enrichment analyses performed over the main clusters identified in *wt* and *ko* networks of (**a**) liver and (**b**) spleen networks. Gene ratio is defined by the number of genes used as input for the enrichment analyses associated with a particular GO term divided by the total number of input genes.

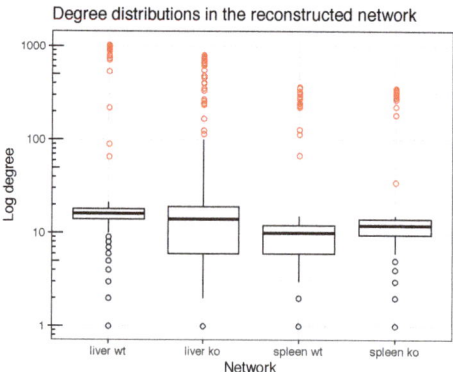

Figure 6. Boxplots representative of the degree distributions for each one of the four reconstructed networks. Identified hubs, according to the $Q3 + 1.5 \times IQR$ criterion, are highlighted in red. The degree cutoffs, above which nodes would be considered as hubs, were 24, 39, 21 and 21, respectively for liver *wt*, liver *ko*, spleen *wt* and spleen *ko* networks. Note degree is represented in a log scale given that the reconstructed networks present a scale-free topology.

5. Discussion

In this work four gene networks were reconstructed to model the genetic response MHV infection in two tissues, liver and spleen, and in two different genetic backgrounds, *wild type* and *Ly6E*$^{\Delta HSC}$. Samples were initially explored in order to design an inference rationale. Not only did the designed approach reveal major differences between the genetic programs in each organ, but also, between different subgroups of samples, in a time-series-like manner. Noticeably, disparities between *wt* and *Ly6E*$^{\Delta HSC}$ samples were observed in both tissues, and differential expression analyses revealed relevant differences in terms of the immune response generated. Hereby, our results predict the impact of *Ly6E ko* on HSC, which resulted in an impaired immune response compared to the *wt* situation.

5.1. Exploratory Analyses Revealed a Time-Series Llike Behaviour on Raw Data, Assisting Network Reconstruction

Overall, results indicate that the reconstruction rationale, elucidated from exploratory findings, is suitable for the modeling of the viral progression. Regarding the variance in gene expression in response to virus, PCA and K-medoid clustering revealed strong differences between samples corresponding to liver spleen, respectively (Figure 2a). These differences set the starting point for the modeling approach, in which samples corresponding to each organ were analyzed independently. This *modus operandi* is strongly supported by the tropism that viruses exhibit for certain tissues, which ultimately results in a differential viral incidence and charge depending on the organ [82]. In particular, the liver is the target organ of MHV, identified as the main disease site [83]. On the other hand, the role of the spleen in innate and adaptive immunity against MHV has been widely addressed [84,85]. The organization of this organ allows blood filtration for the presentation of antigens to cognate lymphocytes by the antigen presenting cells (APCs), which mediate the immune response exerted by T and B cells [86].

As stated before, PCA revealed differences between the three sample groups on each organ: control and MHV-infected at 3 and 5 d p.i. Interestingly, between-groups differences are specially clear for liver samples (Figure 2b), whereas spleen samples are displayed in a continuum-like way. This becomes more evident in organ-wise PCA (Figure 2), and was later confirmed by the exploration of the top 500 most variable genes and differential expression analyses (Figure A2). Furthermore, clear differences between *wt* and *Ly6E*$^{\Delta HSC}$ samples are observed in none of these analyses, although the examination of the differential expression and network reconstruction did exposed divergent immune responses for both genotypes.

5.2. Differential Expression Analyses Revealed Significant Changes between Wild Type and Knockout Samples

The differential expression analyses revealed the progressive genetic response to virus for both organs and genotypes (Figures 3a and 4). In a *wt* genetic background, MHV infection causes an overall rise in the expression level of certain genes, as most DEG in cases vs. control samples are upregulated. However, in a *Ly6E*$^{\Delta HSC}$ genetic background, this upregulation is not as prominent as in a *wt* background, significantly reducing the number of upregulated genes (Figure 3b). Besides, the number of DEG in each comparison varies from *wt* to *Ly6E*$^{\Delta HSC}$ samples.

Attending at the DEG in the performed comparisons, for both the *wt* and *ko* genotypes, liver cases at 3 d p.i. are more similar to liver cases at 5 d p.i. than to liver controls, since the number of DEG between the first two measuring points is significantly lower than the number of DEG between control and case samples at 3 d p.i. (Figure 4a,b). A different situation occurs in the spleen, where *wt* cases at 3 d p.i. are closer to control samples (Figure 4c), whereas *ko* cases at 3 d p.i. seem to be more related to cases at 5 d p.i. (Figure 4d). This was already suggested by hierarchical clustering in the analysis of the top 500 most variable genes, and could be indicative of a different progression of the infection impact on both organs, which could be modulated by gene *Ly6E*, at least for the spleen samples.

Moreover, the results of the DEG analyses indicate that the sole *knockout* of gene *Ly6E* in HSC considerably affects the upregulating genetic program normally triggered by viral infection in *wild type* individuals (in both liver and spleen). Interestingly, there are some genes in each organ and genotype that are differentially expressed in every comparison between the possible three sample types, controls, cases at 3 d p.i. and cases at 5 d p.i. These genes, which we termed highly DEG, could be linked to the progression of the infection, as changes in their expression level occur with days post injection, according to the data. The rest of the DEG, show an uprise or fall when comparing two sample types, which does not change significantly in the third sample type. Alternatively, highly DEG, shown in Table A6, exhibited three different expression patterns: (i) Their expression level, initially low, rises from control to cases at 3 d p.i. and then rises again in cases at 5 d p.i. (ii) Their expression level, initially high in control samples, falls at 3 d p.i. and falls even more at 5 d p.i cases. (iii) Their expression level, initially low, rises from control to cases at 3 d p.i. but then falls at cases at 5 d p.i., when it is still higher than the initial expression level. These expression patterns, which are shown in Figure A9, might be used to keep track of the disease progression, differentiating early from late infection stages.

In some cases, these genes exhibited inconsistent expression levels, specially at 5 d p.i. cases, which indicates the need for further experimental designs targeting these genes. Highly DEG could be correlated with the progression of the disease, as in regulation types (i) and (ii) or by contrast, be required exclusively at initial stages, as in regulation type (iii). Notably, genes *Gm10800* and *Gm4756* are predicted genes which, to date, have been poorly described. According to the STRING database [79], *Gm10800* is associated with gene *Lst1* (Leukocyte-specific transcript 1 protein), which has a possible role in modulating immune responses. In fact, *Gm10800* is homologous to human gene PIRO (Progranulin-Induced-Receptor-like gene during Osteoclastogenesis), related to bone homeostasis [87,88]. Thus, we hypothesize that bone marrow-derived cell lines, including erythrocytes and leukocytes (immunity effectors), could also be regulated by *Gm10800*. On the other hand, *Gm4756* is not associated to any other gene according to STRING. Protein *Gm4756* is homologous to Human protein DHRS7 (dehydrogenase/reductase SDR family member 7) isoform 1 precursor. Nonetheless and to the best of our knowledge, these genes have not been previously related to *Ly6E*, and could play a role in the immune processes mediated by this gene.

Finally, highly DEG were not found exclusively present in *wt* nor *ko* networks, instead, these were common nodes of these networks for each organ. This suggests that highly DEG might be of core relevance upon MHV infection, with a role in those processes independent on $Ly6E^{\Delta HSC}$. Besides, genes *Hykk*, *Ifit3* and *Ifit3b*; identified as highly DEG throughout liver $Ly6E^{\Delta HSC}$ samples were also identified as hubs in the liver *ko* network. Also gene *Saa3*, highly DEG across spleen $Ly6E^{\Delta HSC}$ samples was considered a hub in the spleen *ko* network. Nevertheless, these highly DEG require further experimental validation.

5.3. The Ablation of Ly6E in HSC Results in Impaired Immune Response as Predicted by Enrichment Analyses

The enrichment analyses of the identified clusters at each network revealed that most GO terms are not shared between the two genotypes (Figure 5), despite the considerable amount of shared genes between the two genotypes for a same organ. The network reconstructed from liver *wt* samples reflects a strong response to viral infection, involving leukocyte migration or cytokine and interferon signaling among others. These processes, much related to immune processes, are not observed in its *ko* counterpart.

The liver *wt* network presented four clusters (Figure A5a). Its cluster 1 regulates processes related to leukocyte migration, showing the implication of receptor ligand activity and cytokine signaling, which possibly mediates the migration of the involved cells. Cluster 2 is related to interferon-gamma for the response to MHV, whereas cluster 3 is probably involved in the inflammatory response mediated by pro-inflammatory cytokines. Last, cluster 4 is related to cell extravasation, or the leave of blood cells from blood vessels, with the participation of gene *Nipal1*. The positive regulation observed across all clusters suggests the activation of these processes. Overall, hub genes in this network have been related to the immune response to viral infection, as the innate immune response to the virus is the mediated by interferons. Meanwhile, the liver *ko* network showed three main clusters (Figure A5b). Its cluster 1 would also be involved in defense response to virus, but other processes observed in the liver *wt* network, like leukocyte migration or cytokine activity, are not observed in this cluster nor the others. Cluster 2 is then related to the catabolism of small molecules and cluster 3 is involved in acids biosynthesis. These processes are certainly ambiguous and do not correspond the immune response observed in the *wt* situation, which suggests a decrease in the immune response to MHV as a result of *Ly6E* ablation in HSC.

On the other hand, spleen *wt* samples revealed high nuclear activity potentially involving nucleosome remodeling complexes and changes in DNA accessibility. Histone modification is a type of epigenetic modulation which regulates gene expression. Taking into account the central role of the spleen in the development of immune responses, the manifested relevance of chromatin organization could be accompanied by changes in the accessibility of certain DNA regions with implications in the spleen-dependent immune response. This is supported by the reduced reaction capacity in the first days post-infection of $Ly6E^{\Delta HSC}$ samples compared to *wt*, as indicated by the number of DEG between control and cases at 3 d p.i for these genotypes. The spleen *wt* network displayed three clusters (Figure A5c). Cluster 1, whose genes were all upregulated in $Ly6E^{\Delta HSC}$ samples at 5 d p.i. compared to mock infection, is mostly involved in nucleosome organization and chromatin remodelling, together with cluster 3. Cluster 2 would also be related to DNA packaging complexes, possibly in response to interferon, similarly to liver networks. Instead, in spleen *ko* most genes take part in processes related to the extracellular matrix. In the spleen *ko* network, four clusters were identified (Figure A5d). Cluster 1 is related to the activation of an immune response, but also, alongside with clusters 2 and 4, to the extracellular matrix, possibly in relation with collagen, highlighting its role in the response to MHV. Cluster 3 is implied in protease binding. The dramatic shut down in the *ko* network of the nuclear activity observed in the spleen *wt* network, leads to the hypothesis that the chromatin remodeling activity observed could be related to the activation of certain immunoenhancer genes, modulated by gene *Ly6E*. In any case, further experimental validation of these results would provide meaningful insights in the face of potential therapeutic approaches (See Appendix A for more details).

The exploration of nodes memebership, depending on whether these exclusively belonged to *wt* or *ko* networks or, by contrast, were present in both networks, helped to understand the impairment caused by $Ly6E^{\Delta HSC}$. In this sense, GO enrichment analyses over these three defined categories of the nodes in the liver networks revealed that genes at their intersection are mainly related to cytokine production, leukocyte migration and inflammatory response regulation, in accordance to the phenotype described for MHV-infection [89]. However, a differential response to virus is observed in *wt* mice compared to *Ly6E*-ablated. The nodes exclusively present at the *wt* liver network are related to processes like regulation of immune effector process, leukocyte mediated immunity or adaptive immune response. These processes, which are found at a relatively high gene ratio, are not represented by nodes exclusively present in the liver *ko* network. Additionally, genes exclusively present at the *wt* network and the intersection network are upregulated in case samples with respect to controls (Figure A6a), which suggests the activation of the previously mentioned biological processes. On the other hand, genes exclusively-present at the liver *ko* networks, mostly down-regulated, were found to be associated with catabolism.

As for the spleen networks, genotype-wise GO enrichment results revealed that the previously-mentioned intense nuclear activity involving protein-DNA complexes and nucleosome assembly is mostly due to *wt*-exclusive genes. Actually, these biological processes could be pinpointing cell replication events. Analogously to the liver case, genes that were found exclusively present in the *wt* network and the intersection network are mostly upregulated, whereas in the case of *ko*-exclusive genes the upregulation is not that extensive. Interestingly, the latter are mostly related to extracellular matrix (ECM) organization, which suggest the relevance of *Ly6E* on these. Other lymphocyte antigen-6 (LY-6) superfamily members have been related to ECM remodelling processes such as the Urokinase receptor (*uPAR*), which participates in the proteolysis of ECM proteins [90]. However and to the best of our knowledge, the implications of *Ly6E* in ECM have not been reported.

The results presented are in the main consistent with those by Pfaender et al. [54], who observed a loss of genes associated with the type I IFN response, inflammation, antigen presentation, and B cells in infected $Ly6E^{\Delta HSC}$ mice. Genes *Stat1* and *Ifit3*, selected in their work for their high variation in absence of *Ly6e*, were identified as hub genes in the networks reconstructed from liver *wild type* and *knockout* samples, respectively. It is to be noticed that our approach significantly differs to the one carried out in the original study. In this particular case, we consider that the reconstruction of GCN enables a more comprehensive analysis of the data, potentially finding the key genes involved in the immune response onset and their relationships with other genes. For instance, the transcriptomic differences between liver and spleen upon *Ly6E* ablation become more evident using GCN.

Altogether, the presented results show the relevance of gene *Ly6E* in the immune response against the infection caused by MHV. The disruption of *Ly6E* significantly reduced the immunogenic response, affecting signaling and cell effectors. These results, combining *in vivo* and *in silico* approaches, deepen in our understanding of the immune response to viruses at the gene level, which could ultimately assist the development of new therapeutics. For example, basing on these results, prospective studies on *Ly6E* agonist therapies could be inspired, with the purpose of enhancing the gene expression level via gene delivery. Given the relevance of *Ly6E* in SARS-CoV-2 according to previous studies [54,91], the overall effects of *Ly6E* ablation in HSCs upon SARS-CoV-2 infection, putting special interest in lung tissue, might show similarities with the deficient immune response observed in the present work.

6. Conclusions

In this work we have presented an application of co-expression gene networks to analyze the global effects of *Ly6E* ablation in the immune response to MHV coronavirus infection. To do so, the progression of the MHV infection on the genetic level was evaluated in two genetic backgrounds: wild type mice (*wt*, Ly6Efl/fl) and Ly6E *knockout* mutants (*ko*, $Ly6E^{\Delta HSC}$) mice. For these, viral progression was assessed in two different organs, liver and spleen.

The proposed reconstruction rationale revealed significant differences between MHV-infected *wt* and $Ly6E^{\Delta HSC}$ mice for both organs. In addition we observed that MHV infection triggers a progressive genetic response of upregulating nature in both liver and spleen. In addition, the results suggest that the ablation of gene *Ly6E* at HSC caused an impaired genetic response in both organs compared to *wt* mice. The impact of such ablation is more evident in the liver, consistently with the disease site. At the same time, the immune response in the spleen, which seemed to be mediated by an intense chromatin activity in the normal situation, is replaced by ECM remodeling in $Ly6E^{\Delta HSC}$ mice.

We infer that the presence of *Ly6E* limits the damage in the above mentioned target sites. We believe that the characterization of these processes could motivate the efforts towards novel antiviral approaches. Finally, in the light of previous works, we hypothesize that *Ly6E* ablation might show analogous detrimental effects on immunity upon the infection caused by other viruses including SARS-CoV, MERS and SARS-CoV-2. In future works, we plan to investigate whether the over-expression of *Ly6E* in *wt* mice has an enhancement effect in immunity. In this direction, *Ly6E* gene mimicking (agonist) therapies could represent a promising approach in the development of new antivirals.

Author Contributions: Conceptualization, F.M.D.-C. and F.G.-V.; methodology, F.M.D.-C. and F.G.-V.; software, F.M.D.-C. and F.G.-V.; validation, F.M.D.-C. and F.G.-V.; Visualization, F.M.D.-C., F.G.-V., M.G.-T., F.D.; data curation, F.M.D.-C. and M.G.-T.; writing-original draft preparation, F.M.D.-C., D.S.R.-B., F.G.-V. and M.G.-T.; writing-review and editing, F.M.D.-C., F.G.-V., M.G.-T., D.S.R.-B. and F.D.; supervision, F.G.-V. and F.D.; project administration, F.G.-V. All authors have read and agreed to the published version of the manuscript.

Funding: This work was supported by Pablo de Olavide University: Scholarships for Tutored Research, V Pablo de Olavide University's Research and Transfer Plan 2018-2020 (Grant No. PPI1903).

Conflicts of Interest: The authors declare no conflict of interest.

Appendix A. Figures and Tables

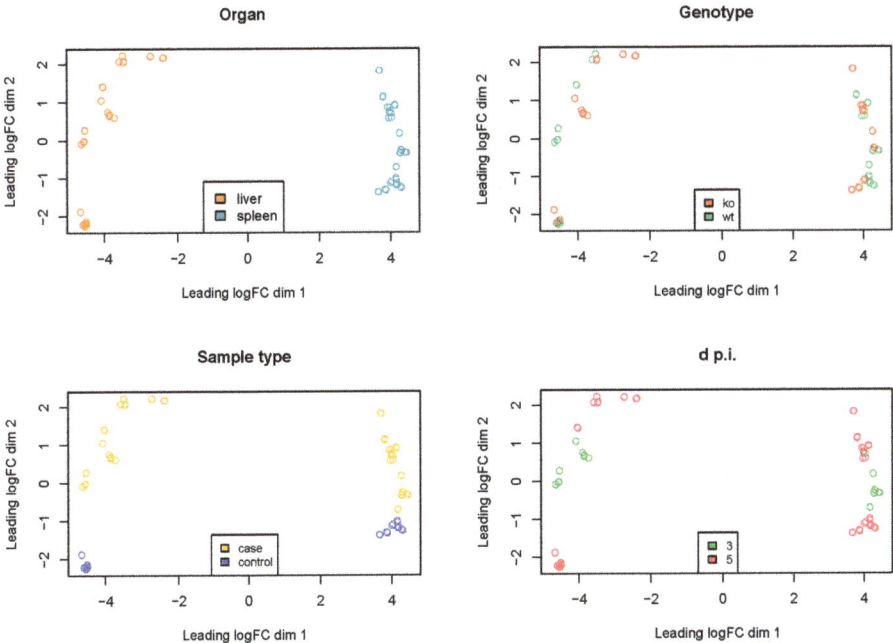

Figure A1. Multidimensional Scaling (MDS) plots showing main differences between individual samples according to the four features these present: organ procedence, genotype, sample type (mock infection or MHV-infected) and days post injection.

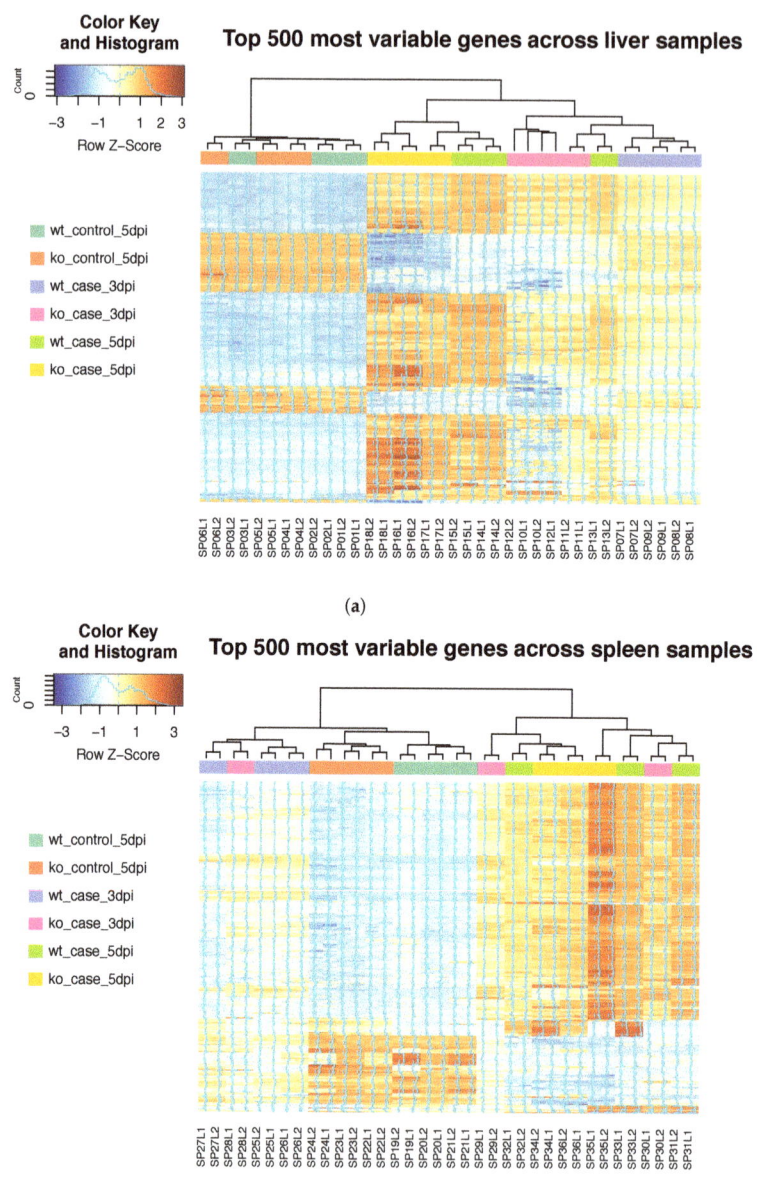

Figure A2. Top 500 most variable genes in (**a**) liver and (**b**) spleen samples. Log2-normalization was applied over the Counts per Million (CPMs) in order to properly compare distributions. Variance estimation reaffirms the homogenity of control vs. case samples. Overall, differences are also observed between 3 and 5 d p.i. case samples.

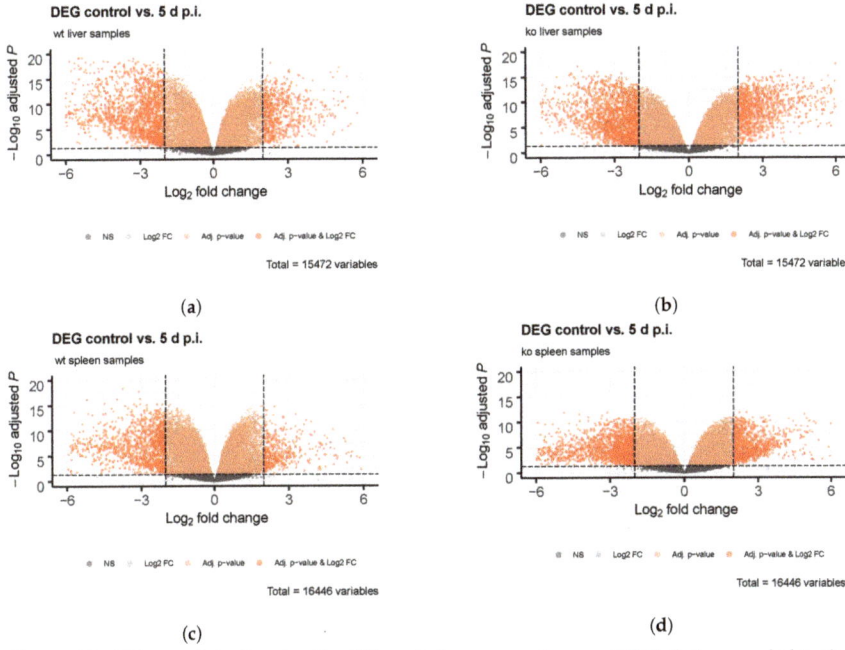

Figure A3. Volcano plots showing the differentially-expressed genes (DEG) that proceeded to the analyses. DEG were filtered by log2FC ≥ 2 and adjusted p value ≤ 0.05. These comparisons were performed both organ and genotype-wise: (**a**) liver *wt*, (**b**) liver *ko*, (**c**) spleen *wt*, (**d**) spleen *ko*. ko, $Ly6E^{\Delta HSC}$.

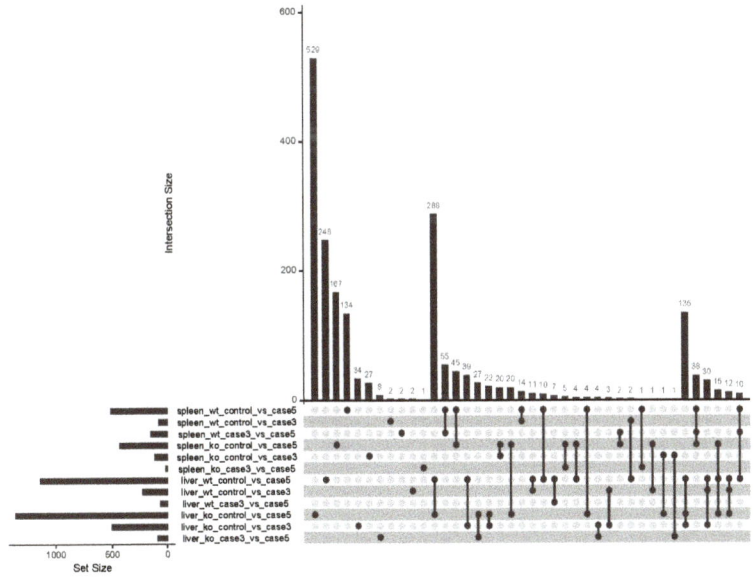

Figure A4. UpSet plot representing the commonalities between the 12 differentially-expressed genes (DEG) groups identified in differential expression analyses. The comparison of controls vs. samples at 5 d p.i. comprised the greatest number of genes for all sample types.

Table A1. Number of DEG used as input to EnGNet for network reconstruction and their latter distribution in inferred networks. Genes that were not assigned to a cluster (or were comprised in minoritary clusters) were not taken into consideration for enrichment analyses.

	Liver wt	Liver ko	Spleen wt	Spleen ko
Input genes	1133	1153	506	426
Network genes	1118	1300	485	403
Cluster 1	262	284	180	109
Cluster 2	218	379	255	190
Cluster 3	579	624	36	77
Cluster 4	59			25
Unconnected/minor clustered	0	13	14	2

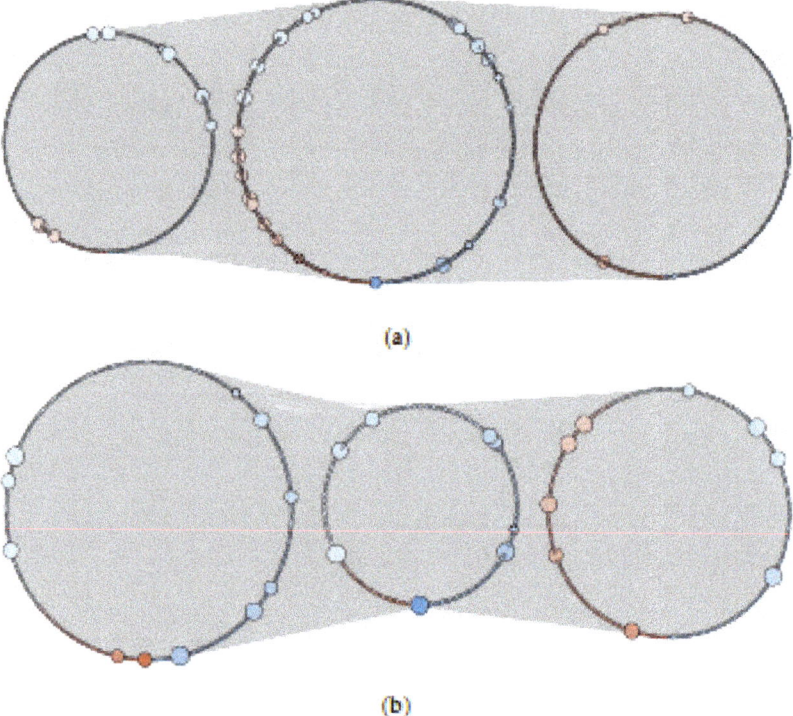

Figure A5. Inferred networks for (**a**) liver *wt* (1118 nodes, 16,281 edges, 4 clusters), (**b**) liver *ko* (1300 nodes, 15,727 edges, 3 clusters), (**c**) spleen *wt* (485 nodes, 4042 edges, 3 clusters), (**d**) spleen *ko* (403 nodes, 4220 edges, 4 clusters). Nodes are colored according to log2FC, upregulated genes in blue, downregulated genes in red. Clusters are numbered from left to right. Node size is represented according to node's degree. Edge transparency is represented according to edge weight. Networks are displayed using the yfiles organic layout [92].

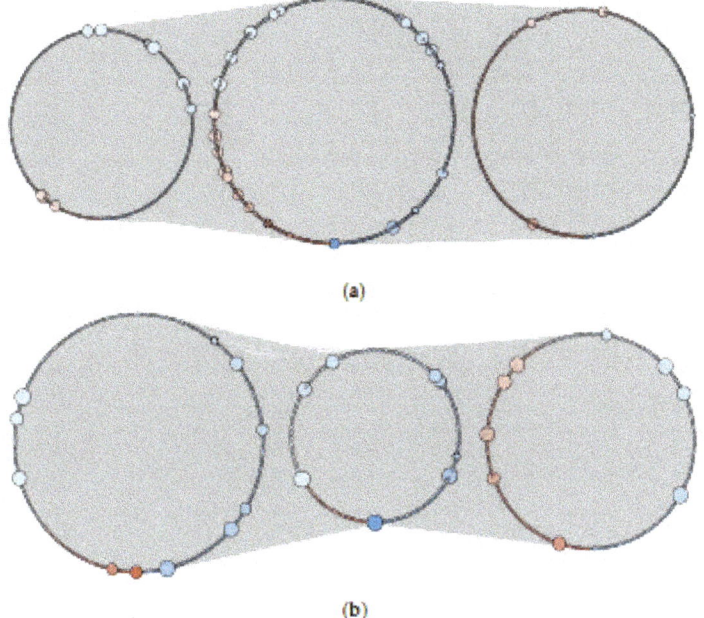

(a)

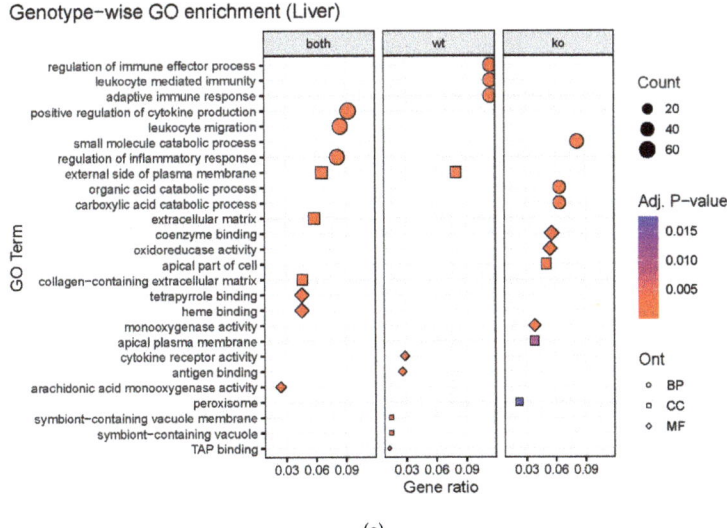

(b)

Figure A6. Networks resulting from the organ-wise merging of (**a**) *wt* and (**b**) *ko* samples. From left to right, nodes are displayed in circles depending on whether genes are contained exclusively at the *wt*, in the intersection between the *ko* and *wt* networks and in the *ko* network exclusively. Nodes are sorted and colored according to log2FC, upregulated genes in blue, downregulated genes in red. Node size is represented according to node's degree.

(a)

Figure A7. *Cont.*

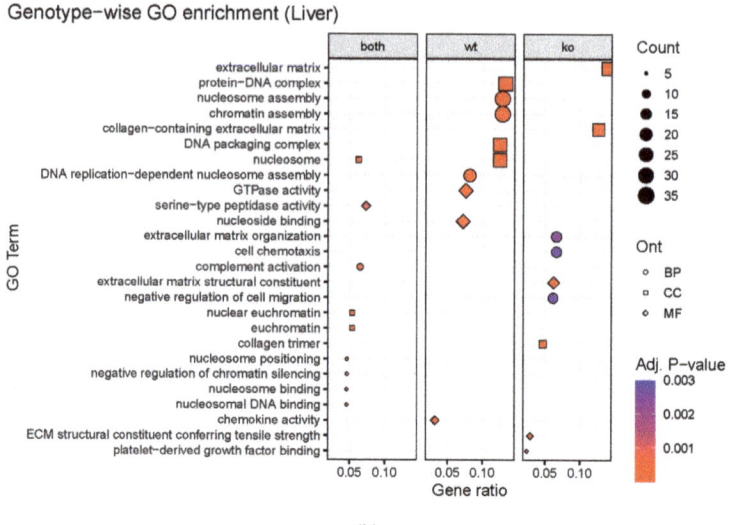

(b)

Figure A7. Enrichment analyses based on node exclusiveness of (**a**) liver and (**b**) spleen networks. *wt* refers to nodes exclusively present at those networks reconstructed from *wt* samples; *ko* refers to nodes exclusively present at networks reconstructed from $Ly6E^{\Delta HSC}$ samples; *both* addresses shared nodes between *wt* and *ko* networks. Gene ratio is defined by the number of genes used as input for the enrichment analyses associated with a particular GO term divided by the total number of input genes.

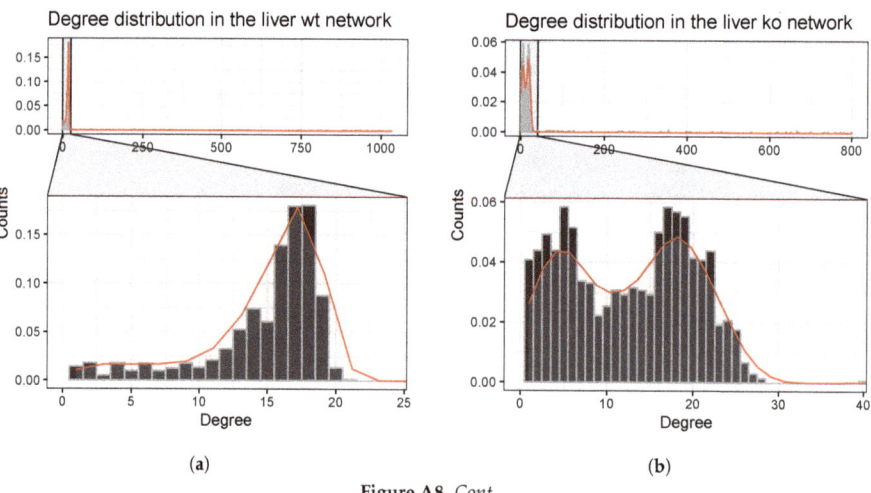

(a)   (b)

Figure A8. *Cont.*

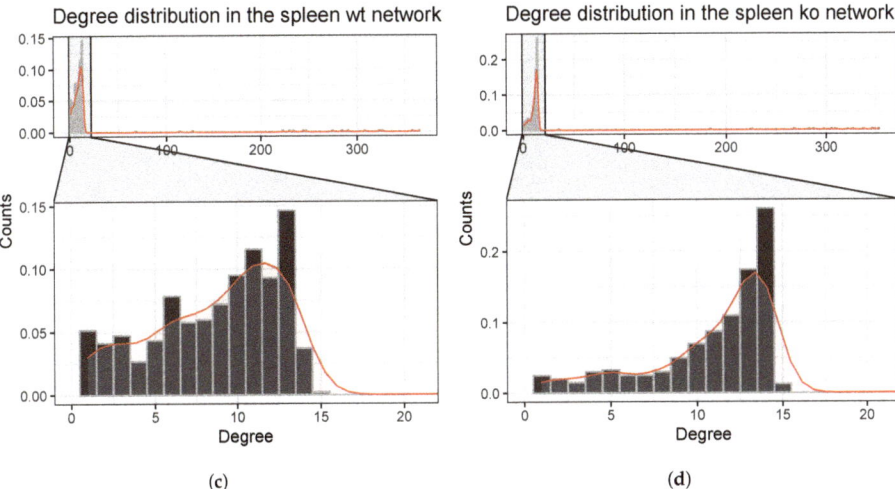

Figure A8. Distribution of node's degree throughout the networks reconstructed from (**a**) liver *wt* samples, (**b**) liver *ko* samples, (**c**) spleen *wt* samples and (**d**) spleen *ko* samples. The distribution trendline is shown in red. Nodes that are not present in the zoomed area are considered hubs. Note degree distributions do not fit a normal distribution (Shapiro–Wilk normality test, p-value < 0.05).

Table A2. Hubs identified in the network reconstructed from liver *wt* samples. Degree cutoff: 24. Reg. regulation.

Ensembl ID	Cluster	Degree	Reg.	Symbol	Description
ENSMUSG00000034593	1	1033	up	Myo5a	myosin VA
ENSMUSG00000000982	3	1006	up	Ccl3	chemokine (C-C motif) ligand 3
ENSMUSG00000030745	2	997	up	Il21r	interleukin 21 receptor
ENSMUSG00000032322	3	989	up	Pstpip1	proline-serine-threonine phosphatase-interacting protein 1
ENSMUSG00000079227	3	975	up	Ccr5	chemokine (C-C motif) receptor 5
ENSMUSG00000031304	3	957	up	Il2rg	interleukin 2 receptor, gamma chain
ENSMUSG00000069268	3	940	up	Hist1h2bf	histone cluster 1, H2bf
ENSMUSG00000027071	1	938	down	P2rx3	purinergic receptor P2X, ligand-gated ion channel, 3
ENSMUSG00000019232	3	929	down	Etnppl	ethanolamine phosphate phospholyase
ENSMUSG00000032643	3	921	up	Fhl3	four and a half LIM domains 3
ENSMUSG00000033763	3	904	down	Mtss2	MTSS I-BAR domain containing 2
ENSMUSG00000032094	1	887	up	Cd3d	CD3 antigen, delta polypeptide
ENSMUSG00000050896	3	883	up	Rtn4rl2	reticulon 4 receptor-like 2
ENSMUSG00000067219	4	801	down	Nipal1	NIPA-like domain containing 1
ENSMUSG00000110439	3	780	down	Mup22	major urinary protein 22
ENSMUSG00000004105	2	743	down	Angptl2	angiopoietin-like 2
ENSMUSG00000081650	1	713	up	Gm16181	-
ENSMUSG00000050395	2	538	up	Tnfsf15	tumor necrosis factor (ligand) superfamily, member 15

Table A2. *Cont.*

Ensembl ID	Cluster	Degree	Reg.	Symbol	Description
ENSMUSG00000038067	1	220	up	Csf3	colony stimulating factor 3 (granulocyte)
ENSMUSG00000026104	2	90	up	Stat1	signal transducer and activator of transcription 1
ENSMUSG00000037965	2	66	up	Zc3h7a	zinc finger CCCH type containing 7 A

Table A3. Hubs identified in the network reconstructed from liver $Ly6E^{\Delta HSC}$ samples. Degree cutoff: 39. Reg. regulation.

Ensembl ID	Cluster	Degree	Reg.	Symbol	Description
ENSMUSG00000029445	2	800	down	Hpd	4-hydroxyphenylpyruvic acid dioxygenase
ENSMUSG00000037071	3	781	down	Scd1	stearoyl-Coenzyme A desaturase 1
ENSMUSG00000041773	3	773	up	Enc1	ectodermal-neural cortex 1
ENSMUSG00000075015	3	760	up	Gm10801	-
ENSMUSG00000021250	3	742	up	Fos	FBJ osteosarcoma oncogene
ENSMUSG00000031618	3	735	down	Nr3c2	nuclear receptor subfamily 3, group C, member 2
ENSMUSG00000022419	1	732	down	Deptor	DEP domain containing MTOR-interacting protein
ENSMUSG00000033610	3	700	down	Pank1	pantothenate kinase 1
ENSMUSG00000024349	3	667	up	Tmem173	transmembrane protein 173
ENSMUSG00000006519	3	666	up	Cyba	cytochrome b-245, alpha polypeptide
ENSMUSG00000035878	3	666	down	Hykk	hydroxylysine kinase 1
ENSMUSG00000054630	2	652	down	Ugt2b5	UDP glucuronosyltransferase 2 family, polypeptide B5
ENSMUSG00000041757	3	639	down	Plekha6	pleckstrin homology domain containing, family A member 6
ENSMUSG00000053398	3	620	up	Phgdh	3-phosphoglycerate dehydrogenase
ENSMUSG00000022025	3	555	down	Cnmd	chondromodulin
ENSMUSG00000029659	2	482	up	Medag	mesenteric estrogen dependent adipogenesis
ENSMUSG00000062380	2	461	up	Tubb3	tubulin, beta 3 class III
ENSMUSG00000069309	3	408	up	Hist1h2an	histone cluster 1, H2an
ENSMUSG00000034285	3	399	down	Nipsnap1	nipsnap homolog 1
ENSMUSG00000027654	3	355	up	Fam83d	family with sequence similarity 83, member D
ENSMUSG00000073435	2	355	down	Nme3	NME/NM23 nucleoside diphosphate kinase 3
ENSMUSG00000021062	2	336	up	Rab15	RAB15, member RAS oncogene family
ENSMUSG00000037852	3	271	up	Cpe	carboxypeptidase E
ENSMUSG00000096201	2	260	up	Gm10715	-
ENSMUSG00000022754	2	245	up	Tmem45a	transmembrane protein 45a
ENSMUSG00000038233	1	239	down	Gask1a	golgi associated kinase 1A

Table A3. *Cont.*

Ensembl ID	Cluster	Degree	Reg.	Symbol	Description
ENSMUSG00000043456	2	236	up	Zfp536	zinc finger protein 536
ENSMUSG00000095891	2	168	up	Gm10717	-
ENSMUSG00000096688	1	126	down	Mup17	major urinary protein 17
ENSMUSG00000099398	2	115	up	Ms4a14	membrane-spanning 4-domains, subfamily A, member 14
ENSMUSG00000025002	1	99	down	Cyp2c55	cytochrome P450, family 2, subfamily c, polypeptide 55
ENSMUSG00000074896	1	91	up	Ifit3	interferon-induced protein with tetratricopeptide repeats 3
ENSMUSG00000062488	1	86	up	Ifit3b	interferon-induced protein with tetratricopeptide repeats 3B
ENSMUSG00000029417	1	78	up	Cxcl9	chemokine (C-X-C motif) ligand 9
ENSMUSG00000057465	1	77	up	Saa2	serum amyloid A 2
ENSMUSG00000050908	2	69	up	Tvp23a	trans-golgi network vesicle protein 23A
ENSMUSG00000030142	1	63	up	Clec4e	C-type lectin domain family 4, member e
ENSMUSG00000038751	1	61	down	Ptk6	PTK6 protein tyrosine kinase 6
ENSMUSG00000068606	1	40	up	Gm4841	predicted gene 4841

Table A4. Hubs identified in the network reconstructed from spleen *wt* samples. Degree cutoff: 21. Reg. regulation.

Ensembl ID	Cluster	Degree	Reg.	Symbol	Description
ENSMUSG00000019505	2	365	up	Ubb	ubiquitin B
ENSMUSG00000094777	2	358	up	Hist1h2ap	histone cluster 1, H2ap
ENSMUSG00000057729	3	326	up	Prtn3	proteinase 3
ENSMUSG00000056071	1	323	up	S100a9	S100 calcium binding protein A9 (calgranulin B)
ENSMUSG00000025403	2	308	up	Shmt2	serine hydroxymethyltransferase 2 (mitochondrial)
ENSMUSG00000023132	2	290	up	Gzma	granzyme A
ENSMUSG00000078920	2	284	up	Ifi47	interferon gamma inducible protein 47
ENSMUSG00000037894	1	274	up	H2afz	H2A histone family, member Z
ENSMUSG00000035472	2	247	down	Slc25a21	solute carrier family 25 (mitochondrial oxodicarboxylate carrier), member 21
ENSMUSG00000009350	1	244	up	Mpo	myeloperoxidase
ENSMUSG00000103254	1	234	up	Ighv1-15	-
ENSMUSG00000069274	1	230	up	Hist1h4f	histone cluster 1, H4f
ENSMUSG00000028328	2	223	down	Tmod1	tropomodulin 1
ENSMUSG00000094322	1	128	up	Ighv9-4	-
ENSMUSG00000094124	1	114	up	Ighv1-74	-
ENSMUSG00000094546	1	68	up	Ighv1-26	-

Table A5. Hubs identified in the network reconstructed from spleen $Ly6E^{\Delta HSC}$ samples. Degree cutoff: 21. Reg. regulation

Ensembl ID	Cluster	Degree	Reg.	Symbol	Description
ENSMUSG00000027715	2	353	up	Ccna2	cyclin A2
ENSMUSG00000024742	3	349	up	Fen1	flap structure specific endonuclease 1
ENSMUSG00000024640	2	347	up	Psat1	phosphoserine aminotransferase 1
ENSMUSG00000040026	2	338	up	Saa3	serum amyloid A 3
ENSMUSG00000039713	2	327	down	Plekhg5	pleckstrin homology domain containing, family G (with RhoGef domain) member 5
ENSMUSG00000075289	4	322	down	Carns1	carnosine synthase 1
ENSMUSG00000067610	2	309	down	Klri1	killer cell lectin-like receptor family I member 1
ENSMUSG00000031503	1	305	up	Col4a2	collagen, type IV, alpha 2
ENSMUSG00000095700	3	298	up	Ighv10-3	-
ENSMUSG00000076613	3	287	up	Ighg2b	-
ENSMUSG00000051079	2	282	down	Rgs13	regulator of G-protein signaling 13
ENSMUSG00000036027	2	268	down	1810046K07Rik	RIKEN cDNA 1810046K07 gene
ENSMUSG00000027962	1	225	up	Vcam1	vascular cell adhesion molecule 1
ENSMUSG00000049130	1	184	up	C5ar1	complement component 5a receptor 1
ENSMUSG00000066861	1	35	up	Oas1g	2'-5' oligoadenylate synthetase 1G

Table A6. Highly DEG. List of DEG that are differentially-expressed for every of the comparisons performed: control vs. cases at 3 d p.i., control vs. cases at 5 d p.i. and cases at 3 vs. 5 d p.i. Memb, membership to the group of samples genes belong; ko, $Ly6E^{\Delta HSC}$ samples. Reg. Type refers to the three expression patterns observed, described in Section 5.

Ensembl ID	Symbol	Description	Memb.	Reg. Type
ENSMUSG00000032487	Ptgs2	prostaglandin-endoperoxide synthase 2	liver *wt*	1
ENSMUSG00000029816	Gpnmb	glycoprotein (transmembrane) nmb	liver *wt*	1
ENSMUSG00000035385	Ccl2	chemokine (C-C motif) ligand 2	liver *wt*	1
ENSMUSG00000035373	Ccl7	chemokine (C-C motif) ligand 7	liver *wt*	1
ENSMUSG00000015437	Gzmb	granzyme B	liver *wt*	1
ENSMUSG00000038037	Socs1	suppressor of cytokine signaling 1	liver *wt*	1
ENSMUSG00000026839	Upp2	uridine phosphorylase 2	liver *ko*	2
ENSMUSG00000075014	Gm10800	-	liver *ko*	1
ENSMUSG00000040660	Cyp2b9	cytochrome P450, family 2, subfamily b, polypeptide 9	liver *ko*	2
ENSMUSG00000056978	Hamp2	hepcidin antimicrobial peptide 2	liver *ko*	2
ENSMUSG00000073940	Hbb-bt	hemoglobin, beta adult t chain	liver *ko*	2
ENSMUSG00000052305	Hbb-bs	hemoglobin, beta adult major chain	liver *ko*	2
ENSMUSG00000025473	Adam8	a disintegrin and metallopeptidase domain 8	liver *ko*	1
ENSMUSG00000056973	Ces1d	carboxylesterase 1D	liver *ko*	2
ENSMUSG00000025317	Car5a	carbonic anhydrase 5a, mitochondrial	liver *ko*	2
ENSMUSG00000050578	Mmp13	matrix metallopeptidase 13	liver *ko*	1
ENSMUSG00000049723	Mmp12	matrix metallopeptidase 12	liver *ko*	1

Table A6. Cont.

Ensembl ID	Symbol	Description	Memb.	Reg. Type
ENSMUSG00000035878	Hykk	hydroxylysine kinase 1	liver *ko*	2
ENSMUSG00000069917	Hba-a2	hemoglobin alpha, adult chain 2	liver *ko*	2
ENSMUSG00000009350	Mpo	myeloperoxidase	liver *ko*	1
ENSMUSG00000109482	Gm4756	-	liver *ko*	2
ENSMUSG00000060807	Serpina6	serine (or cysteine) peptidase inhibitor, clade A, member 6	liver *ko*	2
ENSMUSG00000079018	Ly6c1	lymphocyte antigen 6 complex, locus C1	liver *ko*	1
ENSMUSG00000074896	Ifit3	interferon-induced protein with tetratricopeptide repeats 3	liver *ko*	3
ENSMUSG00000062488	Ifit3b	interferon-induced protein with tetratricopeptide repeats 3B	liver *ko*	3
ENSMUSG00000032808	Cyp2c38	cytochrome P450, family 2, subfamily c, polypeptide 38	liver *ko*	2
ENSMUSG00000025004	Cyp2c40	cytochrome P450, family 2, subfamily c, polypeptide 40	liver *ko*	2
ENSMUSG00000042248	Cyp2c37	cytochrome P450, family 2, subfamily c, polypeptide 37	liver *ko*	2
ENSMUSG00000067225	Cyp2c54	cytochrome P450, family 2, subfamily c, polypeptide 54	liver *ko*	2
ENSMUSG00000054827	Cyp2c50	cytochrome P450, family 2, subfamily c, polypeptide 50	liver *ko*	2
ENSMUSG00000001131	Timp1	tissue inhibitor of metalloproteinase 1	liver *ko*	1
ENSMUSG00000015437	Gzmb	granzyme B	spleen *wt*	1
ENSMUSG00000022584	Ly6c2	lymphocyte antigen 6 complex, locus C2	spleen *wt*	1
ENSMUSG00000040026	Saa3	serum amyloid A 3	spleen *ko*	1

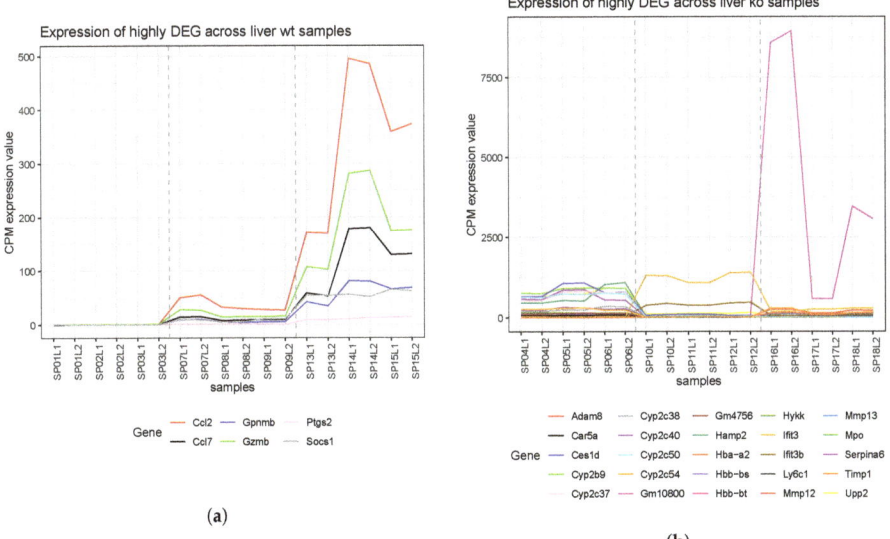

(a)

(b)

Figure A9. Cont.

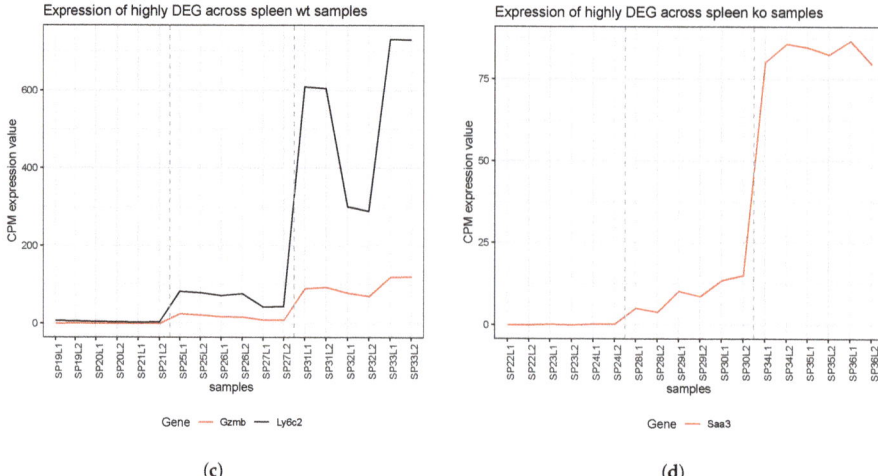

(c)   (d)

Figure A9. CPM-normalized expression values of highly DEG identified across (**a**) liver *wt* samples, (**b**) liver *ko* samples, (**c**) spleen *wt* samples and (**d**) spleen *ko* samples. Dashed lines separate samples from the three groups under study: controls, cases at 3 d p.i. and cases at 5 d p.i. Note sample order within same group is exchangeable.

Appendix B. Validation of the Reconstruction Method

The reconstruction method employed in this case study was validated against other thee well-known inference methods: *ARACNe* [93], *WGCNA* [94] and *wTO* [95]. The output of each reconstruction method, using default values (including *EnGNet*) was compared to a gold standard (GS), retrieved from the *STRING* database.

Four different GSs were taken into consideration, since these were reconstructed from the DEG that were identified in the comparison of control vs. case samples at 5 d p.i., as shown in Section 4.2. These DEG were mapped to the *STRING* database gene identifiers selecting *Mus musculus* as model organism (taxid: 10090). A variable percentage of DEG (6–20%) could not be assigned to a STRING identifier, and were thus removed from the analysis. The interactions exclusively concerning the resulting DEG in each case were retrieved from the STRING database. These interaction networks would serve as GSs. The mentioned DEG (without unmapped identifiers) would also serve as input for the four reconstruction methods to be compared.

The *ARACNe* networks were inferred using the Spearman correlation coefficient following the implementations in the *minet* [96] R package. In this case, mutual information values were normalized and scaled in the range 0–1. On the other hand, the *WGCNA* networks were reconstructed following the original tutorial provided by the authors [97]. The power was defined as 5. Additionally, the *wTO* networks were built using Pearson correlation in accordance to the documentation. Absolute values were taken as relationship weights. Finally, *EnGNet* networks were inferred using the default parameters described in the original article by Gómez-Vela et al. [33]. For the comparison, the Receiver operating characteristic (ROC)-curve was estimated using the *pROC* [98] R package. ROC curves are shown in Figure A10.

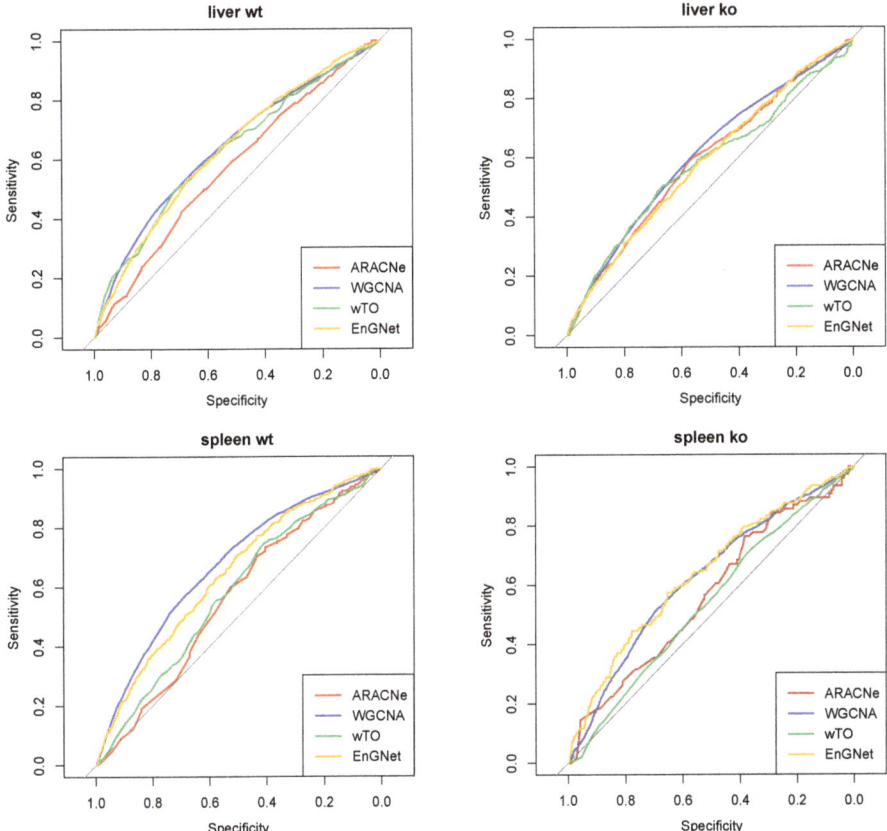

Figure A10. Receiver operating characteristic (ROC) curves for the four datasets obtained in our study using different reconstruction methods. Sensitivity is the true positive rate: $TP/(TP+FN)$. Specificity is the true negative rate: $TN/(TN+FP)$. TP, true positive; TN, true negative; FN, false negative; FP, false positive.

The area under the ROC curve (AUC) was also computed in each case for the quantitative comparison of the methods, as shown in Figure A11a. The AUC compares the reconstruction quality of each method against random prediction. An AUC ≈ 1 corresponds to the perfect classifier whereas am AUC ≈ 0.5 approximates to a random classifier. Thus, the higher the AUC, the better the predictions. On average, *EnGNet* provided the best AUC results, whilst maintaining a good discovery rate. In addition, *EnGNet* provided relatively scarce networks compared to *WGCNA*, as shown in Figure A11b. This is considered of relevance given that sparseness is a main feature of gene networks [7].

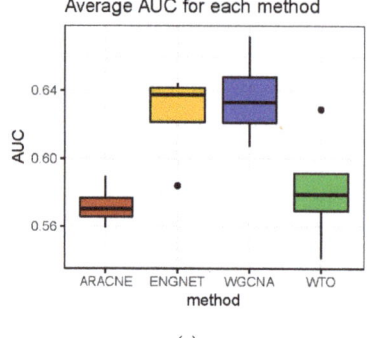
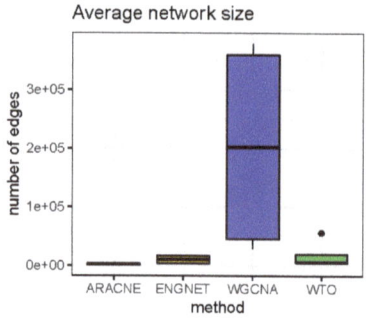

(a) (b)

Figure A11. (**a**) Comparison of the average area under the ROC curve (AUC) for the four reconstruction methods under comparison across the four used datasets. On average, EnGNet outperformed the other three methods in terms of AUC. (**b**) Size comparison of the inferred networks. EnGNet exhibited competitive results in terms of network size, providing considerably sparser networks than WGCNA's.

References

1. Corman, V.M.; Muth, D.; Niemeyer, D.; Drosten, C. Hosts and Sources of Endemic Human Coronaviruses. *Adv. Virus Res.* **2018**, *100*, 163–188. [PubMed]
2. Prentice, E.; McAuliffe, J.; Lu, X.; Subbarao, K.; Denison, M.R. Identification and characterization of severe acute respiratory syndrome coronavirus replicase proteins. *J. Virol.* **2004**, *78*, 9977–9986. [CrossRef] [PubMed]
3. Sheahan, T.P.; Sims, A.C.; Zhou, S.; Graham, R.L.; Pruijssers, A.J.; Agostini, M.L.; Leist, S.R.; Schäfer, A.; Dinnon, K.H.; Stevens, L.J.; et al. An orally bioavailable broad-spectrum antiviral inhibits SARS-CoV-2 in human airway epithelial cell cultures and multiple coronaviruses in mice. *Sci. Transl. Med.* **2020**, *12*, eabb5883. [CrossRef]
4. Voit, E. *A First Course in Systems Biology*; Garland Science: New York, NY, USA, 2017.
5. Delgado, F.M.; Gómez-Vela, F. Computational methods for Gene Regulatory Networks reconstruction and analysis: A review. *Artif. Intell. Med.* **2019**, *95*, 133–145. [CrossRef] [PubMed]
6. Gómez-Vela, F.; Lagares, J.A.; Díaz-Díaz, N. Gene network coherence based on prior knowledge using direct and indirect relationships. *Comput. Biol. Chem.* **2015**, *56*, 142–151. [CrossRef]
7. Hecker, M.; Lambeck, S.; Toepfer, S.; Van Someren, E.; Guthke, R. Gene regulatory network inference: data integration in dynamic models—A review. *Biosystems* **2009**, *96*, 86–103. [CrossRef] [PubMed]
8. Gómez-Vela, F.; Rodriguez-Baena, D.S.; Vázquez-Noguera, J.L. Structure Optimization for Large Gene Networks Based on Greedy Strategy. *Comput. Math. Methods Med.* **2018**, *2018*, 9674108. [CrossRef] [PubMed]
9. Zhang, Q.; Ding, Z.; Wan, L.; Tong, W.; Mao, J.; Li, L.; Hu, J.; Yang, M.; Liu, B.; Qian, X. Comprehensive analysis of the long noncoding RNA expression profile and construction of the lncRNA-mRNA co-expression network in colorectal cancer. *Cancer Biol. Ther.* **2020**, *21*, 157–169. [CrossRef]
10. Díaz-Montaña, J.J.; Gómez-Vela, F.; Díaz-Díaz, N. GNC–app: A new Cytoscape app to rate gene networks biological coherence using gene–gene indirect relationships. *Biosystems* **2018**, *166*, 61–65. [CrossRef]
11. Kumari, S.; Nie, J.; Chen, H.S.; Ma, H.; Stewart, R.; Li, X.; Lu, M.Z.; Taylor, W.M.; Wei, H. Evaluation of gene association methods for coexpression network construction and biological knowledge discovery. *PLoS ONE* **2012**, *7*, e50411. [CrossRef]
12. de Siqueira Santos, S.; Takahashi, D.Y.; Nakata, A.; Fujita, A. A comparative study of statistical methods used to identify dependencies between gene expression signals. *Brief. Bioinform.* **2013**, *15*, 906–918. [CrossRef]
13. Liesecke, F.; Daudu, D.; Dugé de Bernonville, R.; Besseau, S.; Clastre, M.; Courdavault, V.; de Craene, J.O.; Crèche, J.; Giglioli-Guivarc'h, N.; Glévarec, G.; et al. Ranking genome-wide correlation measurements improves microarray and RNA-seq based global and targeted co-expression networks. *Sci. Rep.* **2018**, *8*, 10885. [CrossRef] [PubMed]

14. Marbach, D.; Costello, J.C.; Küffner, R.; Vega, N.M.; Prill, R.J.; Camacho, D.M.; Allison, K.R.; Aderhold, A.; Bonneau, R.; Chen, Y.; et al. Wisdom of crowds for robust gene network inference. *Nat. Methods* **2012**, *9*, 796–804. [CrossRef] [PubMed]
15. Song, L.; Langfelder, P.; Horvath, S. Comparison of co-expression measures: mutual information, correlation, and model based indices. *BMC Bioinform.* **2012**, *13*, 328. [CrossRef] [PubMed]
16. Villaverde, A.F.; Ross, J.; Morán, F.; Banga, J.R. MIDER: Network inference with mutual information distance and entropy reduction. *PLoS ONE* **2014**, *9*, e96732. [CrossRef]
17. Zhang, X.; Bai, J.; Yuan, C.; Long, L.; Zheng, Z.; Wang, Q.; Chenand, F.; Zhou, Y. Bioinformatics analysis and identification of potential genes related to pathogenesis of cervical intraepithelial neoplasia. *J. Cancer* **2020**, *11*, 2150–2157. [CrossRef]
18. Sehrawat, A.; Gao, L.; Wang, Y.; Bankhead, A.; McWeeney, S.K.; King, C.J.; Schwartzman, J.; Urrutia, J.; Bisson, W.H.; Coleman, D.J.; et al. LSD1 activates a lethal prostate cancer gene network independently of its demethylase function. *Proc. Natl. Acad. Sci. USA* **2018**, *115*, E4179–E4188. [CrossRef]
19. Sandor, C.; Beer, N.L.; Webber, C. Diverse type 2 diabetes genetic risk factors functionally converge in a phenotype-focused gene network. *PLoS Comput. Biol.* **2017**, *13*, e1005816. [CrossRef]
20. Wang, L.; Huang, J.; Jiang, M.; Sun, L. Survivin (BIRC5) cell cycle computational network in human no-tumor hepatitis/cirrhosis and hepatocellular carcinoma transformation. *J. Cell. Biochem.* **2011**, *112*, 1286–1294. [CrossRef]
21. He, D.; Liu, Z.P.; Honda, M.; Kaneko, S.; Chen, L. Coexpression network analysis in chronic hepatitis B and C hepatic lesions reveals distinct patterns of disease progression to hepatocellular carcinoma. *J. Mol. Cell Biol.* **2012**, *4*, 140–152. [CrossRef]
22. Nogales, A.; Martínez-Sobrido, L. Reverse genetics approaches for the development of influenza vaccines. *Int. J. Mol. Sci.* **2017**, *18*, 20. [CrossRef] [PubMed]
23. Rajoriya, N.; Combet, C.; Zoulim, F.; Janssen, H.L. How viral genetic variants and genotypes influence disease and treatment outcome of chronic hepatitis B. Time for an individualised approach? *J. Hepatol.* **2017**, *67*, 1281–1297. [CrossRef] [PubMed]
24. Wong, H.H.; Fung, T.S.; Fang, S.; Huang, M.; Le, M.T.; Liu, D.X. Accessory proteins 8b and 8ab of severe acute respiratory syndrome coronavirus suppress the interferon signaling pathway by mediating ubiquitin-dependent rapid degradation of interferon regulatory factor 3. *Virology* **2018**, *515*, 165–175. [CrossRef] [PubMed]
25. Schneider, W.M.; Chevillotte, M.D.; Rice, C.M. Interferon-stimulated genes: a complex web of host defenses. *Annu. Rev. Immunol.* **2014**, *32*, 513–545. [CrossRef] [PubMed]
26. Luo, L.; McGarvey, P.; Madhavan, S.; Kumar, R.; Gusev, Y.; Upadhyay, G. Distinct lymphocyte antigens 6 (Ly6) family members Ly6D, Ly6E, Ly6K and Ly6H drive tumorigenesis and clinical outcome. *Oncotarget* **2016**, *7*, 11165. [CrossRef] [PubMed]
27. Yu, J.; Liu, S.L. Emerging Role of LY6E in Virus–Host Interactions. *Viruses* **2019**, *11*, 1020. [CrossRef]
28. Liu, H.C.; Niikura, M.; Fulton, J.; Cheng, H. Identification of chicken lymphocyte antigen 6 complex, locus E (LY6E, alias SCA2) as a putative Marek's disease resistance gene via a virus-host protein interaction screen. *Cytogenet. Genome Res.* **2003**, *102*, 304–308. [CrossRef]
29. Stier, M.T.; Spindler, K.R. Polymorphisms in Ly6 genes in Msq1 encoding susceptibility to mouse adenovirus type 1. *Mamm. Genome* **2012**, *23*, 250–258. [CrossRef]
30. Yu, J.; Liang, C.; Liu, S.L. Interferon-inducible LY6E protein promotes HIV-1 infection. *J. Biol. Chem.* **2017**, *292*, 4674–4685. [CrossRef]
31. Mar, K.B.; Rinkenberger, N.R.; Boys, I.N.; Eitson, J.L.; McDougal, M.B.; Richardson, R.B.; Schoggins, J.W. LY6E mediates an evolutionarily conserved enhancement of virus infection by targeting a late entry step. *Nat. Commun.* **2018**, *9*, 1–14. [CrossRef]
32. Hackett, B.A.; Cherry, S. Flavivirus internalization is regulated by a size-dependent endocytic pathway. *Proc. Natl. Acad. Sci. USA* **2018**, *115*, 4246–4251. [CrossRef] [PubMed]
33. Gómez-Vela, F.; Delgado-Chaves, F.M.; Rodríguez-Baena, D.S.; García-Torres, M.; Divina, F. Ensemble and Greedy Approach for the Reconstruction of Large Gene Co-Expression Networks. *Entropy* **2019**, *21*, 1139. [CrossRef]

34. Giulietti, M.; Occhipinti, G.; Principato, G.; Piva, F. Identification of candidate miRNA biomarkers for pancreatic ductal adenocarcinoma by weighted gene co-expression network analysis. *Cell. Oncol.* **2017**, *40*, 181–192. [CrossRef]
35. Ray, S.; Hossain, S.M.M.; Khatun, L.; Mukhopadhyay, A. A comprehensive analysis on preservation patterns of gene co-expression networks during Alzheimer's disease progression. *BMC Bioinform.* **2017**, *18*, 579. [CrossRef]
36. Medina, I.R.; Lubovac-Pilav, Z. Gene co-expression network analysis for identifying modules and functionally enriched pathways in type 1 diabetes. *PLoS ONE* **2016**, *11*, e0156006.
37. van Dam, S.; Vosa, U.; van der Graaf, A.; Franke, L.; de Magalhaes, J.P. Gene co-expression analysis for functional classification and gene–disease predictions. *Brief. Bioinform.* **2018**, *19*, 575–592. [CrossRef] [PubMed]
38. Argilaguet Marqués, J.; Pedragosa Marín, M.; Esteve-Codina, A.; Riera Domínguez, M.G.; Vidal, E.; Peligero Cruz, C.; Casella, V.; Andreu Martínez, D.; Kaisho, T.; Bocharov, G.A.; et al. Systems analysis reveals complex biological processes during virus infection fate decisions. *Genome Res.* **2019**, *29*, 907–919. [CrossRef] [PubMed]
39. Ghobadi, M.Z.; Mozhgani, S.-H.; Farzanehpour, M.; Behzadian, F. Identifying novel biomarkers of the pediatric influenza infection by weighted co-expression network analysis. *Virol. J.* **2019**, *16*, 124. [CrossRef] [PubMed]
40. Michlmayr, D.; Pak, T.R.; Rahman, A.H.; Amir, E.A.D.; Kim, E.Y.; Kim-Schulze, S.; Suprun, M.; Stewart, M.G.; Thomas, G.P.; Balmaseda, A.; et al. Comprehensive innate immune profiling of chikungunya virus infection in pediatric cases. *Mol. Syst. Biol.* **2018**, *14*, e7862. [CrossRef]
41. Pedragosa, M.; Riera, G.; Casella, V.; Esteve-Codina, A.; Steuerman, Y.; Seth, C.; Bocharov, G.; Heath, S.C.; Gat-Viks, I.; Argilaguet, J.; et al. Linking cell dynamics with gene coexpression networks to characterize key events in chronic virus infections. *Front. Immunol.* **2019**, *10*, 1002. [CrossRef] [PubMed]
42. Ray, S.; Hossain, S.M.M.; Khatun, L. Discovering preservation pattern from co-expression modules in progression of HIV-1 disease: An eigengene based approach. In Proceedings of the 2016 International Conference on Advances in Computing, Communications and Informatics (ICACCI), Jaipur, India, 21–24 September 2016; pp. 814–820.
43. McDermott, J.; Mitchell, H.; Gralinski, L.; Eisfeld, A.J.; Josset, L.; Bankhead, A., 3rd; Neumann, G.; Tilton, S.C.; Schäfer, A.; Li, C.; et al. The effect of inhibition of PP1 and TNFα signaling on pathogenesis of SARS coronavirus. *BMC Syst. Biol.* **2016**, *10*, 93. [CrossRef] [PubMed]
44. Pan, K.; Wang, Y.; Pan, P.; Xu, G.; Mo, L.; Cao, L.; Wu, C.; Shen, X. The regulatory role of microRNA-mRNA co-expression in hepatitis B virus-associated acute liver failure. *Ann. Hepatol.* **2019**, *18*, 883–892. [CrossRef]
45. Sungnak, W.; Huang, N.; Bécavin, C.; Berg, M.; Queen, R.; Litvinukova, M.; Talavera-López, C.; Maatz, H.; Reichart, D.; Sampaziotis, F.; et al. SARS-CoV-2 entry factors are highly expressed in nasal epithelial cells together with innate immune genes. *Nat. Med.* **2020**, *26*, 681–687. [CrossRef] [PubMed]
46. De Albuquerque, N.; Baig, E.; Ma, X.; Zhang, J.; He, W.; Rowe, A.; Habal, M.; Liu, M.; Shalev, I.; Downey, G.P.; et al. Murine hepatitis virus strain 1 produces a clinically relevant model of severe acute respiratory syndrome in A/J mice. *J. Virol.* **2006**, *80*, 10382–10394. [CrossRef] [PubMed]
47. Ding, Z.; Fang, L.; Yuan, S.; Zhao, L.; Wang, X.; Long, S.; Wang, M.; Wang, D.; Foda, M.F.; Xiao, S. The nucleocapsid proteins of mouse hepatitis virus and severe acute respiratory syndrome coronavirus share the same IFN-β antagonizing mechanism: attenuation of PACT-mediated RIG-I/MDA5 activation. *Oncotarget* **2017**, *8*, 49655. [CrossRef]
48. Case, J.B.; Li, Y.; Elliott, R.; Lu, X.; Graepel, K.W.; Sexton, N.R.; Smith, E.C.; Weiss, S.R.; Denison, M.R. Murine hepatitis virus nsp14 exoribonuclease activity is required for resistance to innate immunity. *J. Virol.* **2018**, *92*, e01531-17. [CrossRef]
49. Gorman, M.J.; Poddar, S.; Farzan, M.; Diamond, M.S. The interferon-stimulated gene Ifitm3 restricts West Nile virus infection and pathogenesis. *J. Virol.* **2016**, *90*, 8212–8225. [CrossRef] [PubMed]
50. Loughner, C.; Bruford, E.; McAndrews, M.; Delp, E.E.; Swamynathan, S.; Swamynathan, S.K. Organization, evolution and functions of the human and mouse Ly6/uPAR family genes. *Hum. Genom.* **2016**, *10*, 10. [CrossRef] [PubMed]
51. Mar, K.B.; Eitson, J.; Schoggins, J. Interferon-stimulated gene LY6E enhances entry of diverse RNA viruses. *J. Immunol.* **2016**, *196*, 217.7.

52. Giotis, E.S.; Robey, R.C.; Skinner, N.G.; Tomlinson, C.D.; Goodbourn, S.; Skinner, M.A. Chicken interferome: avian interferon-stimulated genes identified by microarray and RNA-seq of primary chick embryo fibroblasts treated with a chicken type I interferon (IFN-α). *Vet. Res.* **2016**, *47*, 75. [CrossRef] [PubMed]
53. Kumar, N.; Mishra, B.; Mehmood, A.; Athar, M.; Mukhtar, M.S. Integrative Network Biology Framework Elucidates Molecular Mechanisms of SARS-CoV-2 Pathogenesis. *bioRxiv* **2020**. [CrossRef]
54. Pfaender, S.; Mar, K.B.; Michailidis, E.; Kratzel, A.; Hirt, D.; V'kovski, P.; Fan, W.; Ebert, N.; Stalder, H.; Kleine-Weber, H.; et al. LY6E impairs coronavirus fusion and confers immune control of viral disease. *bioRxiv* **2020**. [CrossRef]
55. Robinson, M.D.; McCarthy, D.J.; Smyth, G.K. edgeR: a Bioconductor package for differential expression analysis of digital gene expression data. *Bioinformatics* **2010**, *26*, 139–140. [CrossRef] [PubMed]
56. Davis, S.; Meltzer, P.S. GEOquery: a bridge between the Gene Expression Omnibus (GEO) and BioConductor. *Bioinformatics* **2007**, *23*, 1846–1847. [CrossRef]
57. Bullard, J.H.; Purdom, E.; Hansen, K.D.; Dudoit, S. Evaluation of statistical methods for normalization and differential expression in mRNA-Seq experiments. *BMC Bioinform.* **2010**, *11*, 94. [CrossRef]
58. Huber, W.; Carey, V.J.; Gentleman, R.; Anders, S.; Carlson, M.; Carvalho, B.S.; Bravo, H.C.; Davis, S.; Gatto, L.; Girke, T.; et al. Orchestrating high-throughput genomic analysis with Bioconductor. *Nat. Methods* **2015**, *12*, 115. [CrossRef]
59. Zhu, A.; Ibrahim, J.G.; Love, M.I. Heavy-tailed prior distributions for sequence count data: removing the noise and preserving large differences. *Bioinformatics* **2019**, *35*, 2084–2092. [CrossRef]
60. Alvarez, J.M.; Riveras, E.; Vidal, E.A.; Gras, D.E.; Contreras-López, O.; Tamayo, K.P.; Aceituno, F.; Gómez, I.; Ruffel, S.; Lejay, L.; et al. Systems approach identifies TGA 1 and TGA 4 transcription factors as important regulatory components of the nitrate response of A rabidopsis thaliana roots. *Plant J.* **2014**, *80*, 1–13. [CrossRef]
61. Delgado-Chaves, F.M.; Gómez-Vela, F.; García-Torres, M.; Divina, F.; Vázquez Noguera, J.L. Computational Inference of Gene Co-Expression Networks for the identification of Lung Carcinoma Biomarkers: An Ensemble Approach. *Genes* **2019**, *10*, 962. [CrossRef]
62. Contreras-Lopez, O.; Moyano, T.C.; Soto, D.C.; Gutiérrez, R.A. Step-by-step construction of gene co-expression networks from high-throughput arabidopsis RNA sequencing data. In *Root Development*; Springer: Berlin/Heidelberg, Germany, 2018; pp. 275–301.
63. Ritchie, M.E.; Phipson, B.; Wu, D.; Hu, Y.; Law, C.W.; Shi, W.; Smyth, G.K. limma powers differential expression analyses for RNA-sequencing and microarray studies. *Nucleic Acids Res.* **2015**, *43*, e47. [CrossRef]
64. Law, C.W.; Chen, Y.; Shi, W.; Smyth, G.K. voom: Precision weights unlock linear model analysis tools for RNA-seq read counts. *Genome Biol.* **2014**, *15*, R29. [CrossRef]
65. Genovese, C.R.; Roeder, K.; Wasserman, L. False discovery control with p-value weighting. *Biometrika* **2006**, *93*, 509–524. [CrossRef]
66. Csardi, G.; Nepusz, T. The igraph software package for complex network research. *InterJournal Complex Syst.* **2006**, *1695*, 1–9.
67. Smoot, M.E.; Ono, K.; Ruscheinski, J.; Wang, P.L.; Ideker, T. Cytoscape 2.8: new features for data integration and network visualization. *Bioinformatics* **2011**, *27*, 431–432. [CrossRef] [PubMed]
68. Gustavsen, J.A.; Pai, S.; Isserlin, R.; Demchak, B.; Pico, A.R. RCy3: Network biology using Cytoscape from within R. *F1000Research* **2019**, *8*, 1774. [CrossRef] [PubMed]
69. Li, W.; Wang, M.; Sun, J.; Wang, Y.; Jiang, R. Gene co-opening network deciphers gene functional relationships. *Mol. Biosyst.* **2017**, *13*, 2428–2439. [CrossRef] [PubMed]
70. Su, G.; Kuchinsky, A.; Morris, J.H.; States, D.J.; Meng, F. GLay: Community structure analysis of biological networks. *Bioinformatics* **2010**, *26*, 3135–3137. [CrossRef] [PubMed]
71. Morris, J.H.; Apeltsin, L.; Newman, A.M.; Baumbach, J.; Wittkop, T.; Su, G.; Bader, G.D.; Ferrin, T.E. clusterMaker: A multi-algorithm clustering plugin for Cytoscape. *BMC Bioinform.* **2011**, *12*, 436. [CrossRef] [PubMed]
72. Doncheva, N.T.; Assenov, Y.; Domingues, F.S.; Albrecht, M. Topological analysis and interactive visualization of biological networks and protein structures. *Nat. Protoc.* **2012**, *7*, 670. [CrossRef] [PubMed]
73. Flock, T.; Hauser, A.S.; Lund, N.; Gloriam, D.E.; Balaji, S.; Babu, M.M. Selectivity determinants of GPCR–G-protein binding. *Nature* **2017**, *545*, 317–322. [CrossRef] [PubMed]

74. Dovoedo, Y.; Chakraborti, S. Boxplot-based outlier detection for the location-scale family. *Commun. Stat. Simul. Comput.* **2015**, *44*, 1492–1513. [CrossRef]
75. Yang, J.; Rahardja, S.; Fränti, P. Outlier detection: how to threshold outlier scores? In Proceedings of the International Conference on Artificial Intelligence, Information Processing and Cloud Computing, Sanya, China, 19–21 December 2019; pp. 1–6.
76. Consortium, G.O. Gene ontology consortium: going forward. *Nucleic Acids Res.* **2015**, *43*, D1049–D1056. [CrossRef] [PubMed]
77. Yu, G.; Wang, L.G.; Han, Y.; He, Q.Y. clusterProfiler: An R package for comparing biological themes among gene clusters. *OMICS J. Integr. Biol.* **2012**, *16*, 284–287. [CrossRef] [PubMed]
78. Huang, D.; Sherman, B.T.; Lempicki, R.A. Systematic and integrative analysis of large gene lists using DAVID bioinformatics resources. *Nat. Protoc.* **2009**, *4*, 44. [CrossRef]
79. Szklarczyk, D.; Morris, J.H.; Cook, H.; Kuhn, M.; Wyder, S.; Simonovic, M.; Santos, A.; Doncheva, N.T.; Roth, A.; Bork, P.; et al. The STRING database in 2017: quality-controlled protein–protein association networks, made broadly accessible. *Nucleic Acids Res.* **2016**, *45*, D362–D368. [CrossRef]
80. Gibson, S.M.; Ficklin, S.P.; Isaacson, S.; Luo, F.; Feltus, F.A.; Smith, M.C. Massive-scale gene co-expression network construction and robustness testing using random matrix theory. *PLoS ONE* **2013**, *8*, e55871. [CrossRef]
81. Milenković, T.; Pržulj, N. Uncovering biological network function via graphlet degree signatures. *Cancer Inform.* **2008**, *6*, CIN-S680. [CrossRef]
82. Baron, S.; Fons, M.; Albrecht, T. Viral pathogenesis. In *Medical Microbiology*, 4th ed.; University of Texas Medical Branch at Galveston: Galveston, TX, USA, 1996.
83. Deng, X.; Chen, Y.; Mielech, A.M.; Hackbart, M.; Kesely, K.R.; Mettelman, R.C.; O'Brien, A.; Chapman, M.E.; Mesecar, A.D.; Baker, S.C. Structure-Guided Mutagenesis Alters Deubiquitinating Activity and Attenuates Pathogenesis of a Murine Coronavirus. *J. Virol.* **2020**. [CrossRef]
84. Khan, H.A.; Ahmad, M.Z.; Khan, J.A.; Arshad, M.I. Crosstalk of liver immune cells and cell death mechanisms in different murine models of liver injury and its clinical relevance. *Hepatobiliary Pancreat. Dis. Int.* **2017**, *16*, 245–256. [CrossRef]
85. Wu, D.; Wang, H.; Yan, W.; Chen, T.; Wang, M.; Han, M.; Wu, Z.; Wang, X.; Ai, G.; Xi, D.; et al. A disparate subset of double-negative T cells contributes to the outcome of murine fulminant viral hepatitis via effector molecule fibrinogen-like protein 2. *Immunol. Res.* **2016**, *64*, 518–530. [CrossRef]
86. Lewis, S.M.; Williams, A.; Eisenbarth, S.C. Structure and function of the immune system in the spleen. *Sci. Immunol.* **2019**, *4*. [CrossRef] [PubMed]
87. Oh, J.; Kim, J.Y.; Kim, H.S.; Oh, J.C.; Cheon, Y.H.; Park, J.; Yoon, K.H.; Lee, M.S.; Youn, B.S. Progranulin and a five transmembrane domain-containing receptor-like gene are the key components in receptor activator of nuclear factor κB (RANK)-dependent formation of multinucleated osteoclasts. *J. Biol. Chem.* **2015**, *290*, 2042–2052. [CrossRef] [PubMed]
88. Dougall, W.C.; Glaccum, M.; Charrier, K.; Rohrbach, K.; Brasel, K.; De Smedt, T.; Daro, E.; Smith, J.; Tometsko, M.E.; Maliszewski, C.R.; et al. RANK is essential for osteoclast and lymph node development. *Genes Dev.* **1999**, *13*, 2412–2424. [CrossRef]
89. Frattini, P.; Villa, C.; De Santis, F.; Meregalli, M.; Belicchi, M.; Erratico, S.; Bella, P.; Raimondi, M.T.; Lu, Q.; Torrente, Y. Autologous intramuscular transplantation of engineered satellite cells induces exosome-mediated systemic expression of Fukutin-related protein and rescues disease phenotype in a murine model of limb-girdle muscular dystrophy type 2I. *Hum. Mol. Genet.* **2017**, *26*, 3682–3698. [CrossRef]
90. Desmedt, S.; Desmedt, V.; Delanghe, J.; Speeckaert, R.; Speeckaert, M. The intriguing role of soluble urokinase receptor in inflammatory diseases. *Crit. Rev. Clin. Lab. Sci.* **2017**, *54*, 117–133. [CrossRef] [PubMed]
91. Zhao, X.; Zheng, S.; Chen, D.; Zheng, M.; Li, X.; Li, G.; Lin, H.; Chang, J.; Zeng, H.; Guo, J.T. LY6E Restricts the Entry of Human Coronaviruses, including the currently pandemic SARS-CoV-2. *bioRxiv* **2020**. [CrossRef]
92. yWorks. Available online: https://www.yworks.com/ (accessed on 16 July 2020.)
93. Margolin, A.A.; Nemenman, I.; Basso, K.; Wiggins, C.; Stolovitzky, G.; Dalla Favera, R.; Califano, A. ARACNE: An algorithm for the reconstruction of gene regulatory networks in a mammalian cellular context. In *BMC Bioinformatics*; Springer: Berlin/Heidelberg, Germany, 2006; Volume 7, p. S7.
94. Langfelder, P.; Horvath, S. WGCNA: An R package for weighted correlation network analysis. *BMC Bioinform.* **2008**, *9*, 559. [CrossRef]

95. Gysi, D.M.; Voigt, A.; de Miranda Fragoso, T.; Almaas, E.; Nowick, K. WTO: An R package for computing weighted topological overlap and a consensus network with integrated visualization tool. *BMC Bioinform.* **2018**, *19*, 392. [CrossRef]
96. Meyer, P.E.; Lafitte, F.; Bontempi, G. minet: AR/Bioconductor package for inferring large transcriptional networks using mutual information. *BMC Bioinform.* **2008**, *9*, 461. [CrossRef]
97. Zhang, B.; Horvath, S. A general framework for weighted gene co-expression network analysis. *Stat. Appl. Genet. Mol. Biol.* **2005**, *4*. [CrossRef] [PubMed]
98. Robin, X.; Turck, N.; Hainard, A.; Tiberti, N.; Lisacek, F.; Sanchez, J.C.; Müller, M. pROC: An open-source package for R and S+ to analyze and compare ROC curves. *BMC Bioinform.* **2011**, *12*, 77. [CrossRef] [PubMed]

© 2020 by the authors. Licensee MDPI, Basel, Switzerland. This article is an open access article distributed under the terms and conditions of the Creative Commons Attribution (CC BY) license (http://creativecommons.org/licenses/by/4.0/).

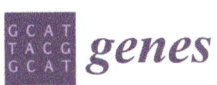

Article

Pitfalls in Single Clone CRISPR-Cas9 Mutagenesis to Fine-Map Regulatory Intervals

Ruoyu Tian [1,†], Yidan Pan [2,3,†], Thomas H. A. Etheridge [3,‡], Harshavardhan Deshmukh [3], Dalia Gulick [1], Greg Gibson [1,*], Gang Bao [2,3,*] and Ciaran M Lee [4,*]

1. Center for Integrative Genomics, Georgia Institute of Technology, Atlanta, GA 30332, USA; rtian@gatech.edu (R.T.); dalia.arafat@biology.gatech.edu (D.G.)
2. Systems, Synthetic, and Physical Biology, Rice University, Houston, TX 77005, USA; yp11@rice.edu
3. Department of Bioengineering, Rice University, Houston, TX 77005, USA; hd16@rice.edu (H.D.); thomasetheridge@alumni.rice.edu (T.H.A.E.)
4. APC Microbiome Ireland, University College Cork, Cork T12 YN60, Ireland
* Correspondence: greg.gibson@biology.gatech.edu (G.G.); gang.bao@rice.edu (G.B.); ciaran.lee@ucc.ie (C.M.L.)
† These authors contributed equally to this work.
‡ Current Affiliation: School of Medicine, University of Texas Health Science Center at San Antonio, TX 78229, USA.

Received: 19 March 2020; Accepted: 22 April 2020; Published: 4 May 2020

Abstract: The majority of genetic variants affecting complex traits map to regulatory regions of genes, and typically lie in credible intervals of 100 or more SNPs. Fine mapping of the causal variant(s) at a locus depends on assays that are able to discriminate the effects of polymorphisms or mutations on gene expression. Here, we evaluated a moderate-throughput CRISPR-Cas9 mutagenesis approach, based on replicated measurement of transcript abundance in single-cell clones, by deleting candidate regulatory SNPs, affecting four genes known to be affected by large-effect expression Quantitative Trait Loci (eQTL) in leukocytes, and using Fluidigm qRT-PCR to monitor gene expression in HL60 pro-myeloid human cells. We concluded that there were multiple constraints that rendered the approach generally infeasible for fine mapping. These included the non-targetability of many regulatory SNPs, clonal variability of single-cell derivatives, and expense. Power calculations based on the measured variance attributable to major sources of experimental error indicated that typical eQTL explaining 10% of the variation in expression of a gene would usually require at least eight biological replicates of each clone. Scanning across credible intervals with this approach is not recommended.

Keywords: eQTL; CRISPR-Cas9; single-cell clone; fine-mapping; power

1. Introduction

Genome-wide association studies (GWAS) over the past decade have been highly successful in identifying tens of thousands of loci influencing disease risk [1-3], but the fine mapping of causal variants has failed to keep pace. Exhaustive studies of Crohn's disease and type 2 diabetes associations, for example, indicate that the average credible interval size for hundreds of loci remains over 100 SNPs, and fewer than 15% of the loci have been reduced to a single high-confidence causal polymorphism [4,5]. This gap in knowledge impedes both the understanding of the biological functions of risk loci and the progress in clinical genetic risk assessment. There are three main challenges to fine mapping. First, the haplotype structure of the human genome ensures that multiple SNPs lie in high linkage disequilibrium (LD) with the peak association signal so that it is rarely possible to promote one variant as causal on statistical evidence alone. Second, it is now clear that at least one-third of loci harbor multiple independent associations, most with overlapping credible intervals [4-6]. Third, the majority of the risk loci are located in non-coding regions of genes [7,8], where they exert their function through regulation of gene expression. Tools for predicting the function of such causal variants generally have low predictive value [9,10].

Moderate-to-high throughput methods are needed to prioritize likely causal variants by experimentally monitoring their effects on gene expression [11]. Two broad classes of approaches have been described: massively parallel reporter assays and genome editing. Massively parallel reporter assays a couple of short segments of potentially regulatory DNA to guide barcodes, which are transcribed following transfection into cells or animals. Sequencing approaches allow identification of under- or over-represented barcodes, indicating differential expression due, for example, to polymorphisms. Genome editing approaches now most commonly use CRISPR-Cas9 to introduce short insertions, deletions, and substitutions into targetable regions across the whole genome. RNA sequencing or other functional readouts, such as fluorescence of a reporter gene, can be used to monitor the impact of specific variants. Recent CRISPRi and CRISPRa pooled screening assays utilize catalytically dead/inactivated Cas9 enzymes (dCas9) that bind to but do not cut the target site. These modified Cas9s have their endonuclease activity removed, but they are still able to bind to the target sites where they contribute to inhibition or activation of gene expression via fused effector domains, such as KRAB (CRISPRi) and VP64 (CRISPRa). They have enabled high-throughput screening of genomic elements, influencing transcription [12] and cellular phenotypes [13–16], with single-cell transcriptome readout. However, the majority of these strategies screen regulatory intervals rather than individual SNPs, so they are not appropriate for fine-mapping causal variants.

Here, we showed the feasibility of gene-centric single-cell clonal analysis, focusing on a handful of genes known to influence the risk of inflammatory bowel disease (IBD) through modulation of gene expression in immune cells. Specifically, we chose to examine four genes with evidence for two independent *cis*-expression Quantitative Trait Loci (eQTL) intervals each, as well as GWAS-significant associations with IBD. The CDGSH iron-sulfur domain 1, *CISD1*, and serologically defined colon cancer antigen 3, *SDCCAG3*, genes are associated with both ulcerative colitis and Crohn's disease [17,18]. The autocrine motility factor receptor, *AMFR*, encodes a glycosylated transmembrane receptor that is also an E3 ubiquitin ligase, knockdown of which in the acute monocytic leukemia cell line, THP-1, induces cell cycle arrest and apoptosis, indicating a critical role for *AMFR* in cell proliferation [19]. *NFXL1* is one of the most up-regulated genes in IL-4 induced macrophages [20].

We used an experimental strategy for targeted SNP evaluation wherein microdeletions targeting candidate eSNPs were introduced by CRISPR-Cas9 and then isolated as single-cell clones on a uniform genetic background. Although homology-directed repair (HDR) would provide a more precise evaluation of allelic replacement, the low efficiency relative to non-homologous end joining (NHEJ) and expectation that indels might have larger effects led us to use NHEJ in these experiments. We chose the HL60 cell line, a pro-myelocytic lineage, which can be induced to undergo differentiation toward neutrophil- or monocyte-like fate, allowing the evaluation of SNP effects in different cell types. Given the challenges in demonstrating conclusively the impacts of a single causal variant, we discussed sources of experimental variance encountered with this strategy, including batch, clonal, and differentiation effects, and used these to derive realistic power estimates for dissection of causal variants. Comparing these estimates with empirically defined eQTL effect sizes, we concluded that this approach is generally incapable of resolving most regulatory associations to single causal variants.

2. Materials and Methods

2.1. eGenes, Candidate eSNPs, and Control SNP Selection

The eGenes *CISD1* and *SDCCAG3* were chosen due to the colocalization of eQTL signals and association with inflammatory bowel disease [21]. *NFXL1* and *AMFR* were included as they are essential for myeloid cell differentiation. Candidate eSNPs were selected from one of at least two independent eQTL credible intervals at each locus identified in a multiple eQTL studies using stepwise conditional regression [6] in two large peripheral blood microarray datasets—the Consortium for the Architecture of Gene Expression (CAGE) [22] and Framingham Heart Study (FHS). They were also confirmed to be eQTL in monocytes [23]. It remains possible that they are not actually active in HL60 cells or their derivatives, and our experiments should be interpreted with this in mind. We also evaluated each SNP in the credible interval with Combined Annotation Dependent Depletion (CADD) score [24] and evolutionary probability (EP) [25]. In each credible interval, we chose the SNP with the lowest p-value, named as "Top SNP", SNPs with low evolutionary probabilities (EP) of the minor allele and (or) high CADD scores, named as "Both" and "High CADD", respectively (Table 1). We also picked SNPs as negative controls with no eQTL signals and in linkage equilibrium with the top SNP, named as "Control". Conditional eQTL profiles can be visualized using our eQTL Hub shiny browser at http://bloodqtlshiny.biosci.gatech.edu/.

Table 1. Guide RNAs and target SNPs. Each guide RNA targets on the "SNP", which is within a credible set of "gene". The effect size (z-score) of each SNP from the eQTLGen browser [26]. "Top SNP" is the SNP with the lowest p-value in the credible set. Several criteria were used to predict the likelihood of candidate SNPs: "High CADD" is the SNP with high CADD (Combined Annotation Dependent Depletion) score that has a high level of deleteriousness of its variants, including Indel variants; "Top" is the SNP with the strongest signal of eQTL-mapping; "Both" is the SNP with both high CADD score and low evolutionary probabilities (EP) of the minor allele; "Control" is the negative control SNP in high linkage disequilibrium (LD) with the top SNP but low CADD and normal EP.

gRNA	Gene	Top SNP	SNP	Z-Score	Type	Genome Location	Coding Region
RG14	SDCCAG3	rs10870171	rs3812594	−34.60	High CADD	Exon of SEC16A	Yes
RG16	CISD1	rs4397793	rs4397793	−23.84	Top	Intron of TFAM	No
RG17	CISD1	rs4397793	rs648138	−70.54	Control	Intergenic of TFAM	No
RG19	CISD1	rs2590375	rs2590363	−100.37	Both	Intron of IPMK	No
RG20	CISD1	rs2590375	rs1416763	−100.27	Both	Intron of CISD1	No
RG26	NFXL1	rs116521751	rs321622	−63.35	Both	Intron of NIPAL1	No
RG34	AMFR	rs8060037	rs8060037	−14.09	Top	Intron of NUDT21	No

2.2. SNP-Targeting and gRNA Screening Design

The chromosomal position of each candidate SNP in reference genome hg19 was obtained from the dbSNP database [27] by searching their RSID. The sequences flanking the targeted SNP were fetched from the NCBI Reference Sequence (RefSeq), providing a gRNA screening window [28]. In each window, all the 19-base sequences followed by the correct *Streptococcus pyogenes* Cas9 protospacer adjacent motif (PAM) sequence (NGG) were collected as candidate gRNAs. gRNAs with GC rate over 80% or less than 10% were filtered out to assure better-cutting performance, and only the gRNAs with a distance of cut site to targeted SNP not more than 10 nucleotides were selected for off-target effect analysis. The in silico predictions of their off-target effects were tested using COSMID [29]. The online tool is available through https://crispr.bme.gatech.edu/.

2.3. Single-Cell Clone Generation

HL60 (ATCC, Manassas, VA, USA, CCL-240) and HL60/S4 (ATCC, Manassas, VA, USA, CRL-3306) cells were grown in suspension at 2×10^5 to 1×10^6 cells/mL in RPMI-1640 with 10% FBS, 2 mM L-glutamine, and 100 µg/mL normocin. After culturing for 18 h to 24 h, cells were pelleted at 200 g for 3 min. Used media was collected and filtered to obtain conditioned media. Bulk cell suspensions were serially diluted on a 96-well plate with conditioned media to facilitate cell growth. Statistically, there were wells that only had a single-cell. Alternatively, some single-cell clones were generated by sorting bulk cells by flow cytometry on a BD FacsAria Fusion with 100-micron nozzle at 37 °C and seeded onto each well of a 96-well plate with the same conditioned media.

2.4. Myeloid Lineage Differentiation

The differentiation of cells into neutrophils was achieved by culturing with 1 µM retinoic acid (RA) [30]. Cells were seeded 18 h before treatment at 2×10^5 cells/mL. HL60 cells were treated for 4 days, and HL60/S4 were treated for 2 days. During differentiation, cell density and viability were checked every 24 h to maintain 2×10^5 to 1×10^6 cells/mL cell density. Additional culture media with RA was added if needed. Cells treated with the same volume of ethanol were used as a negative control.

Differentiation of cells into monocytes was achieved by culturing with 100 nM α1, 25-dihydroxyvitamin D3 (D3) dissolved in ethanol [31]. Cells were seeded at 1.5×10^5 cells/mL at least 18 h before treatment. Both HL60 cells and HL60/S4 were treated for 3 days. During differentiation, alive cell density was checked and normalized every 24 h to maintain 2.5×10^5/mL cell density. Additional culture media with D3 was added if required. Cells treated with the same volume of ethanol were used as negative controls.

2.5. Flow Cytometry

After collection, cells were washed with PBS twice at room temperature. Cells under neutrophil differentiation were then incubated with 7-aminoactinomycin D (7-AAD) (ThermoFisher Scientific, Waltham, MA, USA, cat. No. A1310) and PE-conjugated mouse anti-human CD11b (clone ICRF44) (BD Biosciences, San Jose, CA, USA, cat. No. 557321) or PE-conjugated isotype control mouse mAb (clone: MOPC-21) (Biolegend, San Diego, CA, USA, cat. No. 400112) for 40 min at 4 °C in the dark. Samples were analyzed by BD FacsAria Fusion with a 100-micron nozzle at 4 °C. Cells under monocyte differentiation were incubated with V450 mouse anti-human CD14 (BD Biosciences, San Jose, CA, USA, cat. No. 560349) and adenomatous polyposis coli (APC) mouse anti-human CD71 (BD Biosciences, San Jose, CA, USA, cat. No. 551374) or V450 mouse IgG2b (BD Biosciences, San Jose, CA, USA, cat. No. 560374) and APC mouse IgG1 (BD Biosciences, San Jose, CA, USA, cat. No. 555751) for isotype control. Samples were analyzed by BD FACSMelody at 4 °C. All data were analyzed with FlowJo software v10.6.1 downloaded from https://www.flowjo.com/.

2.6. Immunofluorescence

After collection, cells were washed with PBS twice at room temperature. Then, cells were incubated with Hoechst-33342 (ThermoFisher, Waltham, MA, USA, cat. No. H3570) for 10 to 15 min at 37 °C in the dark. Ten microliters of the cell suspension were used to make a slide, which was sealed with clear nail polish. UV excitation and microscopic imaging were done on an Olympus IX73 inverted microscope system.

2.7. RNA Isolation

Cells were grown in suspension at 2×10^5 to 1×10^6 cells/mL in RPMI-1640 with 10% FBS, 2 mM L-glutamine, and 100 µg/mL normocin. Cells were seeded at 2×10^5 cells/mL 18 h to 24 h before extraction. Each clone had two biological replicates, except bulk HL60/S4. One million cells from each sample were collected by centrifuging at 300 g for 5 min. Total RNA was isolated and purified by RNeasy Plus Mini Kit (Qiagen, Hilden, Germany, cat. Nos. 74,134 and 74,136). Quality control of RNA samples was assessed with a Bioanalyzer 2100 instrument (Agilent, Santa Clara, CA, USA).

2.8. Bulk RNA-Seq and Differential Gene Expression Analysis

cDNA library preparation for single-cell clones was performed using Illumina TruSeq Stranded Sample Preparation, Low Sample (LS) Protocol. Sequencing was performed on an Illumina HiSeq 2500 at Georgia Tech, generating 100 bp paired-end libraries with an average of 51.8 million paired reads per sample. Library preparation for differentiated cells was performed using the NEBNext Ultra II Directional RNA Library Prep Kit for Illumina (New England BioLabs, Ipswich, MA, USA, cat. No. E7760S). Sequencing was performed on Illumina NextSeq, high output, generating 75 bp paired-end libraries with an average of 36 million paired reads per sample. The gene expression data is available at the Gene Expression Omnibus (GEO) under the accession code GSE135507.

RNA-Seq quality control was initiated with Trim Galore, which was used to trim the 13 bp Illumina standard adapter ('AGATCGGAAGAGC') by default, after which quality control was reported by FastQC. Reads were mapped to the hg38 human reference genome by STAR [32], and on average, the mapped reads were 90% of total reads. Aligned sequencing reads were counted with the intersection-strict mode in HTSeq [33] to get read counts for each gene. Scale factors of each sample were computed using the trimmed mean of the M-value (TMM) algorithm in the R package, edgeR [34]. Raw read counts were normalized by scale factors and then transformed into log2 counts per million reads (CPM). Genes were kept if expressed in at least three samples. A total of 11,746 genes were kept in single-cell clone RNA-Seq, while 13,485 genes were kept in differentiated cell RNA-Seq.

Differential gene expression analysis was conducted in edgeR with generalized linear models to contrast the effects of each treatment group. Pairwise comparisons between control and neutrophil derivative, control and monocyte derivative, as well as within each clone of each type of cell, were performed. Likelihood ratio tests were assessed to obtain lists of differentially expressed genes and following Benjamini-Hochberg false discovery rate correction.

Gene ontology analysis was performed using ToppFun [35]. By uploading a list of differentially expressed genes (FDR < 0.001) from the differential gene expression analysis into the website, functional enrichment features were listed, including pathways, Gene Ontology (GO) terms, and phenotypes. Gene ontology analysis was also performed by enrichR [36,37], with four sets of differentially expressed genes (FDR < 0.001) uniquely in HL60 monocyte (968 genes), HL60/S4 monocytes (521 genes), HL60 neutrophils (1462 genes), and HL60/S4 neutrophils (2275 genes).

Principal component analysis (PCA) was performed on 17 single-cell clone samples and 47 differentiated cell samples by "prcomp" function in R, with default settings. Principal variance component analysis (PVCA) was performed in JMP Genomics 8 (SAS Institute, Cary, NC, USA), which sums the weighted proportions of each variance component associated with covariates of interest in order to estimate the overall contribution of biological and technical factors to the gene expression variation. Plots were plotted with R package, ggplot2.

2.9. Variant Calling

Variants were called by GATK [38,39] best practice RNA-seq short variant discovery (SNPs and Indels). Raw RNA-seq reads were mapped to hg19 by STAR [32]. "SplitNCigarReads" was used to split reads that span introns and hard clip mismatching overhangs. Variants were called by "HaplotypeCaller" with default settings. Due to the high false-positive rate of calling variants from RNA-seq data, the "VariantFiltration" function was used to filter potential false-positive calls. Clusters of at least three SNPs within a window of 35 bases were excluded, and calls with read depth lower than 50 were filtered. Moreover, the variant calls were only included if they were consistent in the two biological replicates of the same clone, and only exonic polymorphisms were counted.

2.10. Fluidigm qRT-PCR

Fluidigm real-time qPCR was conducted on a 48 × 48 nanoscale microfluidic chip with 48 EvaGreen probes targeting transcripts of the CRISPR targeted genes, as well as a representative set of lymphoid and myeloid cell marker genes [40], and housekeeping genes. The 48 array samples included single-cell clone CRISPR-edited HL60/S4 from two batches and experimental controls. A total of 2304 qRT-PCR assays with 30 amplification cycles were conducted in parallel according to the manufacturer's protocol. The average Ct value was computed at the exponential phase of each PCR amplification reaction. Since large Ct values correspond, counter-intuitively, to low expression, modified expression values were computed as the Ct values subtracted from 30 (the maximum number of PCR cycles), and the negative outputs were set as 0. This results in a range from null to 30, where each increment, in theory, represents a doubling of initial transcript abundance. To clean up the data, samples with more than 40 unexpressed genes and probes expressed in less than 5 samples were removed. Processed expression data and sample phenotypic information are provided in Tables S1 and S2, respectively. We noted that numerous studies have established the high sensitivity of Fluidigm relative to standard qRT-PCR [41–43] and that all expression levels were in the normal range of detection and not subject to drop-out seen with very low abundance transcripts.

2.11. Plasmid Construction

The SpyCas9 expressing plasmid pX330-U6-Chimeric_BB-CBh-hSpCas9 [44] (Addgene plasmid #42230) was a gift from Dr. Feng Zhang. The pX330 vector was digested by BbsI. For each designed gRNA sequence, a pair of annealed oligos was cloned into the vector before the gRNA scaffold and after the U6 promoter. All clones were validated by Sanger sequencing (Eurofins Genomics, Louisville, KY, USA).

2.12. CRISPR-Edited Single-Cell Clones Generation

A total of 2×10^5 HL60/S4 clone 3 cells and 1 µg of pX330 plasmid per nucleofection reaction (program CA-137, solution SF) were electroporated using the Lonza Nucleofector 4-D based on the manufacturer's protocol. One microgram of pmaxGFP™ vector per nucleofection reaction was co-transfected as the reporter. The cells were cultured at 37 °C for 72 h after nucleofection, and the GFP-positive cells were sorted individually by BD FACSMelody to make single-cell clones following standard protocols. Post-sorting, cells were grown for a week before harvesting and DNA extraction. DNA was extracted using Quick-DNA Miniprep Plus Kit (Zymo Research, Irvine, CA, USA, cat. No. D3024) following the manufacturer's protocol. For each target locus, a PCR product was amplified from the genomic DNA of cells modified by CRISPR-Cas9 and analyzed by Sanger sequencing (Eurofins Genomics, Louisville, KY, USA). The genotype of clones selected in this study is shown in Table S3a, and the number of clones screened and the mutations observed per clone are shown in Table S3b.

2.13. Power Simulation Studies

Power analysis was performed using the mixed model power expression utility in JMP Genomics (SAS Institute, Cary, NC, USA). We created a design file with duplicates of 10 guide RNAs and designated one guide as the causal variant. Additional random effect options for representing batch effects (distributing the guides across into two batches of 5) and clone effects (where the causal variant was represented by two different clones) allowed modeling of the impact of these additional sources of variance. We assessed power at $\alpha = 0.05, 0.01$, and 0.001 for effect sizes of the causal variant in increments of 0.1 standard deviation units (sdu) between 0 and 2, assuming experiments with 2, 4, 8, or 16 replicates of each guide. Batch and clone effects were assumed to be 0.1 or 0.2 sdu. For additional analysis, three of the guides were assumed to affect gene expression, modeling the situation where multiple linked variants account for an eQTL effect.

3. Results

3.1. Effect of Clonal Variability on Gene Expression in HL60 Cells

Since genetic screens are best performed in uniform genetic backgrounds under conditions where environmental variation can be carefully controlled, we started by evaluating the magnitude of the effect of biological and technical factors on gene expression in HL60 cells. HL60 is a pro-myeloid cell line derived from a person with acute promyelocytic leukemia [45,46]. It is known to be homozygous for a *TP53* deletion and a *CDKN2A* premature stop codon and heterozygous for an *NRAS* missense substitution. The main factors of interest were (i) batch effects, (ii) HL60 sub-type, (iii) clonal heterogeneity, and (iv) differentiation status. A derivative known as HL60/S4 has been isolated, which is reported to more efficiently differentiate into myeloid derivatives, such as neutrophils and macrophages [47]. Given the almost 40 years in culture, we reasoned that point mutations that are likely to affect overall gene expression might have accumulated, and, to control this, we isolated three single-cell clones (labeled 1 through 3) of HL60 and four single-cell clones (labeled a through d) of HL60/S4. Differences in growth rates among clones and relative to the bulk parental line were noted.

Clonal variability in gene expression was monitored by bulk RNA-seq of two batches for each of the seven single-cell clones and two parental lines. Figure 1a plots the first two principal components (PC) of expression of 11,746 expressed genes detected with an average depth of over 50 million paired-end 100 bp reads per sample. PC1 separated the two HL60 sub-types unambiguously, and 85% of the variance attributable to the first five PC (86.8% of total variance) was between HL60 and HL60/S4 cells. Individual clones separated along PC2 with relatively little separation between replicates, with the parental lines taking intermediate values. Just 14% of the variance was among clones, but residual replicate effects accounted for less than 1% of it (Figure 1b). These results confirmed that single-cell clones were likely genetically differentiated, implying that, as far as possible, CRISPR-Cas9 editing should be performed on a purified clone.

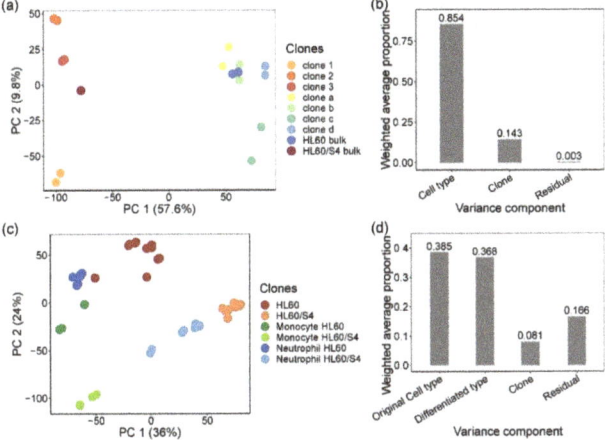

Figure 1. Heterogeneity of gene expression in single-cell clones and myeloid lineage differentiated clones. (**a**) Principal component analysis (PCA) of bulk RNA sequencing of parental single-cell clones and bulk cells. PCA was performed on a normalized log2 CPM count expression matrix of 17 samples from HL60- and HL60/S4-generated single-cell clones. Each dot represents 17 samples, two biological replicates for each clone and bulk, except for HL60/S4 bulk. Samples are colored by clones: warm color dots are samples from HL60/S4 cell lines, while cold color dots are samples from HL60 cell lines. PC1 separated samples by cell type, explaining 57.6% of the total variation. PC2 separated samples by clones, representing 9.8% of the total variation. (**b**) Principal variance component analysis showed the weighted average proportion of each variance component—cell type (85.4%), clone (14.3%), and residual (0.3%)—all of which explained variance captured by the first five principal components (86.8% of total variance). The majority of the total expression variance of single-cell clones was explained by cell type and clone variance components. (**c**) Principal component analysis of bulk RNA sequencing of myeloid lineage differentiated clones, performed by normalized log2 counts per million (CPM) expression matrix. Each dot represents 47 samples from differentiated monocytes and neutrophils and undifferentiated control cells, two biological replicates for each stimulation on each clone. Clone d was excluded due to sequencing error. Samples are colored by cell type and differentiation lineages: monocytes are green, neutrophils are blue, and control cells are red. To distinguish the original cell type of each sample, HL60 cells are dark colors, and HL60/S4 cells are light colors. (**d**) Principal variance component analysis showed the weighted average proportion of each variance component—original cell type (38.5%), differentiated type (36.8%), clone (8.1%), and residual (16.6%)—all of which explained variance captured by the first five principal components (83.9% of total variance). The 16.6% of unexplained variance might be from the variance of biological replicates and cultural differences between two labs.

The extent of genetic differentiation of single-cell clones was evaluated by calling genotypes directly from the RNA-seq data. Given that false-positive calls are elevated due to errors induced by the reverse transcriptase during cDNA preparation, and that allele-specific expression causes SNP ratios not observed in genomic DNA sequence data, we applied variant hard filtering in GATK. Clusters of at least three SNPs within a window of 35 bases were excluded, the variant calls were only included if they were consistent in the two biological replicates of the same clone, and only exonic polymorphisms were counted. On average, each of the HL60 single-cell clones differed from the bulk consensus sequence at 103 of the 7482 single nucleotide variants (SNVs) (1.38%), passing our hard filters. A little over fifty percent more divergence and 166 of 7104 SNVs (2.34%) were uniquely observed in HL60/S4 pairwise clonal comparisons with the bulk HL60/S4 consensus. Furthermore, approximately 3% of the total SNVs were different in the comparison of bulk HL60/S4 and HL60 lines and their derivatives, indicating that there was considerable genetic variability both between the two lines and in single-cell clones. Similar findings have been reported [48] in an analysis of somatic mutation accumulation in a cancer cell line.

Next, we asked how consistent chemical-induced differentiation is across clones. Each of the single-cell clones, with the exception of HL60/S4 clone d, was treated with 1 µM retinoic acid for 4 days (HL60) or 2 days (HL60/S4) in order to generate neutrophil-like cells or with 100 nM α1,25-dihydroxyvitamin D3 for 3 days in order to generate monocyte-like cells. Figure S1 shows characteristics of the cells stained with Hoechst to monitor changes in the morphology of the nucleus, 7-AAD to monitor cell viability, and CD11b, a neutrophil marker. Growth conditions were chosen to optimize the balance of cell differentiation and viability, which also varied among clones. As previously reported [47], HL60/S4 cells more readily differentiated toward neutrophil fate than did HL60 cells. Figure S2 confirms initiation of CD14 expression, as well as the loss of CD71, both markers of monocyte fate, to similar degrees in both bulk HL60 and HL60/S4, though variation among clones of HL60 was also seen (also Table S4a,b), including variability of cell surface marker expression at baseline.

As with the untreated clones, gene expression was again observed to vary substantially between the two sub-types and among clones, with a generally uniform response to treatment and relatively small differences between replicates (Figure 1c). In a joint analysis, HL60/S4 cells tended to have more positive values of PC1 and negative values of PC2 than HL60, and the overall cell-type accounted for 38.5% of the variance captured by the first five PC (83.9% of total variance). Neutrophils occupied an intermediate position between monocytes and undifferentiated cells along both PC axes, and cell fate captured 36.8% of the variance. At baseline, HL60/S4 cells appeared to be more divergent from the derived neutrophil-like and, especially, monocyte-like cells than were HL60 from their derivatives. Clonal differences remained significantly higher than replicate effects.

In total, 5885 and 3319 genes (FDR < 0.0001) were identified that were differentially expressed before and after monocyte and neutrophil lineage differentiation across all clones of two cell types—HL60 and HL60/S4—respectively.

After differentiation, HL60/S4-derived monocyte cells were more transcriptionally divergent from their parental cells than were HL60-derived monocytes: 7381 monocytic differentially expressed genes were detected in HL60/S4, compared with 4167 genes in HL60. *B2M*, a neutrophil-specific differentiation marker, was one of the 4167 genes that were differentially expressed in the neutrophil-derived clone a, clone b, and HL60 bulk cells. There were 5079 differentially expressed genes in the monocyte derivatives of HL60, including the transcription factors *CEBPE*, specifically in clone c derivatives, and *PU.1* in clone b derivatives. Similar gene markers were also documented in a time course of myeloid differentiation [45], although we observed a higher number of differentially expressed genes at the terminal differentiated stage of monocytes than neutrophils, whereas the opposite pattern was found at 6 h post-differentiation [49].

Differences in the degree of inter-clonal differentiation were also detected (Figure S3). For the monocyte derivatives, 1781 genes were differentially expressed relative to undifferentiated cells in all of the clones of the two cell types, and these were enriched in cell cycle, neutrophil degranulation, and rRNA processing pathways. On the other hand, 968 genes were uniquely differentially expressed in the HL60 clonal comparisons, also showing enrichment for neutrophil degranulation and innate immune system pathways. Gene ontology (GO) and pathway analysis was performed by Toppfun, and the significant GO terms and pathways (Bonferroni corrected p-value < 0.00001) for these 968 genes are listed in Figure S4. Similarly, for neutrophil lineage differentiation, 413 differentially expressed genes were shared by HL60 and HL60/S4, enriched for neutrophil degranulation, innate immune system activity, interleukin-10 signaling, chemokine signaling, and cytokine signaling pathways. There were 1462 and 2275 clonal-specific differentially expressed genes in HL60 clones and HL60/S4 clones, respectively, engaging pathways involved in cell cycle and mitochondrial function, and translation and rRNA processing were also enriched. Significant GO terms and pathways (Bonferroni corrected p-value < 0.00001) for HL60 and HL60/S4 are shown in Figures S5 and S6, respectively. Gene ontology enrichment analysis of uniquely differentially expressed genes was also performed using the gene set enrichment tool Enrichr [36,37], with results summarized in Figure S7.

Taken together these results implied that single-cell clones differ in basal gene expression, and although they respond similarly to treatment with retinoic acid or vitamin D3, clonal differences need to be accounted for when evaluating the effect of CRISPR-Cas9 mutagenesis of regulatory regions of target genes.

3.2. Isolation and Evaluation of CRISPR-Edited Single-Cell Clones

We selected seven SNPs in four genes for our initial evaluation of the effect of NHEJ-based CRISPR mutagenesis in HL60/S4 clone 3 as a uniform genetic background. *SDCCAG3*, *NFXL1*, and *AMFR* were each targeted for a single peak eQTL SNP detected by whole blood gene expression, whereas *CISD1* was targeted with four SNPs in one credible eQTL interval. Potential off-target sites of each gRNA with up to two mismatches are provided in Table S5. With genome-wide bioinformatic screening, none of the potential off-target sites were located in coding regions, and the gRNAs had no extra perfect match other than the designed target site. Bulk transfection efficiency was 24.8% based on the percentage of cells expressing GFP signal. GFP-positive cells were considered capable of uptaking plasmid vectors and were single-cell sorted to enrich the edited cells. Of all expanded GFP-positive single-cell clones, 23 out of 166 had obtained Indels, eight of which had removed the target SNP at both allelic copies, while the remainder affected sequences immediately adjacent to the target SNP or only had SNP removal in one allele.

RNA-seq would be prohibitively expensive for comparing gene expression on the scale of dozens of multiple replicated clones, so we next evaluated the potential of high throughput nanoscale quantitative RT-PCR to detect subtle differences in transcript abundance. A 48 × 48 Fluidigm chip was designed, facilitating the measurement of 48 genes (including the four targets, housekeeping controls, and various markers of expression in diverse immune cell type) in 48 samples. The HL60/S4 parental cell line and eight clones were chosen for profiling, one for each guide RNA, and each was grown in duplicate in suspension for 18–24 h, with half the sample frozen down for storage, and the other half used for RNA preparation from fresh cells.

For ease of interpretation, we subtracted the Ct value for each measurement from the number of PCR cycles, 30, resulting in expression values where high values corresponded to high expression. Figure 2a shows that this resulted in a bimodal distribution of gene expression measures, with the smaller peak representing low-abundance transcripts. There was a major difference in the profiles of the frozen and fresh cells, accounting for almost two-thirds of the variance explained by the first five PCs (99.1%) (Figure 2b). To correct for this batch effect, we used Combat, which also standardized the data to a mean of zero and standard deviation of one (Figure 2c). On this scale, most of the variance was now among samples, whereas 9% of first five PCs (99.1%) distinguished clones by which gene was targeted, and 9% was due to differences among gRNAs for *CISD1* (Figure 2d). This implied either that single-gene knockouts affected the expression of a substantial number of other genes, in each clone, or that there was substantial variability among clones that by chance correlated with the nature of the guide RNA. We also observed that normalized *CISD1* expression was lower in cells edited by each of the four gRNAs targeting *CISD1* than in the untreated control parental cell line (Figure 2e). Clone RG17 affected a control SNP in high LD with the peak eQTL but with low CADD score [24,50] and high evolutionary probability [25] of the alternate allele and was the only clone not significantly different from the parental line. However, since it is unlikely that each of the other three sites causally influences gene expression, this result served as a further caution that the process of transfection with CRISPR reagents itself might influence cell growth and gene activity.

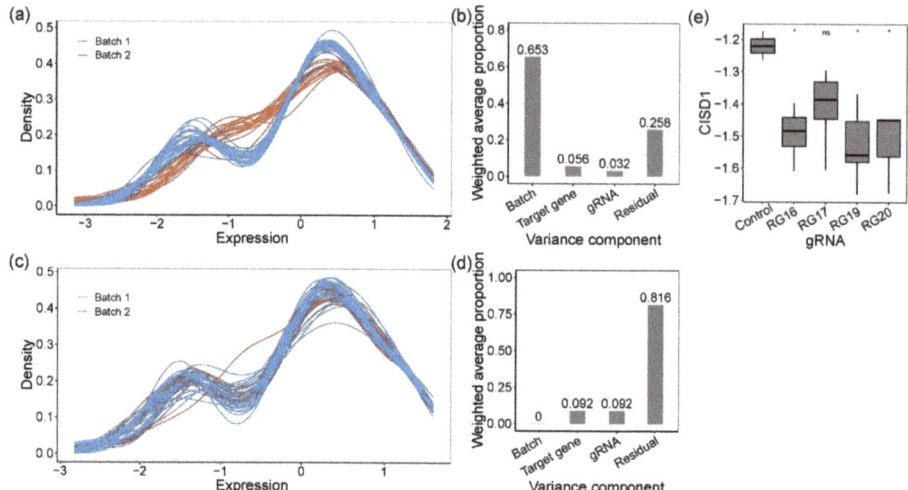

Figure 2. Quantification of gene expression by Fluidigm qRT-PCR and analysis of the variance components. Kernel density plot of standardized gene expression from each sample, color-coded by batches, before (**a**) and after (**c**) removing batch effect. Before (**b**) and after (**d**) batch effect correction, principal variance component analysis showed the weighted average proportion of each variance component: batch 65.3%, 0%, respectively; target gene 5.6%, 9.2%, respectively; gRNA 3.2%, 9.2%, respectively; residual 25.8%, 81.6%, respectively. All of the components explained variance captured by the first five principal components (99.1% and 99.1% of the total variance, respectively). (**e**) Expression of *CISD1*. Pairwise *t*-tests were used to evaluate the difference between CRISPR-Cas9-edited samples (RG16, RG17, RG19, and RG20) and negative controls. RG16, RG19, and RG20 were significantly different from the negative control. * denotes *p*-value < 0.05; ns, not significant.

Similarly, inconsistent results were obtained for the other three genes, as summarized in Figure 3 and Figure S8. Each panel shows box-and-whisker plots for each of the seven guide RNAs and control HL60/S4 cells, with the mean and interquartile range of nine single-cell clones measured with two different PCR probes for three of the genes and one for *SDCCAG3*. In no case was the expression the most extreme for the guide RNA corresponding to the linked gene. For example, *AMFR* expression was highest in cells carrying a mutation in the RG16 guide, disrupting a candidate regulatory site in *CISD1*, whereas *AMFR* expression itself was, on average, the closest to expression in the control cells. Disregarding the control, there were also no cases where the appropriate guide RNA was significantly different from the remaining guides. These results implied either that the selected SNPs were not causal or that the effect sizes of causal variants were too small relative to the observed experimental variability to detect differential expression.

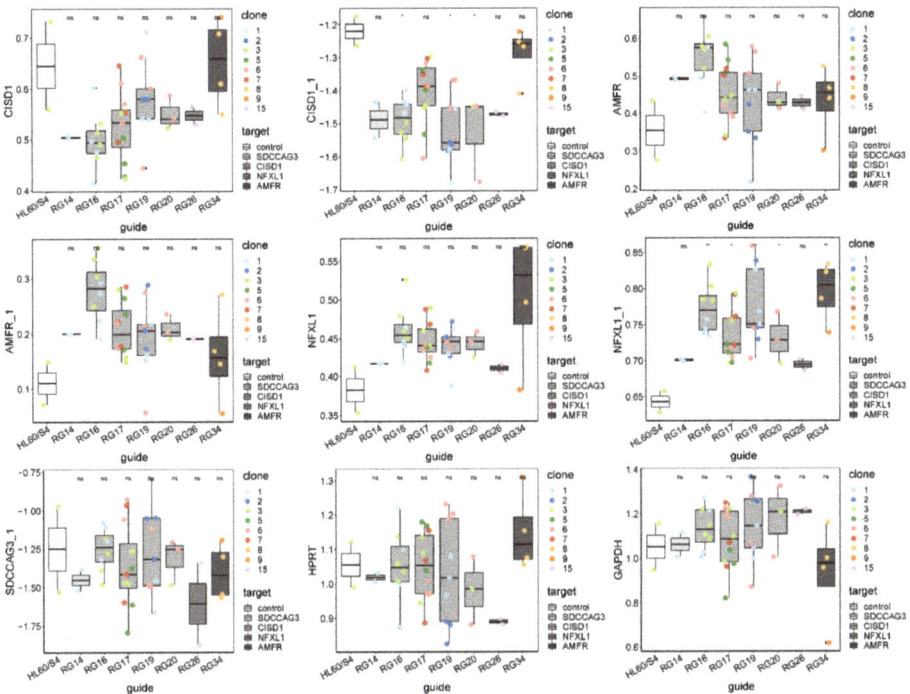

Figure 3. Quantification of all targeted gene expression in all CRISPR-Cas9-edited single-cell clones by Fluidigm qRT-PCR (Tables S1 and S2). *HPRT* and *GAPDH* are housekeeping controls. Single-cell clones were grouped by guide RNA, and the expression of seven probes is shown as boxplot across all clones within each guide RNA group. Clones with the same genotype in each guide RNA group are colored-coded. A pairwise t-test was done to test the difference between CRISPR-Cas9-edited clones and HL60/S4 negative control. * denotes p-value < 0.05; ns, not significant.

3.3. Simulation Studies to Establish Power of Fluidigm-Based Single-Cell Regulatory Assessment

We used these results to guide our design and interpretation of power calculations for experiments designed to determine the effect of single regulatory site disruption. Our baseline scenario assumed targeting of 10 polymorphisms in a single credible interval in which a single eQTL was assumed to account for at least 10% of the variance in transcript abundance at the locus. Such an eQTL corresponded to a difference of approximately 1 standard deviation unit (sdu) in a quantitative assay, such as Fluidigm qRT-PCR or RNA-seq. Given that most single-cell CRISPR-edited clones are heterozygous, it also corresponded to a substitution effect whereby the mutant allele increased or decreased the measured transcript by 1 sdu. We used the mixed model power calculator in JMP-Genomics (Cary, NC) to evaluate the sample size needed to detect an effect of this magnitude, given varying levels of clonal variation, batch effects, and mutation differences.

For the baseline scenario, where there are neither batch nor clonal effects, 80% power to demonstrate that one SNP had an effect that was at least 1 sdu different from the other nine SNPs was achieved with eight replicates of each of the ten clones (Figure 4a,f). Sixteen replicates would enable detection of an effect as small as 0.7 sdu, but four replicates would only be powered to detect a substitution effect of 1.5 sdu. However, the experimental data indicated that individual clones generally did vary, as a consequence of genetic background effects if the transfected cell line was not isogenic, or due to growth differences among aliquots. Modeling these differences as a random effect of just 0.2 sdu among the ten clones demonstrated a dramatic reduction in power to detect the main effect (Figure 4b,g). With eight replicates, only an effect size of 1.7 sdu was reliably detected, though 40% power was still obtained for an effect size of 1 sdu. Doubling the size of the experiment only slightly improved the power, whereas four replicates only facilitated the detection of effect sizes of 2 sdu. If we further considered the scenario with a batch effect whereby half the clones had an additional random effect of 0.2 sdu (perhaps because they were grown at a different time), then power reduced yet again, as expected (Figure 4c,h).

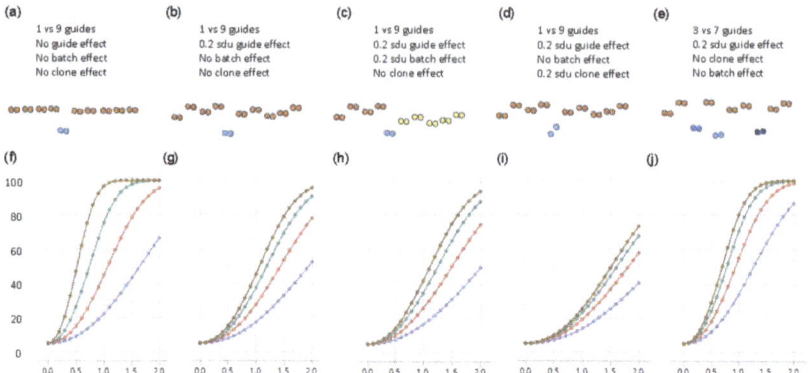

Figure 4. Power curves of Fluidigm-based single-cell clone regulatory assessment of simulation studies. (**a**–**e**) diagrams of five different scenarios and the corresponding panels (**f**–**j**) show the power calculations for exceeding a nominal *p*-value of 0.05, with blue, red, green, and brown curves representing 2, 4, 8, and 16 technical replicates of each clone, respectively. The *y*-axis is the power from 0 to 100 percent, and the *x*-axis is the effect size of eQTL in the standard deviation unit.

A perhaps more realistic scenario is where different edits of the same polymorphic site also have different impacts on gene expression. This could either be because the precise nature of the deletion matters or because the independent clones have slightly different growth properties. We modeled this scenario by allowing for two different clones representing the causal variant, also with a 0.2 sdu random effect difference, the same as the effect of the other nine guide RNAs. In this case (Figure 4d,i), 80% power was never achieved, so it would take greater levels of replication, at least, of the putative causal variant to see a substitution effect in the range of 1 sdu.

A related situation was where more than one of the polymorphisms in the credible interval was responsible for the eQTL effect—for example, three sites in high LD might each account for 0.33 sdu, summing to a combined effect of 1 sdu. To model this, we set three of the guide RNAs to be causal, with the other seven non-functional but retained 0.2 sdu differences among clones. Figure 4e,j show that power was greater than the same scenario with one causal variant and approximately the same as with one causal variant and no differences among the remaining clones. Power was actually greater with fewer replicates (red and blue curves), but, with eight replicates, 80% power still only detected an effect size of 1 sdu, which was three times larger than the presumed individual effect sizes of the contributing causal variants.

4. Discussion

Multiple studies have recently reported good success in mapping regulatory intervals using high throughput approaches in human cells. A previous study [51] scanned across over 100 kb of regulatory DNA in the *TP53* and *ESR1* genes using positive selection for proliferation to enrich cells with aberrantly low expression of the target transcription factors, defining several intervals enriched for signals that overlap with transcription factor binding sites. This approach is, however, dependent on the ability to select on the locus, and similar to methods that sort on the basis of an engineered selectable fluorescence protein [52], only identifies high-impact sites without necessarily discriminating effects of polymorphic sites. Another approach [53] used CRISPRa to map enhancer elements by virtue of activation of regulatory protein-DNA interactions, filtering a handful of short DNA stretches from hundreds of kb of intergenic sequence in the *IL-2RA* gene, but again without the ability to resolve which of the SNPs in a credible interval are responsible for an eQTL. Expression CROP-seq is powered to fine-map eSNPs with 10%–20% effect size within credible intervals by characterizing hundreds of CRISPR/Cas9 genetically mutated single-cell transcriptomes in parallel [54]. Tewhey et al. first demonstrated the utility of massively parallel reporter assays, including the ability to discriminate between alleles at a pre-defined site [55]. Their results and findings from others [56,57] implied that at least 5% of all polymorphisms in regulatory DNA had the potential to regulate target gene expression. The concern remains though that such effects may be artifacts of short reporter genes assayed outside the context of chromatin and complex regulatory interactions.

Our approach instead borrows from classical quantitative genetic screens in model organisms, such as Drosophila and yeast. The objective was to create a panel of genetic perturbations in an isogenic background, evaluating the quantitative impact of each variant relative to the frequency distribution of effects of all other perturbations. For example, *p*-element insertion screens cleanly identified dozens of genes, influencing aging, bristle number, and aspects of fly behavior [58,59]. Closer to our experiments, another study [60] engineered a tiling path across the regulatory region of the *TDH3* gene in *Saccharomyces cerevisiae* and used flow cytometry to quantify gene expression of hundreds of strains, drawing inferences about the impact of stabilizing selection on transcription. We reasoned that a similar approach should be powerful for moderate-sized laboratories without extensive experience in human cell culture. Even though we, and others, have successfully documented regulatory effects of CRISPR-Cas9-mutagenized candidate mutations of large effect [61,62], the results here applied to typical moderate-effect size eQTL do not support this as a general protocol. The remainder of the discussion deals with multiple constraints on the effectiveness of single-cell clone-based screening to dissect credible regulatory intervals in human cell lines.

The first constraint is variability in the mutability of targeted regulatory sites. Our approach was mainly limited in three ways: the requirement of nearby PAM sequences and the short distance between the cut site and targeted SNP, the variable efficiency of different gRNAs, and the distinct Indel pattern for each SNP-targeted gRNA. We started with a list of 250 candidate polymorphisms, approximately 10 each in two independent eQTL intervals of 13 genes, but discovered that only two-thirds of these were suitable CRISPR targets, either because there was no nearby PAM sequence or the target was in repetitive DNA for which it was not possible to design a guide RNA with a unique target sequence. Up to 20% of the remaining sites were predicted to have high probability off-target sites elsewhere in the genome, which might not matter for a scan of *cis*-acting effects but was not ideal. Subsequently, we chose 10 sites as a pilot and screened an average of 24 single-cell clones for each site (23.9 ± 6.7) by Sanger sequencing of the targeted region. As shown in Table S3b, the pilot group had an average of four clones, each with Indels on both alleles (3.8 ± 1.8). The ratio of clones with Indels on both alleles varied from 0% (RG11) to 25% (RG16) so that the theoretical maximum SNP removal rate was different in each gRNA-treated group. RG14, 17, 19, 20, and 34 all had designed cut <5 bp to the targeted SNP, but their percentage of SNP removal on both alleles varied from 0% to 16%, which could be due to variations in the size of Indel mutations, as previously observed [63]. That is to say, many of the CRISPR-induced mutations removed or inserted one or a few nucleotides either side of the polymorphic site without disrupting the polymorphism itself. We concluded that obtaining at least four different clones for a minimum of 20 sites associated with a credible eQTL interval would typically require screening of 500 clones following various iterations of guide RNA design, with less than 100% success and at considerable expense. Allelic replacement by CRISPR-mediated homologous repair would be even more difficult. There are more potential optimizations that may help researchers deal with this constraint. Further optimization can be done in transfection, such as the co-transfection ratio of two plasmids. It is possible that different cell lines would have higher efficiency of mutagenesis.

Other CRISPR/Cas9 delivery methods, such as lentivirus transduction, can also be beneficial for more efficient screening.

The second constraint is clonal variability. We started by addressing a major concern with human cell lines, which is the mutational accumulation in culture. Previous studies [48] showed that tumor cell lines diverge genetically in as few as a dozen passages, resulting in divergent drug responses and gene expression profiles. Accordingly, single-cell cultures of HL60 and the derivative HL60/S4 cell lines are different at the DNA sequence level and have significantly different transcriptomes, both with and without chemical stimulation of differentiation. For a considerable proportion of genes, these differences are of a similar order of magnitude as expected eQTL effects, namely, 20% to 50% differences in normalized abundance. While this observation strongly supports the decision to mutagenize a single-cell clone, genetic differences may not actually be the major source of clonal variation. Mammalian, including human, cells are much more difficult to culture than yeast or bacteria, as thawed aliquots of frozen lines are well known to differ in growth rates and viability. The technical replicates in Figure 1 were all grown in parallel, so did not capture this type of batch effect, which we had not sought to quantify. However, we noted that the parallel culture of the nine mutant clones analyzed was made difficult by variable growth rates and that some thaws failed to grow at all, requiring the expansion of new aliquots. Consequently, batch effects of single-cell clones are a hidden but likely considerable source of gene expression variability.

A third constraint is an expense. Assuming that the cost of RNA sequencing, including cell culture, RNA preparation, library construction, and quality control, could be reduced to $100 a sample using, for example, 3' tagging, an experiment with eight replicates of 20 clones would still cost $16,000. Instead, we adopted a nanoscale quantitative RT-PCR approach, the 48 × 48 Fluidigm array. Each of the data points in Figure 3 was actually the average of four technical replicate qRT-PCR reactions on one plate at the cost of just $1.20 per assay (not including culture and RNA preparation). Technical repeatability is very high with repeated measures typically within 10%, also allowing measurement of dozens of genes simultaneously, so Fluidigm, or similar methods like Nanostring, provides a feasible approach in theory.

However, the fourth constraint, statistical power, emerged as the most serious impediment. A typical eQTL explains between 10% and 20% of the variance in expression of the gene it influences, which corresponds approximately to each allele increasing or decreasing transcript abundance between 0.5 and 1 standard deviation units. We modeled the power to detect such an effect in 80% of experiments, given the variance components observed in our experiments, and found that in the best-case scenario, eight biological replicates would be needed to reliably detect a 1 sdu effect. However, with the addition of modest batch effects, subtle guide RNA differences within a locus, and small differences between different mutations induced by the same clone, power dropped considerably. All such effects are apparent in Figure 3, suggesting that the single clone analyses, while demonstrably capable of discriminating very large regulatory effects of 2 or more sdu, are not generally likely to be detected with this approach. It is possible that cell lines other than HL60 may provide more repeatable results than those described here, which may improve power under some circumstances. In this sense, independent valuation of the magnitude of batch effects for different cell lines under different growth conditions may be advisable, though we doubt that it will make single-cell mutagenesis an optimal screening approach.

Finally, a fifth constraint is an assumption that each eQTL can be reduced to a single eSNP. This is the parsimonious assumption and fits readily with the conception that regulatory SNPs exert their effects by altering the binding affinity for a specific transcription factor. Even though most eQTL span 100 or more polymorphisms in a credible interval, the general assumption is that prioritizing variants according to functional criteria and evolutionary conservation, using scores, such as CADD or LINSIGHT, reduces the search space to fewer than ten candidates. However, given that these variants are in tight linkage disequilibrium with similar frequencies [10], if they have similar functional scores, then it is possible that the observed univariate eQTL effect is actually due to the summation of two or smaller contributing effects. Under this scenario, the power to detect multiple causal variants is also reduced.

These considerations and the overwhelmingly negative results of our experiments lead us to the recommendation not to pursue single clone-based profiling as a general approach to the fine mapping of regulatory variants. Despite the conceptual limitation that effects are evaluated outside the context of normal chromatin, massively parallel reporter assays seem to be more powerful and subject to less experimental constraint.

Supplementary Materials: The following are available online at http://www.mdpi.com/2073-4425/11/5/504/s1, Figure S1: Characteristics of neutrophils by immunofluorescence and flow cytometry analysis, Figure S2: Characteristics of monocytes by flow cytometry analysis, Figure S3: Venn diagram of differential expressed genes, Figure S4: Gene ontology and pathway analysis of differential expression genes in HL60 monocyte derivatives, Figure S5: Gene ontology and pathway analysis of differential expression genes in HL60 neutrophil derivatives; Figure S6: Gene ontology and pathway analysis of differential expression genes in HL60/S neutrophil derivatives, Figure S7: Gene ontology enrichment analysis of differential expression genes in HL60 and HL60/S4 monocyte and neutrophil derivatives, Figure S8: Quantification of all targeted gene expression normalized by GAPDH in all CRISPR-Cas9-edited single-cell clones by Fluidigm qRT-PCR, Table S1: Fluidigm qRT-PCR normalized expression data, Table S2: Fluidigm qRT-PCR samples phenotype, Table S3a: Genotype of single-cell clones used in this study, Table S3b: The number of sequenced single-cell clones, clones with Indels, and clones with SNP removal at both alleles, Table S4a: Monocyte differentiation efficiencies of HL60, HL60/S4, and HL60 clones; drug-treated groups are in duplicates, Table S4b: CD11b+/7-AAD- cell proportion of differentiated neutrophils and negative control cells analyzed by flow cytometry, Table S5: Off-target analysis of gRNA designs with up to two mismatches.

Author Contributions: Conceptualization, G.G., G.B.; Formal analysis, R.T., Y.P.; Data curation, R.T., Y.P., T.H.A.E., H.D., D.G.; Writing—Original draft preparation, R.T., Y.P.; Writing—Review and editing, G.G., C.M.L.; Funding acquisition, G.G., G.B. All authors have read and agreed to the published version of the manuscript.

Funding: This research was funded by the National Institute of Health, project number: 1R01HG008146-01A.

Conflicts of Interest: The authors declare no conflict of interest.

References

1. Altshuler, D.; Daly, M.J.; Lander, E.S. Genetic mapping in human disease. *Science* **2008**, *322*, 881–888. [CrossRef] [PubMed]
2. Hindorff, L.A.; Sethupathy, P.; Junkins, H.A.; Ramos, E.M.; Mehta, J.P.; Collins, F.S.; Manolio, T.A. Potential etiologic and functional implications of genome-wide association loci for human diseases and traits. *Proc. Natl. Acad. Sci. USA* **2009**, *106*, 9362–9367. [CrossRef] [PubMed]
3. Visscher, P.M.; Wray, N.R.; Zhang, Q.; Sklar, P.; McCarthy, M.I.; Brown, M.A.; Yang, J. 10 years of GWAS discovery: biology, function, and translation. *Am. J. Hum. Genet.* **2017**, *101*, 5–22. [CrossRef] [PubMed]
4. Huang, H.; Fang, M.; Jostins, L.; Mirkov, M.U.; Boucher, G.; Anderson, C.A.; Andersen, V.; Cleynen, I.; Cortes, A.; Crins, F. Fine-mapping inflammatory bowel disease loci to single-variant resolution. *Nature* **2017**, *547*, 173. [CrossRef] [PubMed]
5. Mahajan, A.; Taliun, D.; Thurner, M.; Robertson, N.R.; Torres, J.M.; Rayner, N.W.; Payne, A.J.; Steinthorsdottir, V.; Scott, R.A.; Grarup, N. Fine-mapping type 2 diabetes loci to single-variant resolution using high-density imputation and islet-specific epigenome maps. *Nat. Genet.* **2018**, *50*, 1505. [CrossRef]
6. Zeng, B.; Lloyd-Jones, L.R.; Montgomery, G.W.; Metspalu, A.; Esko, T.; Franke, L.; Vosa, U.; Claringbould, A.; Brigham, K.L.; Quyyumi, A.A. Comprehensive Multiple eQTL Detection and Its Application to GWAS Interpretation. *Genetics* **2019**, *212*, 302091. [CrossRef]
7. Gusev, A.; Lee, S.H.; Trynka, G.; Finucane, H.; Vilhjálmsson, B.J.; Xu, H.; Zang, C.; Ripke, S.; Bulik-Sullivan, B.; Stahl, E. Partitioning heritability of regulatory and cell-type-specific variants across 11 common diseases. *Am. J. Hum. Genet.* **2014**, *95*, 535–552. [CrossRef]
8. Bulik-Sullivan, B.; Finucane, H.K.; Anttila, V.; Gusev, A.; Day, F.R.; Loh, P.-R.; Duncan, L.; Perry, J.R.; Patterson, N.; Robinson, E.B. An atlas of genetic correlations across human diseases and traits. *Nat. Genet.* **2015**, *47*, 1236. [CrossRef]
9. Li, M.J.; Pan, Z.; Liu, Z.; Wu, J.; Wang, P.; Zhu, Y.; Xu, F.; Xia, Z.; Sham, P.C.; Kocher, J.-P.A. Predicting regulatory variants with composite statistic. *Bioinformatics* **2016**, *32*, 2729–2736. [CrossRef]
10. Liu, L.; Sanderford, M.D.; Patel, R.; Chandrashekar, P.; Gibson, G.; Kumar, S. Biological relevance of computationally predicted pathogenicity of noncoding variants. *Nat. Commun.* **2019**, *10*, 330. [CrossRef]
11. Huo, Y.; Li, S.; Liu, J.; Li, X.; Luo, X.-J. Functional genomics reveal gene regulatory mechanisms underlying schizophrenia risk. *Nat. Commun.* **2019**, *10*, 670. [CrossRef] [PubMed]

12. Gasperini, M.; Hill, A.J.; McFaline-Figueroa, J.L.; Martin, B.; Kim, S.; Zhang, M.D.; Jackson, D.; Leith, A.; Schreiber, J.; Noble, W.S. A Genome-wide framework for mapping gene regulation via cellular genetic screens. *Cell* **2019**, *176*, 377–390.e19. [CrossRef] [PubMed]
13. Adamson, B.; Norman, T.M.; Jost, M.; Cho, M.Y.; Nuñez, J.K.; Chen, Y.; Villalta, J.E.; Gilbert, L.A.; Horlbeck, M.A.; Hein, M.Y. A multiplexed single-cell CRISPR screening platform enables systematic dissection of the unfolded protein response. *Cell* **2016**, *167*, 1867–1882.e21. [CrossRef] [PubMed]
14. Dixit, A.; Parnas, O.; Li, B.; Chen, J.; Fulco, C.P.; Jerby-Arnon, L.; Marjanovic, N.D.; Dionne, D.; Burks, T.; Raychowdhury, R. Perturb-Seq: Dissecting molecular circuits with scalable single-cell RNA profiling of pooled genetic screens. *Cell* **2016**, *167*, 1853–1866.e17. [CrossRef]
15. Jaitin, D.A.; Weiner, A.; Yofe, I.; Lara-Astiaso, D.; Keren-Shaul, H.; David, E.; Salame, T.M.; Tanay, A.; van Oudenaarden, A.; Amit, I. Dissecting immune circuits by linking CRISPR-pooled screens with single-cell RNA-seq. *Cell* **2016**, *167*, 1883–1896.e15. [CrossRef]
16. Datlinger, P.; Rendeiro, A.F.; Schmidl, C.; Krausgruber, T.; Traxler, P.; Klughammer, J.; Schuster, L.C.; Kuchler, A.; Alpar, D.; Bock, C. Pooled CRISPR screening with single-cell transcriptome readout. *Nat. Methods* **2017**, *14*, 297. [CrossRef]
17. Anderson, C.A.; Boucher, G.; Lees, C.W.; Franke, A.; D'Amato, M.; Taylor, K.D.; Lee, J.C.; Goyette, P.; Imielinski, M.; Latiano, A. Meta-analysis identifies 29 additional ulcerative colitis risk loci, increasing the number of confirmed associations to 47. *Nat. Genet.* **2011**, *43*, 246. [CrossRef]
18. Jostins, L.; Ripke, S.; Weersma, R.K.; Duerr, R.H.; McGovern, D.P.; Hui, K.Y.; Lee, J.C.; Schumm, L.P.; Sharma, Y.; Anderson, C.A. Host–microbe interactions have shaped the genetic architecture of inflammatory bowel disease. *Nature* **2012**, *491*, 119. [CrossRef]
19. Wang, Y.; Ma, L.; Wang, C.; Sheng, G.; Feng, L.; Yin, C. Autocrine motility factor receptor promotes the proliferation of human acute monocytic leukemia THP-1 cells. *Int. J. Mol. Med.* **2015**, *36*, 627–632. [CrossRef]
20. Czimmerer, Z.; Varga, T.; Poliska, S.; Nemet, I.; Szanto, A.; Nagy, L. Identification of novel markers of alternative activation and potential endogenous PPARγ ligand production mechanisms in human IL-4 stimulated differentiating macrophages. *Immunobiology* **2012**, *217*, 1301–1314. [CrossRef]
21. Marigorta, U.M.; Denson, L.A.; Hyams, J.S.; Mondal, K.; Prince, J.; Walters, T.D.; Griffiths, A.; Noe, J.D.; Crandall, W.V.; Rosh, J.R.; et al. Transcriptional risk scores link GWAS to eQTLs and predict complications in Crohn's disease. *Nat. Genet.* **2017**, *49*, 1517–1521. [CrossRef]
22. Lloyd-Jones, L.R.; Holloway, A.; McRae, A.; Yang, J.; Small, K.; Zhao, J.; Zeng, B.; Bakshi, A.; Metspalu, A.; Dermitzakis, M. The genetic architecture of gene expression in peripheral blood. *Am. J. Hum. Genet.* **2017**, *100*, 228–237. [CrossRef] [PubMed]
23. Fairfax, B.P.; Humburg, P.; Makino, S.; Narambhai, V.; Wong, D.; Laou, E.; Jostins, L.; Plant, K.; Andrews, R.; McGee, C.; et al. Innate immune activity conditions the effect of regulatory variants upon monocyte gene expression. *Science* **2014**, *343*, 1246949. [CrossRef]
24. Kircher, M.; Witten, D.M.; Jain, P.; O'Roak, B.J.; Cooper, G.M.; Shendure, J. A general framework for estimating the relative pathogenicity of human genetic variants. *Nat. Genet.* **2014**, *46*, 310. [CrossRef] [PubMed]
25. Liu, L.; Tamura, K.; Sanderford, M.; Gray, V.E.; Kumar, S. A molecular evolutionary reference for the human variome. *Mol. Biol. Evol.* **2015**, *33*, 245–254. [CrossRef]
26. Westra, H.J.; Peters, M.J.; Esko, T.; Yaghootkar, H.; Schurmann, C.; Kettunen, J.; Christiansen, M.W.; Fairfax, B.P.; Schramm, K.; Powell, J.E.; et al. Systematic identification of trans eQTLs as putative drivers of known disease associations. *Nat. Genet.* **2013**, *45*, 1238–1243. [CrossRef] [PubMed]
27. Sherry, S.T.; Ward, M.-H.; Kholodov, M.; Baker, J.; Phan, L.; Smigielski, E.M.; Sirotkin, K. dbSNP: The NCBI database of genetic variation. *Nucleic Acids Res.* **2001**, *29*, 308–311. [CrossRef] [PubMed]
28. Pruitt, K.D.; Tatusova, T.; Maglott, D.R. NCBI reference sequences (RefSeq): A curated non-redundant sequence database of genomes, transcripts and proteins. *Nucleic Acids Res.* **2006**, *35*, D61–D65. [CrossRef] [PubMed]
29. Cradick, T.J.; Qiu, P.; Lee, C.M.; Fine, E.J.; Bao, G. COSMID: A web-based tool for identifying and validating CRISPR/Cas off-target sites. *Mol. Ther. Nucleic Acids* **2014**, *3*, e214. [CrossRef]
30. Breitman, T.; Selonick, S.E.; Collins, S.J. Induction of differentiation of the human promyelocytic leukemia cell line (HL-60) by retinoic acid. *Proc. Natl. Acad. Sci. USA* **1980**, *77*, 2936–2940. [CrossRef]
31. Okazaki, T.; Bell, R.M.; Hannun, Y.A. Sphingomyelin turnover induced by vitamin D3 in HL-60 cells. Role in cell differentiation. *J. Biol. Chem.* **1989**, *264*, 19076–19080. [PubMed]

32. Dobin, A.; Davis, C.A.; Schlesinger, F.; Drenkow, J.; Zaleski, C.; Jha, S.; Batut, P.; Chaisson, M.; Gingeras, T.R. STAR: Ultrafast universal RNA-seq aligner. *Bioinformatics* **2013**, *29*, 15–21. [CrossRef] [PubMed]
33. Anders, S.; Pyl, P.T.; Huber, W. HTSeq—A Python framework to work with high-throughput sequencing data. *Bioinformatics* **2015**, *31*, 166–169. [CrossRef] [PubMed]
34. Robinson, M.D.; McCarthy, D.J.; Smyth, G.K. edgeR: A Bioconductor package for differential expression analysis of digital gene expression data. *Bioinformatics* **2010**, *26*, 139–140. [CrossRef] [PubMed]
35. Chen, J.; Bardes, E.E.; Aronow, B.J.; Jegga, A.G. ToppGene Suite for gene list enrichment analysis and candidate gene prioritization. *Nucleic Acids Res.* **2009**, *37*, W305–W311. [CrossRef] [PubMed]
36. Chen, E.Y.; Tan, C.M.; Kou, Y.; Duan, Q.; Wang, Z.; Meirelles, G.V.; Clark, N.R.; Ma'ayan, A. Enrichr: Interactive and collaborative HTML5 gene list enrichment analysis tool. *BMC Bioinform.* **2013**, *14*, 128. [CrossRef]
37. Kuleshov, M.V.; Jones, M.R.; Rouillard, A.D.; Fernandez, N.F.; Duan, Q.; Wang, Z.; Koplev, S.; Jenkins, S.L.; Jagodnik, K.M.; Lachmann, A. Enrichr: A comprehensive gene set enrichment analysis web server 2016 update. *Nucleic Acids Res.* **2016**, *44*, W90–W97. [CrossRef]
38. McKenna, A.; Hanna, M.; Banks, E.; Sivachenko, A.; Cibulskis, K.; Kernytsky, A.; Garimella, K.; Altshuler, D.; Gabriel, S.; Daly, M. The Genome Analysis Toolkit: A MapReduce framework for analyzing next-generation DNA sequencing data. *Genome Res.* **2010**, *20*, 1297–1303. [CrossRef]
39. Van der Auwera, G.A.; Carneiro, M.O.; Hartl, C.; Poplin, R.; Del Angel, G.; Levy-Moonshine, A.; Jordan, T.; Shakir, K.; Roazen, D.; Thibault, J. From FastQ data to high-confidence variant calls: The genome analysis toolkit best practices pipeline. *Curr. Protoc. Bioinform.* **2013**, *43*, 11.10.11–11.10.33.
40. Preininger, M.; Arafat, D.; Kim, J.; Nath, A.P.; Idaghdour, Y.; Brigham, K.L.; Gibson, G. Blood-informative transcripts define nine common axes of peripheral blood gene expression. *PLoS Genet.* **2013**, *9*, e1003362. [CrossRef]
41. Jang, J.S.; Simon, V.A.; Feddersen, R.M.; Rakhshan, F.; Schultz, D.A.; Zschunke, M.A.; Lingle, W.L.; Kolbert, C.P.; Jen, J. Quantitative miRNA expression analysis using fluidigm microfluidics dynamic arrays. *BMC Genom.* **2011**, *12*, 144. [CrossRef] [PubMed]
42. Coudray-Meunier, C.; Fraisse, A.; Martin-Latil, S.; Delannoy, S.; Fach, P.; Perelle, S. A novel high-throughput method for molecular detection of human pathogenic viruses using a nanofluidic real-time PCR System. *PLoS ONE* **2016**, *11*, e0147832. [CrossRef] [PubMed]
43. Sanchez-Freire, V.; Ebert, A.D.; Kalisky, T.; Quake, S.R.; Wu, J.C. Microfluidic single-cell real-time PCR for comparative analysis of gene expression patterns. *Nat. Protoc.* **2012**, *7*, 829–838. [CrossRef]
44. Cong, L.; Ran, F.A.; Cox, D.; Lin, S.; Barretto, R.; Habib, N.; Hsu, P.D.; Wu, X.; Jiang, W.; Marraffini, L.A. Multiplex genome engineering using CRISPR/Cas systems. *Science* **2013**, *339*, 819–823. [CrossRef] [PubMed]
45. Collins, S.J.; Gallo, R.C.; Gallagher, R.E. Continuous growth and differentiation of human myeloid leukaemic cells in suspension culture. *Nature* **1977**, *270*, 347. [CrossRef] [PubMed]
46. Gallagher, R.; Collins, S.; Trujillo, J.; McCredie, K.; Ahearn, M.; Tsai, S.; Metzgar, R.; Aulakh, G.; Ting, R.; Ruscetti, F. Characterization of the continuous, differentiating myeloid cell line (HL-60) from a patient with acute promyelocytic leukemia. *Blood* **1979**, *54*, 713–733. [CrossRef]
47. Leung, M.-F.; Sokoloski, J.A.; Sartorelli, A.C. Changes in microtubules, microtubule-associated proteins, and intermediate filaments during the differentiation of HL-60 leukemia cells. *Cancer Res.* **1992**, *52*, 949–954.
48. Ben-David, U.; Siranosian, B.; Ha, G.; Tang, H.; Oren, Y.; Hinohara, K.; Strathdee, C.A.; Dempster, J.; Lyons, N.J.; Burns, R. Genetic and transcriptional evolution alters cancer cell line drug response. *Nature* **2018**, *560*, 325. [CrossRef]
49. Ramirez, R.N.; El-Ali, N.C.; Mager, M.A.; Wyman, D.; Conesa, A.; Mortazavi, A. Dynamic gene regulatory networks of human myeloid differentiation. *Cell Syst.* **2017**, *4*, 416–429.e3. [CrossRef]
50. Rentzsch, P.; Witten, D.; Cooper, G.M.; Shendure, J.; Kircher, M. CADD: Predicting the deleteriousness of variants throughout the human genome. *Nucleic Acids Res.* **2018**, *47*, D886–D894. [CrossRef]
51. Korkmaz, G.; Lopes, R.; Ugalde, A.P.; Nevedomskaya, E.; Han, R.; Myacheva, K.; Zwart, W.; Elkon, R.; Agami, R. Functional genetic screens for enhancer elements in the human genome using CRISPR-Cas9. *Nat. Biotechnol.* **2016**, *34*, 192. [CrossRef] [PubMed]
52. Rajagopal, N.; Srinivasan, S.; Kooshesh, K.; Guo, Y.; Edwards, M.D.; Banerjee, B.; Syed, T.; Emons, B.J.; Gifford, D.K.; Sherwood, R.I. High-throughput mapping of regulatory DNA. *Nat. Biotechnol.* **2016**, *34*, 167. [CrossRef] [PubMed]

53. Simeonov, D.R.; Gowen, B.G.; Boontanrart, M.; Roth, T.L.; Gagnon, J.D.; Mumbach, M.R.; Satpathy, A.T.; Lee, Y.; Bray, N.L.; Chan, A.Y. Discovery of stimulation-responsive immune enhancers with CRISPR activation. *Nature* **2017**, *549*, 111. [CrossRef] [PubMed]
54. Pan, Y.; Tian, R.; Lee, C.M.; Bao, G.; Gibson, G. Fine-mapping within eQTL Credible Intervals by Expression CROP-seq. *Biol. Meth. Protoc.* **2020**. [CrossRef]
55. Tewhey, R.; Kotliar, D.; Park, D.S.; Liu, B.; Winnicki, S.; Reilly, S.K.; Andersen, K.G.; Mikkelsen, T.S.; Lander, E.S.; Schaffner, S.F. Direct identification of hundreds of expression-modulating variants using a multiplexed reporter assay. *Cell* **2016**, *165*, 1519–1529. [CrossRef] [PubMed]
56. Kreimer, A.; Zeng, H.; Edwards, M.D.; Guo, Y.; Tian, K.; Shin, S.; Welch, R.; Wainberg, M.; Mohan, R.; Sinnott-Armstrong, N.A. Predicting gene expression in massively parallel reporter assays: A comparative study. *Hum. Mutat.* **2017**, *38*, 1240–1250. [CrossRef]
57. Kalita, C.A.; Brown, C.D.; Freiman, A.; Isherwood, J.; Wen, X.; Pique-Regi, R.; Luca, F. High-throughput characterization of genetic effects on DNA–protein binding and gene transcription. *Genome Res.* **2018**, *28*, 1701–1708. [CrossRef]
58. Norga, K.K.; Gurganus, M.C.; Dilda, C.L.; Yamamoto, A.; Lyman, R.F.; Patel, P.H.; Rubin, G.M.; Hoskins, R.A.; Mackay, T.F.; Bellen, H.J. Quantitative analysis of bristle number in Drosophila mutants identifies genes involved in neural development. *Curr. Biol.* **2003**, *13*, 1388–1396. [CrossRef]
59. Magwire, M.M.; Yamamoto, A.; Carbone, M.A.; Roshina, N.V.; Symonenko, A.V.; Pasyukova, E.G.; Morozova, T.V.; Mackay, T.F. Quantitative and molecular genetic analyses of mutations increasing Drosophila life span. *PLoS Genet.* **2010**, *6*, e1001037. [CrossRef]
60. Metzger, B.P.; Yuan, D.C.; Gruber, J.D.; Duveau, F.; Wittkopp, P.J. Selection on noise constrains variation in a eukaryotic promoter. *Nature* **2015**, *521*, 344. [CrossRef]
61. Li, X.; Kim, Y.; Tsang, E.K.; Davis, J.R.; Damani, F.N.; Chiang, C.; Hess, G.T.; Zappala, Z.; Strober, B.J.; Scott, A.J. The impact of rare variation on gene expression across tissues. *Nature* **2017**, *550*, 239. [CrossRef] [PubMed]
62. Zhao, J.; Akinsanmi, I.; Arafat, D.; Cradick, T.; Lee, C.M.; Banskota, S.; Marigorta, U.M.; Bao, G.; Gibson, G. A burden of rare variants associated with extremes of gene expression in human peripheral blood. *Am. J. Hum. Genet.* **2016**, *98*, 299–309. [CrossRef] [PubMed]
63. van Overbeek, M.; Capurso, D.; Carter, M.M.; Thompson, M.S.; Frias, E.; Russ, C.; Reece-Hoyes, J.S.; Nye, C.; Gradia, S.; Vidal, B. DNA repair profiling reveals nonrandom outcomes at Cas9-mediated breaks. *Mol. Cell* **2016**, *63*, 633–646. [CrossRef] [PubMed]

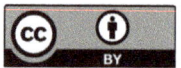

© 2020 by the authors. Licensee MDPI, Basel, Switzerland. This article is an open access article distributed under the terms and conditions of the Creative Commons Attribution (CC BY) license (http://creativecommons.org/licenses/by/4.0/).

MDPI
St. Alban-Anlage 66
4052 Basel
Switzerland
Tel. +41 61 683 77 34
Fax +41 61 302 89 18
www.mdpi.com

Genes Editorial Office
E-mail: genes@mdpi.com
www.mdpi.com/journal/genes